Alcohol and Heart Disease

Alcohol and Heart Disease

Edited by

Ronald R. Watson

Division Health Promotion Sciences
University of Arizona College of Public Health and School of Medicine
Tucson, Arizona, USA

and

Adam K. Myers

Department of Physiology and Biophysics
Georgetown University Medical Center
Washington, DC, USA

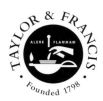

London and New York

First published 2002
by Taylor & Francis
11 New Fetter Lane, London EC4P 4EE

Simultaneously published in the USA and Canada
by Taylor & Francis Inc,
29 West 35th Street, New York, NY 10001

Taylor & Francis is an imprint of the Taylor & Francis Group

© 2002 Taylor & Francis

Typeset in Goudy by
Integra Software Services Pvt. Ltd., Pondicherry, India
Printed and bound in Great Britain by
TJ International Ltd, Padstow, Cornwall

Every effort has been to ensure that the advice and information in this book
is true and accurate at the time of going to press. However, neither the publisher
nor the authors can accept any legal responsibility or liability for any errors or
omissions that may be made. In the case of drug administration, any medical procedure
or the use of technical equipment mentioned within this book, you are strongly
advised to consult the manufacturers's guidelines.

British Library Cataloguing in Publication Data
A catalogue record for this book is available
from the British Library

Library of Congress Cataloging in Publication Data
A catalog record has been requested

ISBN 0–415–27347–1

Contents

Tables

Figures

Contributors

Abdel A. Abdel-Rahman
Department of Pharmacology
The Brody Medical School
East Carolina University
Greenville, NC 27858
USA

Albert D. Arvallo
College of Public Health
University of Arizona
School of Medicine
Tucson, AZ 85724-5155
USA

Mary E. Beckemeier
Department of Internal Medicine
Division of Cardiology
St. Louis University Health Science
   Center
St. Louis, Missouri 63110
USA

Puran S. Bora
Department of Opthalmology and
   Visual Sciences
Kentucky Lions Eye Center
301 E Muhammad Ali
Louisville KY 40202
USA

Paul A. Cahill
School of Biotechnology
Dublin City University
Glasnevin, Dublin 9
Ireland

Simon K.K. Cheung
Section of Cardiology
UMDNJ, Department of Medicine
185 S. Orange Avenue,
Newark NJ 07103-2714
USA

Jules Constant
57 Tillinghast Place, Buffalo
NY 14216
USA

Richard Cooper
Department of Preventive Medicine
   and Epidemiology
Loyola University Stritch
School of Medicine
2160 South First Ave
Maywood, IL 60153
USA

Kabita Das
Department of Physiology & Biophysics
Georgetown University Medical Center
Washingtown, DC 20007
USA

Mark Deeg
Indiana University School of Medicine
Endocrinology (111E)
1481 W. 10th Street,
Indianapolis, IN 46202
USA

M.J. Dunn
Department of Surgery
National Heart and Lung Institute
Imperial College School of Medicine
Heart Science Centre, Harefield Hospital
Harefield, Middlesex UB9 6JH
UK

Mary O. Gray
Department of Cardiology
San Francisco Veterans Affairs
Medical Center
4150 Clement Street
San Francisco, CA 94121
USA

Matti Hillbom
Department of Neurology
Oulu University Hospital
FIN-90220, Oulu
Finland

Leo Hsu
Veterans Affairs Medical Center
GRECC Service
St. Louis, Missouri 63108
USA

R. Hunter
Department of Nutrition
School of Life Sciences
King's College
London
150 Stamford Street
London SE1 8WA
UK

Seppo Juvela
Associate Professor of Neurosurgery
Department of Neurosurgery
Helsinki University Central Hospital
Topeliuksenkatu 5
FIN-02600 Helsinki
Finland

John W. Karanian
OST/CDRH, FDA
8401 Mirkurk Road
Laurel, MD, 20708
USA

Jaana M. Leppälä
Department of Public Health
Finland
11811 Venice Blvd Apt 315
Los Angeles
CA 90066-3944
USA

Youlian Liao
Department of Biometry and Epidemiology
Medical University of South Carolina
135 Rutledge Avenue
Charleston SC 29425
USA

D. Mantle
Department of Neurochemistry
Regional Neurosciences Centre
Newcastle General Hospital
Newcastle Upon Tyne NE4 6BE
UK

Daniel McGee
Department of Biometry and Epidemiology
Medical University of South Carolina
135 Rutledge Avenue
Charleston SC 29425
USA

Daria Mochly-Rosen
Department of Molecular Pharmacology
Standford University of Medicine
Standford, CA
USA

Adam K. Myers
Department of Physiology & Biophysics
Georgetown University Medical Center
Washingtown, DC 20007
USA

Mariann R. Piano
Associate Professor
University of Illinois at Chicago
College of Nursing (MC 802)
845 S. Damen
Chicago, IL 60612
USA

Victor R. Preedy
Molecular and Cellular
Protein Metabolism Laboratory
Department of Nutrition and Dietetics
School of Life Sciences
King's College London,
Stamford Street
London SE1 8WA
UK

Eileen M. Redmond
University of Rochester Medical Center
Department of Surgery
Box SURG
601 Elmwood Ave
Rochester, NY 14642-8410
USA

Timothy J. Regan
Section of Cardiology
UMDNJ, Department of Medicine
185 S. Orange Avenue
Newark NJ 07103-2714
USA

P.J. Richardson
Department of CardiologyKing's College
School of Medicine and Dentistry
Bessemer Road
London, SE5 9PJ, UK

Norman Salem
Laboratory of Membrane Biochemistry
and Biophysics
National Institute on Alcohol Abuse
and Alcoholism
National Institutes of Health
12420 Parklawn Drive
Rockville, MD 20852, USA

Helmut Seitz
Laboratory of Alcohol Research
Liver Disease and Nutrition
and
Department of Medicine
Salem Medical Center
University of Heidelberg
Zeppelinstr. 11–33
HEIDELBERG 69121, Germany

R. Tomas Sepulveda
Arizona Prevention Center
University of Arizona
College of Public Health
Tucson, AZ 85724-5155, USA

A. Gerald Shaper
Department of Primary Care and Pop. Sci.
Royal Free and Univ. College Med. Sch.
Rowland Hill St.
London, NW3 2PF
England

David Solkoff
Arizona Prevention Center
University of Arizona
College of Public Health
Tucson, AZ 85724-5155, USA

S. Goya Wannamettee
Department of Primary Care and Pop. Sci.
Royal Free and Univ. College Med. Sch.
Rowland Hill St.
London, NW3 2PF, England

Ronald R. Watson
Arizona Prevention Center
University of Arizona
College of Public Health
Tucson, AZ 85724-5155, USA

S. Worrall
Alcohol Research Unit
Department of Biochemistry
The University of Queensland
Brisbane, Queensland
QLD 4072, Australia

Jin Zhang
Arizona Prevention Center
University of Arizona
College of Public Health
Tucson, AZ 85724-5155, USA

Qing-Hui Zhang
Department of Physiology & Biophysics
Georgetown University Medical Center
Washingtown, DC 20007
USA

Preface

Alcohol research is in a golden era. With advances in molecular biology, the degree to which genetic makeup predetermines susceptibility to alcohol abuse and alcoholism is being defined. With more powerful tools for data collection and analysis and increased funding in this area, the epidemiology of alcohol consumption and alcohol-related health issues is being better elucidated. With the blossoming of the field of neuroscience, neural mechanisms underlying alcohol addiction and appetitive behavior are being discovered. The importance of this expanding knowledge is underscored by the fact that alcohol is one of the most widely used and abused drugs in most civilizations, and the health costs of alcohol are so great that among drugs of abuse, they are rivaled only by those of tobacco.

Of course, the consideration of alcohol use and abuse presents special problems. Humankind has had a complex relationship with alcohol from the beginning of recorded history. In most societies, some level of alcohol consumption is acceptable, and social and religious rites often incorporate drinking. That alcohol has both detrimental and beneficial effects has always been appreciated. Along with some of the obvious negative effects of intoxication and chronic use, the preservative, antiseptic and anesthetic effects of alcohol, for example, have been known since ancient times. With the flourishing of alcohol research, both the negative and positive aspects are being better defined, but alcohol is a true double-edged sword. Its use in medicine has been invaluable over the centuries, but few health care practitioners today would recommend that a non-drinker take up alcohol consumption for health purposes.

Effects of alcohol on the heart and cardiovascular system follow the same paradigm: its chronic abuse is clearly associated with negative effects, such as hypertension, heart failure, bleeding disorders, atrial fibrillation and stroke. At the same time, it has long been suspected that moderate consumption might be of benefit to cardiovascular health, and in fact, recent, large scale epidemiological studies demonstrate that used in moderation, it might protect against morbidity and mortality associated with coronary artery disease and perhaps thrombotic strokes. Obviously, with coronary artery disease being the most prevalent cause of death in most Western societies, and with stroke also being high on that list, understanding how alcohol affects the heart and blood vessels is an important goal. As alcohol research has gathered steam in recent years, so too has research related to alcohol consumption and cardiovascular health and disease.

It is against this background that this volume was conceived and prepared. In it, leading scientists from across the world and from a broad set of scientific disciplines present the state of knowledge on alcohol and heart disease as well as related background material. The recent advances in the epidemiology of heart disease and drinking are considered, as are the multiple mechanisms underlying the negative effects of drinking on cardiovascular health. Interaction of alcohol with other drugs affecting the heart and circulation is a medically important area that is also discussed. From the public's perspective, one of the most interesting outcomes of alcohol research has been the demonstration that moderate alcoholic beverage consumption may protect against coronary artery disease and associated mortality. Specific components of certain beverages, notably red wine, might have their own beneficial effects, as might ethanol itself. This intriguing area is dealt with in a number of chapters, from a number of perspectives. It is our hope that this volume highlights the excellent work being done in these fascinating areas and serves to stimulate further research into important, related public health questions.

The Editors

Ronald R. Watson, Ph.D., initiated the Specialized Alcohol Research Center at the University of Arizona College of Medicine and had directed the center for 6 years. Dr. Watson has edited 50 books, including 10 on alcohol abuse and 4 on other drugs of abuse. He has worked for several years on research for the U.S. Navy Alcohol and Substance Abuse Program.

Dr. Watson attended the University of Idaho but graduated from Brigham Young University in Provo, Utah with a degree in chemistry in 1966. He completed his Ph.D. degree in 1971 in biochemistry at Michigan State University. His postdoctoral schooling in nutrition and microbiology was completed at the Harvard School of Public Health and included a 2-year postdoctoral research experience in immunology. He was an assistant professor of immunology and did research at the University of Mississippi Medical Center in Jackson from 1973 to 1974. He was an assistant professor of microbiology and immunology at the Indiana University Medical School from 1974 to 1978 and an associate professor at Purdue University in the Department of Food and Nutrition from 1978 to 1982. In 1982, Dr. Watson joined the faculty at the University of Arizona in the Department of Family and Community Medicine. He is also a research professor in the University of Arizona's newly formed College of Public Health. He is a member of the Sarver Heart Center. He has published 450 research papers and review chapters. Dr. Watson currently directs a National Institute of Health grant on alcohol's effects on heart disease in AIDS, a NIDA supplement to it to understand the role of cocaine as a cofactor, and a National Heart, Lung and Blood Institute grant on AIDS and heart dysfunction in mice.

Adam Myers received his Ph.D. in Physiology at Georgetown University (Washington, DC), where he now teaches cardiovascular physiology to medical and graduate students. Dr. Myers is Professor and Director of Graduate Studies in Physiology. His major research interests are in mechanisms of cardiovascular disease and thrombosis, areas in which he has published extensively. He has a long-standing interest in the effects of moderate alcohol consumption on platelets and thrombosis, which is the focus of a chapter in this volume. Dr. Myers is a member of the Research Society on Alcoholism.

Chapter 1

Alcohol and cardiovascular disease: large population studies

Youlian Liao, Daniel McGee and Richard Cooper

INTRODUCTION

As early as the late 18th century, wine, spiritous liquors, and opium were described as the relievers for angina pectoris [1]. In the early decades of the 20th century, an inverse relation was first observed between heavy alcohol intake and atherosclerotic disease [2,3]. A series of studies among alcoholics and problem drinkers later suggested an excess risk of coronary heart disease (CHD) [4,5]. However, problem drinkers are different from other people in a number of ways, making it difficult to generalize this association to the population level. Clinical series and case-control studies collect data on alcohol intake after the outcome of interest has occurred. These studies often have limited data on other traits, which may be associated with developing the end points and also with alcohol intake. After the mid 20th century prospective cohort studies began to be established. Data on alcohol consumption were collected with varying detail at the baseline. This allowed study of the relationship between present alcohol intake and the future occurrence of cardiovascular disease, even though this was not the major aim of the original studies.

The large population prospective studies [6–35] of alcohol and cardiovascular disease, including CHD and stroke, are listed in Table 1.1. If a cohort reported results on the same topic more than once, the most recent data are shown in the table. We excluded studies that described only the relationship between alcohol and total mortality. All cohorts included had a sample size of more than 4,000, the Cancer Prevention Study II of the American Cancer Society enrolling the largest number with nearly 490,000 participants [21]. The studies presented in the table include general population samples from the local communities [6–11,30,32], national representative samples [23], volunteers [20,21,33], screenees or participants in clinical trials [24,25,31], special ethnic [8,9] or occupation groups [12–19,29,35], and persons from medical clinics [26–28,34] or health care subscribers [22]. The majority of cohorts were observed for more than 10 years [6–10,13–17,20,23,26–29,32–35].

MAJOR FINDINGS

Alcohol and nonfatal myocardial infarction or incidence of CHD

Data on the incidence of myocardial infarction or CHD were available for about 40% of the cited cohorts. It is no longer disputed that drinkers as a group have a lower incidence of

Table 1.1 Large population studies examining alcohol intake and cardiovascular disease

[Reference] Cohort	Baseline Year	Sampling Method	Sample Size	Categories of Alcohol Intake	CHD			Death (N)	Stroke + (N)
					Yrs*	Death (N)	Incidence (N)		
[6] Framingham Heart Study	1950	Residents aged 29–62 years in Framingham, MA at exam 2	4,745	0, 1, 2–3, 4–7, 8–19, and 20+ oz/week (men); 0, 1, 2–3, 4–9, and 10+ oz/week (women)	24	1,490			~400
[7]		At exam 2 or exam 7	4,625	oz per month	22		809		288
[8] Honolulu Heart Program	1965–68	Japanese ancestry (men) aged 45 and older residing on the Hawaiian island of Oahu	7,878	None, light (1–14 oz/month), moderate (15–39 oz/month), and heavy (≥40 oz/month)	12				290
[9]	1971–74	Men who survived to exam 3	6,069	Abstainer, light (1–14 ml/day), moderate (15–39 ml/day), and heavy drinker (≥40 ml/day)	15	819		132	70 (death)
[10] Puerto Rico Heart Health Program	1965–68	Male residents aged 35–79 years from three urban and four rural areas of Puerto Rico	9,150	0, 1–14, 15–39, 40–79, and ≥80 g/day	12	1,383	164 (nonfatal MI)	306	
[11] Yugoslavia Cardiovascular Disease Study	1964–65	Male residents aged 35–62 years living in Bosnia and Croatia	11,121	<monthly, monthly to <weekly, weekly to <daily, daily but not drunk last week, and daily and drunk last week	7		164	95	
[12] Nurses' Health Study	1980	Female registered nurses aged 34–59 living in 11 large states	87,526	0, <1.5, 1.5–4.9, 5.0–14.9, 15.0–24.9, and ≥25 g/day	4		200		141
[13]			85,709	0, 0.1–1.4, 1.5–4.9, 5.0–14.9, 15.0–29.9, and ≥30.0 g/day	12	2,658		320	
[14] Physicians Health Study	1981–84	Male physicians aged 40–84 years in an aspirin/B-carotene randomized trial	21,530	<1, 1, 2–4, 5–6 drinks/week, 1 drink/day, and ≥2 drinks/day	11		1,368 (angina) 690 (MI)		
[15]			21,876	<1, 1, 2–4, 5–6, 7–13, and ≥14 drinks/week	11	1,206		185 394 (CVD)	60 (death)
[16]			21,537	<1, 1, 2–4, 5–6 drinks/wk, 1 drink/day, and ≥2 drinks/day	12			141 (Sudden cardiac)	

Study	Year	N	Alcohol consumption categories	No. of categories		Events	Outcome
[17]		21,870	<1, 1, 2–4, 5–6 drinks/week, and ≥1 drink/day	12			679
[18] Physicians Health Study enrollment cohort	1982–83	89,299	rarely/never, 1–3 drinks/month, 1, 2–4, 5–6 drinks/week, 1 drink/day, and ≥2 drinks/day	5	3,216	514 (MI); 1,450 (CVD)	150 (death)
[19] Health Professionals Follow-up Study	1986	44,059	0, 0.1–2.0, 2.1–5.0, 5.1–10.0, 10.1–15.0, 15.1–30.0, 30.1–50.0, and >50.0 g/day	2		350	
[20] American Cancer Society Prospective Study	1959	276,802	None, occasional, 1, 2, 3, 4, 5, 6+ drinks/day, and irregular drinkers	12	42,756	18,771	2,512 (death)
[21] Cancer Prevention Study II	1982	489,626	None, less than daily, 1 drink/day, 2–3 drinks/day, ≥4 drinks/day	9	46,325	10,252	2,379 (death)
[22] Kaiser Permanente Study	1978–85	128,934	Lifelong abstainer, ex-drinker, <1/month, >1/month to <1/day, 1–2/day, 3–5/day, and ≥6 drinks/day	8	4,503	940; 1,685 (CVD)	
[23] NHANES I Epidemiologic Follow-up Study	1971–75	6,788	Lifetime abstainers, current abstainers, <2, 2–7, 8–14, 15–28, 29–42, and >42 drinks/week	15	1,560	552	
[24] Lipid Research Clinics Follow-up Study	1972–76	7,461	0, 1–9, 10–19, 20–29, and 30+ ml/day	9		91; 178 (CVD)	
[25] Post trial follow-up of the Multiple Risk Factor Intervention Trial	1982	11,688	0, 1–7, 8–14, 15–21, and ≥22 drinks/week	4		190	
[26] British Regional Health Study	1978–80	7,272	None, occasional (<1 unit/week), light (1–15 units/week), moderate (16–42 units/week), and heavy (≥6 units/day)	17	1,308	445	

Table 1.1 (Continued)

[Reference] Cohort	Baseline Year	Sampling Method	Sample Size	Categories of Alcohol Intake	Yrs*	CHD Death (N)	CHD Incidence (N)	Death (N)	Stroke + (N)
[27]			7,273	None, occasional, weekend drinker: 1–2, 3–6, or >6 drinks/day, and daily drinker: 1–2, 3–6, or >6 drinks/day	14				216
[28]	1983–85	Survivors at 5 yrs after the initial exam	6,439	Lifelong teetotaller, ex-drinker, occasional (<1/week), light (1–15/week), moderate (16–42/week), and heavy (>42 units/week)	10	929	490	472 (CVD)	
[29] British male physicians	1978	Male British doctors who replied to the 1978 alcohol questionnaire	12,321	None, 1–7, 8–14, 15–21, 22–28, 29–42, and ≥43 units/week	13	3,328		1,061	380 (death)
[30] Social Insurance Institution's Mobile Clinic health Survey (Finland)	1973–76	Men aged 40–64 years in 12 cohorts drawn from 4 geographical regions of Finland	4,532	0, <200 g/month, and ≥200 g/month	5	314		140 89 (Sudden)	
[31] Finnish Cancer Prevention Study	1985–88	Male cigarette smokers aged 50–69 years in a primary cancer prevention trial	26,556	nondrinkers, light (≤24.0 g/day), moderate (24.1–60.0 g/day), and heavy (>60.0 g/day)	6				960
[32] Copenhagen City Heart Study	1976–78	Random, age stratified samples aged 30–79 years	13,285	Never, monthly, weekly, 1–2 drinks/day, and 3–5 drinks/day	11	2,229		1,119 (CVD)	
[33] Swedish Conscripts Study	1969–70	Military conscripts aged 17–21 years	49,618	0, 0.1–14.9, 15–30, ≥30 g/day	25	1,473	279 (MI)		233
[34] Eastern France study	1978–83	Consecutive men aged 40–60 years coming for a comprehensive health appraisal	34,014	0-occasion, 1–21, 22–32, 33–54, 55–76, 77–128, and >128 g/day	13	2,642		284 427 (CVD)	
[35] Japanese male physicians	1965	Male physicians from western Japan	5,135	Non-drinker, ex-drinker, occasional drinker, <54 ml/day, and ≥54 ml/day	19	1,283		184 525 (CVD)	230

* Length of follow-up (years); +Number of incidence cases unless otherwise indicated; CHD=coronary heart disease; CVD=cardiovascular disease; NHANES I=the First National Health and Nutrition Examination Survey.

acute myocardial infarction or CHD than do non-drinkers. However, it is unresolved as to whether there is a dose-response relation between increasing alcohol intake and decreasing incidence and whether there is an increase in risk at the high end of alcohol intake. An inverse relationship between alcohol intake and incidence of CHD was found in the Framingham Heart Study [7], the Yugoslavia Cardiovascular Disease Study [11], the Physicians' Health Study [14], the Health Professional's Follow-up Study [19], and in the middle-aged group (51–64 years) of the Honolulu Heart Program [9]. A clear dose–response relationship among drinkers was not found in the British Regional Health Study [26,28], the Nurses' Health Study [12], and the First National Health and Nutrition Examination Survey Epidemiologic Follow-up Study [23]. The Kaiser Permanente Study of alcohol intake and subsequent hospitalization for acute myocardial infarction showed that compared with lifelong abstainers, a lower risk of hospitalization for CHD was present among those who took alcohol more than monthly to ≥6 drinks per day [36]. There was no apparent difference in the hospitalization rate among the wide ranges of alcohol intake. The majority of studies did not find an increase in the incidence of CHD at the high end of the drinking distribution [9,12,14,26,28,33]. However, among females in the First National Health and Nutrition Examination Survey Epidemiologic Follow-up Study [23], an increased risk was found above 28 drinks per week relative to abstainers. Among males in this study, no upturn in risk was revealed at higher intake. The Honolulu Heart Study reported a higher risk of incident CHD in heavy compared to light male drinkers aged 65 to 75 years [9].

Alcohol and CHD mortality

The observed relationship between alcohol intake and CHD death has been reported to be linear (direct or inverse), L-shaped, U-shaped, or showing no relation. In the 5-year follow-up study of 4,532 middle-aged Finnish men [30], non-drinkers had the lowest CHD mortality. Increased alcohol intake was associated with increased age-adjusted CHD mortality, especially in men with prior CHD. The opposite was reported in the post-trial follow-up of the Multiple Risk Factor Intervention Trial [25]. The original 5-year trial was to determine the effects of multifactor intervention on death from CHD in a population of high-risk men randomly assigned either to a special intervention program or to their usual sources of medical care in the community. The post-trial follow-up was conducted in 11,488 men who did not develop CHD and survived to the end of the trial. A reverse dose–response relationship between alcohol intake and CHD death rate was found [25].

Many studies have found an L-shaped pattern of alcohol–CHD relationship with mortality decreasing with increasing consumption up to a point and then leveling off. This pattern implies that there was no significant up-turn in the trends of CHD mortality among heavy drinkers. These studies include the Framingham Heart Study [6], the Nurses' Health Study [13], Cancer Prevention Study II [21], the Eastern France Study [34], a study among the Japanese male physicians [35], the Physicians Health Study enrollment cohort (death from cardiovascular disease as the endpoint) [18], males from the Kaiser Permanente Study [22], males from the First National Health and Nutrition Examination Survey Epidemiologic Follow-up Study [23], and beer drinkers in the Copenhagen City Heart Study [32].

A U-shaped curve signifies an initial decrease in the CHD death rate followed by an increase at higher levels of alcohol consumption. This relationship was reported in the American Cancer Society Prospective Study [20], the Lipid Research Clinics Follow-up Study (death from cardiovascular disease as the endpoint) [24], the studies on male physicians in the

US [15] and UK [29], females from the Kaiser Permanente Study [22] and from the First National Health and Nutrition Examination Survey Epidemiologic Follow-up Study (12), and spirits drinkers in the Copenhagen City Heart Study [32].

The British Regional Health Study found no convincing evidence that light or moderate drinking has a protective effect on mortality from cardiovascular disease [28]. Lifelong tee-totallers, light, moderate, and heavy drinkers had similar age-adjusted cardiovascular death rates.

Alcohol and sudden cardiac death

Evidence for a strong association between alcohol and sudden death has been reported among problem drinkers [37,38]. Findings among population studies published in the 1980s were, however, inconsistent. A positive association between alcohol consumption and the incidence of sudden coronary death was detected in the cohort of 4,532 Finnish men with or without prior CHD [30]. No association was found in the Puerto Rico Heart Health Program [10], the Yugoslavia Cardiovascular Disease Study [11], and the Framingham Heart Study [39]. The numbers of sudden deaths were small in these reports, however. In the Physicians Health Study, men who consumed light-to-moderate amounts of alcohol (2–6 drinks per week) had a significantly reduced risk of sudden cardiac death compared with those who rarely or never consumed alcohol [16]. Only 3% of the physicians drank 2 or more drinks per day. Men in this open-end category had neither an increase nor a reduction in risk. About 11% of men in the British Regional Heart Study [40] were heavy drinkers who drank more than 6 drinks per day and they had the highest incidence rate of sudden cardiac death in this cohort. This positive association between heavy drinking and the incidence of sudden death was most apparent in men without pre-existing CHD.

Alcohol and stroke

Alcohol was recognized as a possible risk factor for stroke as early as the 17th century [41]. Results gathered from large prospective studies were not available until the late 1970s to early 1980s and the epidemiological evidence has been highly inconsistent. Variations in the reported alcohol–stroke relationship are much greater than for the alcohol–CHD relationship. Increasing alcohol consumption was related to an increased incidence of all strokes (fatal and non-fatal) in men from the Honolulu Heart Program [8], in the Swedish conscripted men [33], and in the male smokers in the Finnish Cancer Prevention Study [31]. Alcohol intake was also associated with an increased total stroke mortality in men from the Yugoslavia Cardiovascular Disease Study [42] and the Japanese male physicians [35]. On the other hand, some studies [17,21] have reported an L-shaped alcohol–stroke relationship. The Cancer Prevention Study II [21] found that men who consumed alcohol less than daily through 4 or more drinks per day had a similar stroke mortality that was lower than the rates for non-drinkers. The Physicians Health Study reported that compared to men who had less than 1 drink per week, those who drank more than this, including up to 1 or more drinks per day, had a reduced risk of stroke [17]. However, several studies [12,18,20,27,29] suggested a J-shaped relationship between alcohol and stroke, i.e., light alcohol consumption may decrease the risk of stroke, higher levels of consumption may increase the risk. The level of alcohol intake at which the risk of stroke increased ranged from 1 drink per day (the Physicians' Health Study enrollment cohort) [18] to around 4 drinks per day (the American Cancer Society Prospective Study) [20] and 6 drinks per day (the British Regional Health Study and the British male physicians) [27,29].

Stroke consists of various subtypes and each stroke subtype has a distinct dose–response relationship with alcohol consumption. A positive linear association between alcohol intake and hemorrhagic stroke (intracerebral hemorrhage or subarachnoid hemorrhage) has consistently been found [8,12,31,35]. The Physicians Health Study is an exception in which no significant relationship existed [17]. The epidemiologic pattern of ischemic stroke and alcohol consumption is uncertain. It has been described as inverse linear [12,17], J-shaped [31,35], and showing no relationship [8].

DISCUSSION

Inherent weakness in observational studies

Consistency is often cited as one of the criteria making an observed association more likely to be causal. However, results from studies with the same design can be wrong or artefactual and remain consistent. Most population studies rely on volunteers. This may bias the study samples toward cooperative persons, who are, perhaps, more health conscious than nonparticipants. The heaviest drinkers are not likely to be included in the large cohort studies and this may diminish the role of heavier drinking in the overall results. Studies on the highly educated and health conscious groups [12–19,29,35] are more likely to miss the up-turn of a J-shaped relationship between alcohol and outcome. The most fundamental weakness in the observational studies is that the preference and quantity of alcohol intake are entirely self-determined by the participants. Hence, all reports on the benefit of small-to-moderate alcohol consumption to cardiovascular disease reduction are referenced to those who are 'self-selected to consume small-to-moderate alcohol'.

Measurements of alcohol intake

Alcohol consumption based on self-reported data consistently account for only 40–60% of alcohol purchases [43]. The greatest problem facing alcohol research is the lack of a reference standard with which to validate self-reported drinking. Collateral reports by significant others do not necessarily provide better information [43]. Biochemical markers, which are useful in the diagnosis of alcoholism and recent drinking, cannot be used to estimate absolute alcohol intake at an individual level. Most observational studies ask the respondents to recall their usual intake over a long period of time, say 1 month or 1 year. This approach is likely to yield information about modal frequencies and quantities and thus underestimate average intake. On the other hand, recalling the actual intake during all actual drinking occasions over a short period of time (e.g., 24 hours) ignores the day-to-day variations in alcohol consumption. Among the five main methods used to assess alcohol intake i.e., quantity frequency, extended quantity frequency, retrospective diary, prospective diary, and 24-hour recalls, the mean level of alcohol intake differs by 20% [44]. When researchers asked specifically about intake of beer, wine, and liquor, this resulted in 20% higher estimates of intake.

Under-reporting of alcohol consumption by respondents is common in epidemiologic studies. If all respondents underestimate their alcohol consumption proportionally, relative risk estimates for any given level of alcohol use would be mislabeled but would have rank-order validity. The hypothesized association between alcohol intake and cardiovascular disease would be found, but safe levels of drinking could not be established since true drinking habits were not known. Alternatively, if response error is not proportional, this will not only affect the existence and the shape of the association between alcohol and health, but also the relative risk could be underestimated, overestimated, or completely spurious. The ultimate effects of response error are unknown, but this issue clearly represents an important potential limitation for all epidemiologic research on alcohol.

The authors of the various studies reported their findings variously in 'standard drinks', grams, fluid ounces, or milliliters, which makes interpretation and comparison of levels of alcohol cited in the different studies difficult. The amount of alcohol in grams in each drink/unit varied from country to country, and study to study, being 8–10 g in the United Kingdom, 9–13 g in the United States, 14 g in Canada, and 21–28 g in Japan [45]. Likewise, the quoted average alcohol content of beer, wine, and spirits varied. Among the 4 studies (the Framingham Study, the Honolulu Heart Study, the Third National Cancer Survey, and the British Regional Heart Study), 'three drinks per day' means anything from 24–48 g of alcohol per day, depending on the country as well as the assumptions made by the authors [45].

Unhealthy abstainers question

A large proportion of abstainers (non-drinkers) are ex-drinkers [46]. Men who were heavier drinkers are more likely to reduce their alcohol consumption as they grow older [46–48]. This is at least in part associated with the accumulating burden of ill-health and medication as people grow older [49]. The British Regional Health Study suggested a strong downward drift from heavy or moderate drinking to occasional drinking or abstinence under the influence of accumulating ill-health not necessarily related to alcohol intake [47]. Ex- and never-drinkers were more frequently unmarried and had the highest prevalence rates of angina, ECG abnormalities, elevated blood pressure, and several other chronic conditions [50,51]. Thus, abstainers may constitute a misleading reference category for the analysis of the relation between alcohol and disease, and for the interpretation of alcohol-related dose–risk relations, leading to underestimates of alcohol-related effects or overestimates of alcohol-related benefits. Since investigating the alcohol–health relationship might not be one of the original study aims of the cohorts, complete alcohol intake histories are often not available. Only a few studies could separate ex-drinkers from life-time abstainers [9,22,28,35]. Hence, many reports conducted alternative analyses by excluding either non-drinkers or persons with pre-existing cardiovascular disease [6,10,12,14–16,18–21,23,24,29,31].

Other confounders

The difficulty of controlling completely for correlates of alcohol use and of cardiovascular disease is obvious. For example, alcohol use is related to age, sex, race/ethnic background, geographical location, smoking, coffee use, educational attainment/socioeconomic status, marital status, adiposity, salt use and other dietary habits, religious affiliation, social network, stress, psychological well-being, and physical activity. People who drink (excluding heavy drinkers) had a better self-perceived health status than did non-drinkers [52]. The differences in self-perceived health status accounted for one-fourth to one-third of the lower risk of subsequent mortality among alcohol drinkers [52]. Health status was also related to people's preference for different alcoholic beverages, such as red and white wine, beer, or liquor. Compared with persons who drank no wine, self-reported suboptimal health was less frequent among both men and women who imbibed 1–4 drinks of wine [53]. Information on many potential confounders was either unavailable in many studies, or very difficult to define, measure, and control.

Drinking patterns and beverage types

Drinking patterns have been studied surprisingly little. Yet, drinking patterns vary and are of obvious health relevance. The frequency of drunkenness, the frequency of hangover and morning drinking have been found to be related to mortality from several causes [54]. Changes in drinking between years may influence mortality [9,55]. Most reports classify participants using a total consumption variable (e.g., drinks per day) based on estimates of customary drinking frequency and amount of alcohol consumed on a typical occasion. This does not quantify variability in drinking frequency or amount consumed; binge drinkers may be classified with controlled, regular drinkers on the basis of their common average daily alcohol intake. Because the health effects of moderate drinking may depend on drinking pattern, failure to differentiate between binge drinkers and regular drinkers may obscure real associations. Type of beverage may have a role even if the amount of ethyl alcohol imbibed is the same. The epidemiological evidence favoring one type of beverage over another is inconsistent, possibly because of large differences in demographics, social habits, diet, smoking, personality, lifestyle, and other behaviors among drinkers [6,19,56,57]. The beverage types differ not only in alcohol concentration but also in the usual drinking pattern. Wine in particular is often taken with food, slowly and with regularity.

What is 'moderate' drinking?

While it is generally agreed that we should do all things in moderation [58], there is less agreement about the precise definition of 'moderate' drinking. Use of different sets of drinking categories in different reports has resulted in different interpretations, and the number and boundaries of categories appears to be determined by the sample size available in the study. Classification of moderate alcohol consumption ranges from a half a drink per day (or less) in some studies, up to six drinks a day in others [59]. Data from the National Health Interview Survey [52] demonstrated that people with different drinking habits perceived 'moderate' drinking differently. Only 25% of men who drink 3 or more drinks per day, in comparison to 56% of other men, considered 2 or fewer drinks per occasion as moderate. Likewise, only 6% of the women who drink at least 2 drinks per day (vs. 27% of other women) perceived moderate drinking as 1 drink or less per occasion. The National Health and Medical Research Council [60] in Australia has recommended responsible, hazardous and harmful levels of alcohol intake for the public. Not exceeding 4 standard drinks per day for men and 2 drinks for women is recommended as 'safe and responsible' drinking. In England, the Royal College of Physicians, Psychiatrists, and General Practitioners [61] advised a 'sensible' limit of alcohol intake of 21 units per week (~16 drinks in the US) for men and 14 units (~11 drinks) for women. The US Dietary Guidelines Advisory Committee [62] on the Dietary Guidelines for Americans defined moderate drinking as no more than 2 drinks per day for men and no more than 1 drink per day for women. There is a very high correlation between the mean level of alcohol consumption in a community and the prevalence of heavy drinkers, such that an increase in consumption of only 15 g per week might be associated with a 10% increase in the prevalence of heavy drinkers [63]. Hence, an appropriate definition of the optimal level of drinking has important public health implications.

Some statistical issues

The non-continuous feature of the measures of drinking habit has limited studies on the alcohol–health relationship to categorical analyses. The categories selected, the number of categories, and the distance between the categories were determined by the available data, the sample sizes and number of outcome events. The clear demonstration of a U- or J-shaped relationship requires a much larger amount of data than is generally appreciated. Some studies have combined all cardiovascular diseases or all types of stroke as the endpoint. This is often necessary because of the small numbers of cases for some of the diagnostic endpoints, but might result in partial cancellation of positive and negative associations. Furthermore, as the result of a loss of power in the categorical analysis, many reports drew conclusions based on visual observation on the trends in relative risks by drinking categories and ignored the results of formal statistical tests.

Another drawback of the categorical approach is the inability to clearly define the alcohol intake level related to minimum risk. On the other hand, treating alcohol intake as a continuous variable and fitting a quadratic function forces the estimated relationship between alcohol and outcome to be symmetric. Over- or under-estimation of the optimal level will occur if the true relationship is asymmetric.

In the study of the alcohol–health relationship, it is sometimes difficult to differentiate a potential confounder from a mediator of a causal outcome. Examples of these factors are blood pressure, lipoproteins, hemostasis, perceived health status, and other indicators of current health. Control strategies in a data analysis initially should not include risk factors that might serve as potential mediators lying in the pathway between alcohol intake and outcome. Failing to control for confounders may inflate the potential benefit of alcohol intake. On the other hand, improper control for mediators may spuriously deflate the potential benefit of alcohol intake. If, for example, alcohol use increases hemorrhagic stroke risk through alcohol-induced hypertension alone, then control for blood pressure would produce a non-significant association between alcohol consumption and stroke.

CONCLUSIONS

Two thirds of Americans report using alcohol and since social drinking is a potentially modifiable behavior, the relation between alcohol consumption and cardiovascular disease is a subject of considerable importance. Although the literature is not unanimous, evidence from large epidemiologic studies leads to the conclusion that moderate alcohol intake decreases risk of non-fatal and fatal CHD and ischemic stroke. The observed differences in the shape of the relationship between various studies might be partly explained by varying distributions of other risk factors and partly by the variation of alcohol intake in the study populations. If heavy drinking was infrequent in a study sample, an L-shaped relationship would be observed instead of a J-shape. If only abstainers and light drinkers were studied, an inverse linear association should appear. If the study sample did not include abstainers, a positive linear trend could emerge.

A randomized, controlled clinical trial is the gold standard to reveal whether the beneficial effect of moderate alcohol intake is in fact due to this alcohol intake or results from some unknown confounding factor that no cohort study, however large, could discover. However, such a trial is unlikely to be performed to establish a direct link between alcohol consumption and health. Prospective observation of representative samples is the available method that comes closest to the ideal. A good start would be to design large cohort studies with the express aim of revealing the effects of alcohol intake on health. The studies presently available have not been designed primarily to this end. The problem of confounding, given the inter-correlation of many lifestyle practices and the imprecision with which they are measured, creates subtle and complex statistical challenges.

Several guidelines for safe and sensible alcohol drinking have been suggested [60–62]. However, individual susceptibility varies with age, sex, drinking patterns, drinking situations, and even genetic and constitutional backgrounds, so that a single guideline for all persons may not be appropriate. The relation between low levels of drinking and cardiovascular disease will vary depending on a person's underlying (i.e., absolute) risk of this disease. The groups most likely to benefit from drinking small amounts of alcohol are those, such as older people, at high absolute risk of CHD and ischemic stroke and at low absolute risk of injury, cirrhosis, and other alcohol-related disease. As a group, young people have a very low absolute risk of CHD and a high absolute risk of injury.

Populations with low mortality from CHD often have high death rates from hemorrhagic stroke, which is strongly positively associated with alcohol consumption [64]. In these countries, 'safe' limits would need to be considerably lower than in most western countries [65]. With steep declines in cardiovascular mortality in many countries, the protective effect of alcohol may have decreased as well, and a downward shift of the optimal level of intake may have occurred. Data from more recent cohorts are needed to answer this question.

Any advice about the consumption of alcohol must take into account not only the relation between alcohol and cardiovascular disease but also the well-known association of heavy consumption of alcohol with a large number of health risks. Public health policy concerning alcohol intake also requires consideration of all aspects of the outcomes of drinking, that is, mortality, morbidity and social, economic and criminal consequences, as well as quality of life.

REFERENCES

1 Heberden W. Some account of a disorder of the breast. *Med. Trans. R. Coll. Physic.* 1786; **2**: 59–67.

2 Cabot RC. Relation of alcohol to arteriosclerosis. JAMA 1904; **43**: 774–775.

3 Leary T. Therapeutic value of alcohol with special consideration of relations of alcohol to cholesterol, and thus to diabetes, to arteriosclerosis, and to gallstones. *N. Engl. J. Med.* 1931; **205**: 231–242.

4 Pell S, D'Alonzo CA. A five-year mortality study of alcoholics. *J. Occupat. Med.* 1973; **15**: 120–125.

5 Robinette CD, Hrubec Z, Fraumeni JF Jr. Chronic alcoholism and subsequent mortality in World War II veterans. *A. J. Epidemiol.* 1979; **109**: 687–700.

6 Friedman LA, Kimball AW. Coronary heart disease mortality and alcohol consumption in Framingham. *Am. J. Epidemiol.* 1986; **124**: 481–489.

7 Gordon T, Kannel WB. Drinking habits and cardiovascular disease: The Framingham Study. *Am. Heart J.* 1983; **105**: 667–673.

8 Donahue RP, Abbott RD, Reed DM, Yano K. Alcohol and hemorrhagic stroke. The Honolulu Heart Program. JAMA 1986; **255**: 2311–2314.

9 Goldberg RJ, Burchfiel CM, Reed DM, Wergowske G, Chiu D. A prospective study of the health effects of alcohol consumption in middle-aged and elderly men. The Honolulu Heart Program. *Circulation* 1994; **89**: 651–659.

10 Kittner SJ, Garcia-Palmieri MR, Costas R Jr, Cruz-Vidal M, Abbott RD, Havlik RJ. Alcohol and coronary heart disease in Puerto Rico. *Am. J. Epidemiol.* 1983; **117**: 538–550.

11 Kozarevic D, Demirovic J, Gordon T, Kaelber CT, McGee D, Zukel WJ. Drinking habits and coronary heart disease: the Yugoslavia Cardiovascular Disease Study. *Am. J. Epidemiol.* 1982; **116**: 748–758.

12 Stampfer MJ, Colditz GA, Willett WC, Speizer FE, Hennekens CH. A prospective study of moderate alcohol consumption and the risk of coronary disease and stroke in women. *N. Engl. J. Med.* 1988; **319**: 267–273.

13 Fuchs CS, Stampfer MJ, Colditz GA, Giovannucci EL, Manson JE, Kawachi I, Hunter DJ, Hankinson SE, Hennekens CH, Rosner B, Speizer FE, Willett WC. Alcohol consumption and mortality among women. *N. Engl. J. Med.* 1995; **332**: 1245–1250.

14 Camargo CA Jr, Stampfer MJ, Glynn RJ, Grodstein F, Gaziano JM, Manson JE, Buring JE, Hennekens CH. Moderate alcohol consumption and risk for angina pectoris or myocardial infarction in U.S. male physicians. *Ann. Intern. Med.* 1997; **126**: 372–375.

15 Camargo CA Jr, Hennekens CH, Gaziano JM, Glynn RJ, Manson JE, Stampfer MJ. Prospective study of moderate alcohol consumption and mortality in US male physicians. *Arch. Intern. Med.* 1997; **157**: 79–85.

16 Albert CM, Manson JE, Cook NR, Ajani UA, Gaziano JM, Hennekens CH. Moderate alcohol consumption and the risk of sudden cardiac death among US male physicians. *Circulation* 1999; **100**: 944–950.

17 Berger K, Ajani UA, Kase CS, Gaziano JM, Buring JE, Glynn RJ, Hennekens CH. Light-to-moderate alcohol consumption and the risk of stroke among U.S. male physicians. *N. Engl. J. Med.* 1999; **341**: 1557–1564.

18 Gaziano JM, Gaziano TA, Glynn RJ, Sesso HD, Ajani UA, Stampfer MJ, Manson JE, Hennekens CH, Buring JE. Light-to-moderate alcohol consumption and mortality in the Physicians' Health Study enrollment cohort. *J. Am. Coll. Cardiol.* 2000; **35**: 96–105.

19 Rimm EB, Giovannucci EL, Willett WC, Colditz GA, Ascherio A, Bosner B, Stampfer MJ. Prospective study of alcohol consumption and risk of coronary disease in men. *Lancet* 1991; **338**: 464–468.

20 Boffetta P, Garfinkel L. Alcohol drinking and mortality among men enrolled in an American Cancer Society Prospective Study. *Epidemiology* 1990; **1**: 342–348.

21 Thun MJ, Peto R, Lopez AD, Monaco JH, Henley SJ, Heath CW, Doll R. Alcohol consumption and mortality among middle-aged and elderly U.S. Adults. *N. Engl. J. Med.* 1997; **337**: 1705–1714.

22 Klatsky AL, Armstrong MA, Friedman GD. Alcohol and mortality. *Ann. Intern. Med.* 1992; **117**: 646–654.

23 Rehm JT, Bondy SJ, Sempos CT, Vuong CV. Alcohol consumption and coronary heart disease morbidity and mortality. *Am. J. Epidemiol.* 1997; **146**: 495–501.

24 Criqui MH, Cowan LD, Tyroler HA, Bangdiwala S, Heiss G, Wallace RB, Cohn R. Lipoproteins as mediators for the effects of alcohol consumption and cigarette smoking on cardiovascular mortality: results from the Lipid Research Clinics Follow-up Study. *Am. J. Epidemiol.* 1987; **126**: 629–637.

25 Suh I, Shaten BJ, Cutler JA, Kuller LH for the Multiple Risk Factor Intervention Trial Research Group. Alcohol use and mortality from coronary heart disease: the role of high-density lipoprotein cholesterol. *Ann. Intern. Med.* 1992; **116**: 881–887.

26 Wannamethee SG, Shaper AG. Type of alcoholic drink and risk of major coronary heart disease events and all-cause mortality. *Am. J. Pub. Health.* 1999; **89**: 685–690.

27 Wannamethee SG, Shaper AG. Patterns of alcohol intake and risk of stroke in middle-aged British men. *Stroke* 1996; **27**: 1033–1039.

28 Wannamethee SG, Shaper AG. Lifelong teetotallers, ex-drinkers and drinkers: Mortality and the incidence of major coronary heart disease events in middle-aged British men. *Int. J. Epidemiol.* 1997; **26**: 523–531.

29 Doll R, Peto R, Hall E, Wheatley K, Gray R. Mortality in relation to consumption of alcohol: 13 years' observations on male British doctors. *BMJ* 1994; **309**: 911–918.

30 Suhonen O, Aromaa A, Reunanen A, Knekt P. Alcohol consumption and sudden coronary death in middle-aged Finnish men. *Acta Med. Scand.* 1987; **221**: 335–341.

31 Leppälä JM, Paunio M, Virtamo J, Fogelholm R, Albanes D, Taylor PR, Heinonen OP. Alcohol consumption and stroke incidence in male smokers. *Circulation* 1999; **100**: 1209–1214.

32 Grønbæk M, Deis A, Sørensen TIA, Becker U, Schnohr P, Jensen G. Mortality associated with moderate intakes of wine, beer, or spirits. *BMJ* 1995; **310**: 1165–1169.

33 Romelsjö A, Leifman A. Association between alcohol consumption and mortality, myocardial infarction, and stroke in 25 year follow up of 49,618 young Swedish men. *BMJ* 1999; **319**: 821–822.

34 Renaud SC, Guéguen R, Schenker J, d'Houtaud A. Alcohol and mortality in middle-aged men from Eastern France. *Epidemiol.* 1998; **9**: 184–188.

35 Kono S, Ikeda M, Tokudome S, Nishizumi M, Kuratsune M. Alcohol and mortality: a cohort study of male Japanese physicians. *Int. J. Epidemiol.* 1986; **15**: 527–532.

36 Klatsky AL, Armstrong MA, Friedman GD. Relations of alcoholic beverage use to subsequent coronary artery disease hospitalizations. *Am. J. Cardiol.* 1986; **58**: 710–714.

37 Dyer AR, Stamler J, Paul O, Berkson DM, Lepper MH, McKean H, Shekelle RB, Lindberg HA, Garside D. Alcohol consumption, cardiovascular risk factors, and mortality in two Chicago epidemiologic studies. *Circulation* 1977; **56**: 1067–1074.

38 Lithel H, Aberg H, Sclines I, Hedstrand H. Alcohol intemperance and sudden death. *BMJ* 1987; **294**: 1456–1458.

39 Gordon T, Kannel WB. Drinking habits and cardiovascular disease: The Framingham Study. *Am. Heart J.* 1983; **105**: 667–673.

40 Wannamethee G, Shaper AG. Alcohol and sudden cardiac death. *Br. Heart J.* 1992; **68**: 443–448.

41 Hillbom ME. What supports the role of alcohol as a risk factor for stroke? *Acta Med. Scand.* (Suppl.) 1987; **717**: 93–106.

42 Kozararevic D, McGee D, Vojvodic N, Racic Z, Dawber T, Gordon T, Zukel W. Frequency of alcohol consumption and morbidity and mortality: The Yugoslavia Cardiovascular Disease Study. *Lancet* 1980; **1**: 613–616.

43 Midanik L. The validity of self-reported alcohol consumption and alcohol problems: a literature review. *Br. J. Addict.* 1982; **77**: 357–382.

44 Feunekes GI, van't Veer P, van Staveren WA, Kok FJ. Alcohol intake assessment: the sober facts. *Am. J. Epidemiol.* 1999; **150**: 105–112.

45 Turner C. How much alcohol is in a 'standard drink'? An analysis of 125 studies. *Br. J. Addiction* 1990; **85**: 1171–1175.

46 Wannamethee G, Shaper AG. Men who do not drink: a report from the British Regional Heart Study. *Int. J. Epidemiol.* 1988; **7**: 307–316.

47 Wannamethee G, Shaper AG. Changes in drinking habits in middle-aged British men. *J. R. Coll. Gen. Pract.* 1988; **38**: 440–442.

48 Rehm J, Sempos CT. Alcohol consumption and all-cause mortality. *Addiction* 1995; **90**: 471–480.

49 Shaper AG. The 'unhealthy abstainers' question is still important (Commentaries). *Addiction* 1995; **90**: 488–490.

50 Shaper AG, Wannamethee G, Walker M. Alcohol and mortality in British men: explaining the U-shaped curve. *Lancet* 1988; **2**: 1267–1273.

51 Marmot M, Brunner E. Alcohol and cardiovascular disease: the status of the U shaped curve. *Br. Med. J.* 1991; **303**: 565–568.

52 Liao Y, McGee DL, Cao G, Cooper RS. Alcohol intake and mortality: findings from the National Health Interview Survey (1988 and 1990). *Am. J. Epidemiol.* 2000; **151**: 651–659.

53 Poikolainen K, Vartiainen E. Wine and good subjective health. *Am. J. Epidemiol.* 1999; **150**: 47–50.

54 Poikolainen K. Inebriation and mortality. *Int. J. Epidemiol.* 1983; **12**: 151–155.

55 Lazarus NB, Kaplan GA, Cohen RD, Leu DJ. Change in alcohol consumption and risk of death from all causes and from ischaemic heart disease. *BMJ* 1991; **303**: 553–556.

56 Rimm EB, Klatsky A, Grobbee D, Stampfer MJ. Review of moderate alcohol consumption and reduced risk of coronary heart disease: is the effect due to beer, wine, or spirits? *BMJ* 1996; **312**: 731–736.

57 Klatsky AL, Armstrong MA, Kipp H. Correlates of alcoholic beverage preference: traits of persons who choose wine, liquor or beer. *Br. J. Addict.* 1990; **85**: 1279–1289.

58 Ellison RC. All things in moderation (Editorials). *Epidemiol.* 1991; **2**: 232–233.

59 Stampfer MJ, Rimm EB, Walsh DC. Alcohol, the heart, and public policy (Commentary). *Am. J. Pub. Health* 1993; **83**: 801–804.

60 National Health and Medical Research Council. *Is There a Safe Level of Daily Consumption of Alcohol for Men and Women? Recommendations Regarding Responsible Drinking Behaviour.* 2nd ed. Canberra, Australia: Australian Government Publishing Service, 1992.

61 Royal College of Physicians, Royal College of Psychiatrists, Royal College of General Practitioners. *Alcohol and the Heart in Perspective: Sensible Limits Reaffirmed.* London, England: RCP, RCPsych, RCGP, 1995.

62 US Department of Agriculture, US Department of Health and Human Services, US Dietary Guideline Committee. *Nutrition and Your Health: Dietary Guidelines for Americans.* 4th ed. Washington, DC: US Government Printing Office, 1995. (US GPO publication no. 1996-402-519) (Home & Garden Bulletin no. 232).

63 Rose G, Day S. The population mean predicts the number of deviant individuals. *BMJ* 1990; **301**: 1031–1034.

64 Usehima H, Ohsaka T, Asakura S. Regional differences in stroke mortality and alcohol consumption in Japan. *Stroke* 1986; **17**: 19–24.

65 Jackson R, Beaglehole R (Commentary). Alcohol consumption guidelines: relative safety vs absolute risks and benefits. *Lancet* 1995; **346**: 716.

Chapter 2

The alcoholic cardiomyopathies: genuine and pseudo

Jules Constant

GENUINE ALCOHOLIC CARDIOMYOPATHY: ASYMPTOMATIC TYPE

There is ample evidence that acute or chronic alcohol ingestion may be a myocardial depressant. There is also evidence that acute or chronic alcohol ingestion may be a skeletal muscle depressant. In one study in asymptomatic alcoholics, almost one third of the men and half of the women showed histologic evidence of deltoid muscle myopathy with accompanying muscle weakness and depression of ejection fraction [1]. Low doses of ethanol, even as little as two cocktails, have been shown to be able to decrease myocardial contractility in normal subjects [2–5]. If the subject is alcoholic or already has some cardiac muscle disease on which alcohol is superimposed, the depressant effect of acute alcohol ingestion is exaggerated [6,7]. Partly responsible for the deleterious effects of alcohol in patients who have cardiac disease is the finding that in such patients alcohol acts as a vasoconstrictor [8]. However, when a decreased afterload is necessary for improving the function of a heart in Class 3 or 4 heart failure, the peripheral vasodilatory effects of a few drinks of a moderate amount of alcohol may not produce any hemodynamic deterioration [9].

Chronic alcoholics without cardiac symptoms have been shown to have slightly depressed myocardial function as shown especially well by systolic time intervals and by the rise in pulmonary artery pressure and end-diastolic pressure with exercise [10–12]. Acute or chronic alcohol ingestion is frequently associated with conduction abnormalities and abnormal T waves, e.g., notched T waves, as well as arrhythmias, especially atrial fibrillation [13–15]. This asymptomatic alcoholic type of cardiomyopathy with slightly decreased myocardial function is not what is generally meant by an alcoholic cardiomyopathy even though in fact it is so. When nutritional deficiencies together with heavy intake of alcohol combine to produce overt congestive heart failure, this produces a genuine type of alcoholic cardiomyopathy known as beriberi heart disease, which may be further divided into two types, an acute hyperkinetic and an acute hypokinetic type. Both types respond to stopping alcohol and taking thiamine and a nutritious diet [16].

GENUINE ALCOHOLIC CARDIOMYOPATHIES: SYMPTOMATIC TYPES

Acute shoshin beriberi

The classic oriental shoshin beriberi (sho=acute damage and shin=heart) first described by Aalsmeer and Wenckebach [17] in 1929, is due to a lack of thiamine. It manifests as a hyperkinetic cardiovascular syndrome with severe congestive failure, stocking-glove cyanosis, acidosis, vascular collapse and death [18]. However, it has had to be modified for the occidental varieties because in the occident the thiamine deficiency has usually combined alcohol with general nutritional deficiencies.

Thiamine deficiency can be produced by either blockage of absorption or excess excretion. Alcohol apparently interferes with thiamine absorption, while diuretics cause excess excretion [19]. Beriberi heart failure has been produced by the long-term use of furosemide which can deplete the body of all water-soluble vitamins including thiamine [20,21].

The acute fulminate variety has been called by the misleading oxymoron 'high output failure'. This is indeed heart failure if the failing heart is defined as one whose function is insufficient to supply the perfusion requirements of the body. With thiamine deficiency there not only is a moderate degree of myocardial dysfunction but also intense vasodilatation, especially in muscles, creating the effect of a total body AV fistula somewhat similar to that produced by amyl nitrite inhalation. Since the degree of failure in beriberi depends on the degree of peripheral vasodilatation, acute fulminant cases are often precipitated by excessive exercise in hot weather or by fever. The edema is presumably secondary to the increase in blood volume and venous pressure necessary to increase the cardiac output and so fill the expanded vascular bed. The increased venous pressure and peripheral edema was given the misnomer of right heart failure [22].

The low peripheral resistance begins to return toward normal within 1 h of the intravenous thiamine administration and may be normal within a few weeks [17]. The return of the afterload to normal often unmasks the accompanying myocardial dysfunction, because the response of the myocardium to thiamine seems to lag behind the response of the peripheral vasculature [17].

Low output hypokinetic beriberi

The chronic alcoholic with severe nutritional deficiency for at least 3 months usually enters hospital with severe reversible congestive heart failure after being on minimal food intake for about 1 week. After a few weeks in hospital with abstention from alcohol and with good nutrition, especially with thiamine supplementation, the heart usually returns to normal size and the congestive heart failure disappears without the need for further drug therapy [16,18]. The symptoms of such patients may be a peripheral neuropathy or Wernicke's encephalopathy [23].

Some low output reversible types of alcoholic cardiomyopathies have been caused by toxic materials added to the alcohol. For example, the Munich 'beer heart' was first described in 1884. This alcoholic cardiomyopathy was considered a mystery when it killed persons in Belgium, Quebec, Omaha and Minneapolis between 1964 and 1966. Disappearance of the syndrome followed almost immediately upon removal of cobalt which had been added to improve the 'head' [24].

Alcoholic versus viral or idiopathic chronic dilated cardiomyopathy (DCM)

The most prevalent confusion with the alcoholic heart disease caused by thiamine and nutritional deficiency is with viral or idiopathic chronic DCM. Between 20 and 35% of all cases of DCM are thought to occur because of excessive ethanol intake [25]. However, in both alcoholic and idiopathic chronic DCM, the clinical picture is similar. In the early stages of both categories of congestive heart failure, the patients often show some response to bedrest, salt restriction, diuretics, and digitalis. Afterwards there is slight-to-moderate cardiac dilatation. Still later the heart becomes markedly enlarged. Once cardiac failure appears, life expectancy can be measured in months or, at the most, a few years. Death is usually from heart failure, uncontrolled arrhythmias, or thromboembolism. In both, the electrocardiogram may show conduction disturbances, nonspecific ST-T abnormalities, and even anterior infarction.

The pathology of the heart in alcoholic patients with chronic DCM is somewhat different from non-alcoholics with chronic DCM. The alcoholics tend to have more myocardial hypertrophy, interstitial fibrosis, and electrical irritability [26,27]. Although gross microscopic examination has not been able to distinguish chronic idiopathic DCM from the chronic DCM found in alcoholics [28], electron microscopy has shown that patients who have also been chronic alcoholics have swelling of the sarcoplasmic reticulum which is more severe and generalized rather than focal [29,30]. However, these differences from the DCM in non-alcoholics do not mean that the severe cardiomyopathy was caused by the alcohol but may only mean that the alcohol, in addition to the other causes of idiopathic DCM, can cause characteristic pathologic changes.

Likewise, even though it is true that patients with chronic DCM due to alcohol have less muscle strength and more histologic findings of skeletal myopathy than patients with idiopathic DCM, this does not prove that the DCM was caused by alcohol [25]. The skeletal pathology may be the result of a combination of congestive heart failure from any cause plus the alcohol.

That alcohol may not be entirely responsible for the chronic DCM in alcoholics is suggested by the lack of correlation between the quantity of alcohol consumed and the development of such DCM [31] and also by the finding that most alcoholics who have been drinking heavily for at least 5 years show no clinical evidence of heart failure. The incidence of chronic DCM in alcoholics is relatively low, at about 12% [25].

After 4 months of daily heavy drinking, an S3 and elevated venous pressure can develop, signs which can revert to normal on stopping the alcohol if this was the sole cause of the failure [16,32,33]. However, many of those with the usual diagnosis of alcoholic cardiomyopathy will not have their congestive heart failure signs disappear merely on stopping the alcohol [34].

There are studies that suggest that alcohol modifies the incidence and course of cardiomyopathies caused by other agents, the most likely being viral [34,35]. It is probable that many cases of so-called idiopathic DCM are viral in origin. In one study of non-alcoholic patients with idiopathic DCM, 30% showed enteroviral RNA on endomyocardial biopsy [35]. Hibbs *et al.* [36] found that electron microscopic examination showed evidence of virus-like particles in the heart of a patient who had an alcoholic cardiomyopathy. It is conceivable that many alcoholics with DCM may have had a mild or forgotten viral infection and their chronic DCM may represent a modified form of burned out viral myocarditis [37]. About one third of patients with a past history of proven Coxsackie viral myocarditis show a depression of myocardial function 2–5 years after the acute episode [38]. In India, about 15% of patients with proven viral myocarditis had persistent heart failure when seen 3 months later [39].

The absence of evidence of a viral etiology is no proof that the idiopathic chronic DCM was not viral in etiology. Considerable evidence indicates that cardiac injury in clinical and experimental cardiotropic Coxsackie B-3 virus-induced myocarditis is mediated by the immune system. In the murine infection, detectable virus is absent in the heart and body fluids even when inflammation and necrosis are maximum. In addition, inoculation of T-lymphocyte-deficient mice with the virus does not result in significant myocarditis even when the virus is isolated from the heart [40]. This suggests that the virus initiates an immune response which produces inflammation and necrosis but the virus does not directly induce significant cardiac injury. It is possible that alcohol influences the myocardial immune response to produce more inflammation and necrosis.

Another clue to the possibility that alcoholics may have a viral pathogenesis for their chronic DCM is a little-known experiment on viral myocarditis in mice. Morin et al. [41] administered Coxsackie B virus to 48 mice. One half received laboratory chow and alcohol and the other half received laboratory chow and sweetened water. At the end of 5 weeks, 80% of the alcohol group showed microscopic cardiac involvement. Only 30% of the non-alcohol group had cardiac lesions ($p = 0.02$). The cardiac involvement in the mice that received the alcohol was not only more frequent but also more severe than in the non-alcohol group [41].

How the damage of a viral attack on the myocardium can be augmented by alcohol is unknown, although there are many possibilities. It has been suggested, for example, that it may be due to the loss of potassium and magnesium from the myocardium or the ability of alcohol to inhibit the active transport of cations across the cell membrane [27,42]. An analogy may be made with the rather similar incidence of liver cirrhosis in chronic alcoholics (about 8%) because this also points to the possibility that an infection caused by a hepatotropic virus may be made more damaging by the presence of alcohol.

However, no matter what the reason for the synergistic effect of alcohol with a viral cardiomyopathy, we are not justified in using the term 'alcoholic cardiomyopathy' for the chronic DCM found in alcoholics that does not respond within a few weeks to good nutrition and withdrawal from alcohol. That term suggests more than we know since it may be a viral cardiomyopathy in an alcoholic. Although an alcoholic is no more likely to have a myotropic viral infection than a non-alcoholic, the virus may have much more chance of producing severe myocardial damage.

Thus, for those alcoholics with either an acute or chronic heart failure syndrome that responds to good nutrition, thiamine, and a withdrawal from alcohol, the term 'alcoholic cardiomyopathy' is appropriate. However, for the alcoholic with a chronic DCM that does not respond to good nutrition and alcohol withdrawal, the preferred terminology is 'idiopathic DCM in an alcoholic'.

REFERENCES

1 Urbano-Marquez A, Estruch R, Fernandez-Sola J, Nocolas JM. The greater risk of cardiomyopathy and myopathy in women compared with men. JAMA 1995; **274**: 149–154.
2 Ahmed SS, Levinson GE, Regan TJ. Altered systolic time intervals with low doses of ethanol in man. *Circulation* 1971; **43–44** (Suppl. II): 119.

3 Child JS, Kovick RB, Levisman JA, Pearce ML. Cardiac effects of acute ethanol ingestion unmasked by autonomic blockade. *Circulation* 1979; **59**: 120–125.

4 Gould L, Reddy CVR, Goswami K, Venkataraman K, Gomprecht RF. Cardiac effects of two cocktails in normal man. *Chest* 1973; **63**: 943–947.

5 Delgado CE, Fortuin NJ, Ross RS. Acute effects of low doses of alcohol on left ventricular function by echocardiography. *Circulation* 1975; **51**: 535–540.

6 Conway N. Haemodynamic effects of ethyl alcohol in patients with coronary heart disease. *Br. Heart J.* 1968; **30**: 638–644.

7 Inasaka T, Sugimoto T, Kaseno K, Uraoka T, Sato K, Ikeda T. Effects of ethanol on the responses of STI to exercise: A study in the normal subjects. *CV Sound Bull.* 1974; p. 373.

8 Gould L. Hemodynamic effects of ethanol in patients with cardiac disease (abstract): *JAMA* 1972; **222**: 1331.

9 Greenberg BH. Acute effects of alcohol in patients with congestive heart failure. *Ann. Intern. Med.* 1982; **97**: 171–175.

10 Gould L, Zahir M, Shariff M, DiLieto M. Cardiac hemodynamics in alcoholic heart disease. *Ann. Intern. Med.* 1969; **71**: 543–553.

11 Slany J. Ergometric studies in chronic alcoholics. *JAMA* 1973; 223–236.

12 Spodick DH, Pigott VM, Chirife R. Preclinical cardiac malfunction in chronic alcoholism. *N. England M. Med.* 1972; **287**: 677–680.

13 Ettinger PO, Wu CF, DelaCruz C Jr, Weisse AB, Ahmed SS, Regan TJ. Arrhythmias and the 'holiday heart': Alcohol associated cardiac rhythm disorder. *Am. Heart J.* 1978; **95**: 555–562.

14 Constant J, Carlisle R. The notched T wave in LVH and alcoholism. *Chest* 1970; **57**: 540.

15 Tofler DB, Saker RM, Rollo KA, Burvill MJ, Stenhouse N. Electrocardiogram of the social drinker in Perth, Western Australia. *Br. Heart J.* 1969; **31**: 306–312.

16 Burch GE, Walsh JJ. Cardiac insufficiency in chronic alcoholism. *Am. J. Cardiol.* 1960; **6**: 864–874.

17 Aalsmeer WC, Wenckebach KF. The heart and circulatory system in beriberi. *Am. Heart J.* 1929; **4**: 630.

18 Attas M, Hanley HG, Stults D, Jones MR, McAllister RG. Fulminant beriberi heart disease with lactic acidosis. *Circulation* 1978; **58**: 566–571.

19 King JF, Easton R, Dunn M. Acute pernicious beriberi heart disease. *Chest* 1972; **61**: 512–517.

20 Kawai C, Wakabayashi A, Hirose K, Yui Y, Itokawa Y. Cardiomyopathies of miscellaneous origin. *World Congress Tokyo*, 1978; 0841.

21 Nishi S, Shinyashiki T, Uchimura S, Tanaka H, Katanazako H, Okura H, Kanehisa T. Electron microscopic observations on cardiomyopathy in thiamine deficient mice. *World Congress Tokyo* 1978; 0841.

22 Constant J. Solving nomenclature problems in cardiology: II. Updating terminology in clinical cardiology. *Cardiology* 1995; **86**: 361–364.

23 Baron JH, Oliver LC. Fulminating beriberi. *Lancet* 1958; **i**: 354–356.

24 Herrell WE. Beer drinkers' disease. *Clin. Med.* 1967; **74**: 15.

25 Fernandez-Sola J, Estruch R, Grau JM, Pare JC, Rubin E, Urbano-Marquez A. The relation of alcoholic myopathy to cardiomyopathy. *Ann. Intern. Med.* 1994; **120**: 529–536.

26 Askanas A, Udoshi M, Sadjadi SA. The heart in chronic alcoholism: A noninvasive study. *Am. Heart J.* 1980; **99**: 9–16.

27 Ballas M, Zoneraich S, Yunis M, Zoneraich O, Rosner F. Noninvasive cardiac evaluation in chronic alcoholic patients with alcohol withdrawal syndrome. *Chest* 1982; **82**: 148–153.

28 Tobin JR, Driscoll JF, Lim MT, Sutton GC, Szanto PB, Gunnar RM. Primary myocardial disease and alcoholism. *Circulation* 1967; **35**: 754–764.

29 Alexander CS. Idiopathic heart disease: Electron microscopic examination of myocardial biopsy specimens in alcoholic heart disease. *Am. J. Med.* 1966; **41**: 229–234.

30 Bulloch RT, Pearce MB, Murphy M, Jenkins BJ, Davis JL. Myocardial lesions in idiopathic and alcoholic cardiomyopathy. *Am. J. Cardiol.* 1972; **29**: 15–25.

31 Burin E. Cardiovascular effects of alcohol. *Pharmacol. Biochem. Behav.* 1980; **13**(Suppl. 1): 37–40.

32 McDonald CD, Burch GE, Walsh JJ. Alcoholic cardiomyopathy managed with prolonged bed rest. *Ann. Intern. Med.* 1971; **74**: 681–691.

33 Regan TJ, Levinson GE, Oldewurtel HA, Frank MJ, Weiss AB, Moschos CB. Ventricular function in noncardiacs with alcoholic fatty liver: Role of ethanol in the production of cardiomyopathy. *J. Clin. Invest.* 1969; **48**: 397–407.

34 Schwartz L, Sample KA, Wigle ED. Severe alcoholic cardiomyopthy reversed with abstention from alcohol. *Am. J. Cardiol.* 1975; **36**: 963–966.

35 Miller H, Abelman WH. Effects of dietary ethanol upon experimental trypanasomal myocarditis. *Proc. Soc. Exp. Biol.* 1967; **126**: 193–198.

36 Hibbs RG, Ferrans VJ, Black WC. Alcoholic cardiomyopathy. An electron microscopic study. *Am. Heart J.* 1965; **69**: 766–769.

37 Paushinger M, Preis S, Triesch A, Doerner A, Schultheil HG. Detection of entoviral RNA in endomyocardial biopsies in patients having chronic myocarditis. *Circulation* 1994; **90**: 1174.

38 Levi GF, Prote C, Quadri A, Ratti S. Coxsackie virus disease and cardiomyopathy. *Am. Heart J.* 1977; **93**: 419–421.

39 Saivani G, Dekate MP, Rao CP. Heart disease caused by Coxsackie virus B infection. *Br. Heart J.* 1975; **37**: 819–823.

40 Huber SA, Lodge PA. Coxsackie virus B-3 myocarditis in mice. *Am. J. Pathol.* 1984; **116**: 21–29.

41 Morin Y, Roy PE, Mohiuddin SM, Taskar PK. The influence of alcohol on viral and isoproterenol cardiomyopathy. *Cardiovasc. Res.* 1969; **3**: 363–368.

42 Regan TJ, Koroxenidis G, Moschos CB. The acute metabolic and hemodynamic responses of the left ventricle to ethanol. *J. Clin. Invest.* 1966; **45**: 270–280.

Chapter 3

Wine and lifestyle: role in cardiovascular disease and premature death

S. Goya Wannamethee and A. Gerald Shaper

INTRODUCTION

Light and moderate drinking has consistently been associated with lower risk of coronary heart disease [1–4]. Several studies have suggested that specific types of drink may have different effects on coronary heart disease (CHD) [5,6]. In recent years, much research has focused on the question of whether wines in particular have specific qualities not associated with other types of alcoholic beverage. Studies have suggested a possible role of antioxidants or bioflavanoids [7,8] and of antithrombotic and platelet activity in wine [9,10]. This has lead investigators to postulate that the protective effect of alcohol is only derived from wine drinking or that wine consumption is most beneficial [5,6]. However, a systematic review of ecological, case-control and prospective studies concluded that all alcoholic drinks were linked with lower risk of CHD but there was no consensus concerning the issue of wine drinking being most beneficial [11]. In many of the study populations reviewed, drinks are limited to one or two alcohol-types. Relatively few investigations have been able to compare the effects of different types of drink within the same study population and not surprisingly the findings have not been consistent [12–20]. It is speculated that the apparent differences in effects of alcoholic beverages may be due to differences in lifestyle or behavioural and drinking patterns associated with beverage type. In support of this argument, data from the British Regional Heart Study, a large prospective study of 7735 middle-aged men drawn from 24 towns, was used to examine the role of lifestyle factors in the differential effects of alcoholic beverages on CHD and mortality. In this chapter, we summarise our findings on the relationships between beer, spirit and wine drinking and risk of major CHD events and of all cause mortality, taking into account the differences in lifestyle and personal characteristics associated with beverage type [20]. We also attempt to evaluate the confounding role of lifestyle factors.

BRITISH REGIONAL HEART STUDY

In 1978–80, research nurses administered to each man a standard questionnaire which included questions on frequency, quantity and type of alcohol consumption, smoking habits and medical history. Several physical measurements were made, and blood samples (non-fasting) were taken for measurement of biochemical and haematological variables. All men were followed up for all-cause mortality and cardiovascular morbidity [21]. Analysis was restricted to men with no recall of a doctor diagnosis of CHD or stroke ($N = 7272$ men) in whom there were 901 major CHD events and 1308 deaths from all causes (595 cardiovascular and 713 non-cardiovascular) during a mean follow-up period of 16.8 years. The men were classified into five groups according to their estimated reported weekly intake: *none*, *occasional* (<1 unit/week), *light* (1–15 units/week); *moderate* (16–42 units/week) and *heavy* (>42 units/day). One UK unit of alcohol (one drink) is defined as half a pint of beer, a single measure of spirits, or a glass of wine (approximately 8–10 g alcohol). Heavy drinking refers to those drinking more than six drinks daily or most days. The men were asked to indicate which type of drink they usually took: (1) beer; (2) spirits; (3) mixed beer and spirits; (4) wine/sherry; or (5) mixed wine and sherry, beer and spirits. In this cohort occasional drinkers, a large and relatively stable group, are used as the baseline category as non-drinkers have been shown to be an inappropriate baseline group for studying the effects of alcohol on health and disease [22,23].

Alcohol intake, type of drink and risk of CHD events and mortality

In Table 3.1, comparison is made between occasional drinkers and regular drinkers (light, moderate and heavy combined) for all men who drank and within each of the five alcohol-type intake categories. Consistent with most other studies the BRHS has shown that all regular drinkers (light, moderate and heavy combined) have significantly lower risk for major

Table 3.1 Age-adjusted rates and fully adjusted (+) relative risks for major CHD events and all cause mortality for all men who drink and by type of drink in 6860 men. Occasional drinkers are used as the reference group within each alcohol-type category [20]

Type of drink	Major CHD events		Total mortality	
	Rate/1000 person-years	Adjusted RR+	Rate/1000 person-years	Adjusted RR+
Beer (N = 4101)				
Occasional	9.4	1.00	13.1	1.00
Regular drinkers	8.0	0.78 (0.63, 0.97)	12.2	0.84 (0.71, 1.01)
Spirits (N = 741)				
Occasional	13.6	1.00	13.9	1.00
Regular drinkers	7.9	0.57 (0.39, 0.85)	11.7	0.86 (0.61, 1.21)
Mixed beer and spirits only (N = 983)				
Occasional	10.8	1.00	11.2	1.00
Regular drinkers	8.0	0.75 (0.50, 1.10)	11.0	1.00 (0.69, 1.44)
Wine (N = 500)				
Occasional	6.0	1.00	7.7	1.00
Regular drinkers	5.8	0.92 (0.51, 1.67)	7.6	0.87 (0.51, 1.48)
Mixed wine/sherry, beer and spirits (N = 535)				
Occasional	5.3	1.00	7.5	1.00
Regular drinkers	5.7	1.23 (0.54, 2.79)	6.6	1.09 (0.55, 2.14)
All Regular vs. occasional drinkers		0.77 (0.66, 0.90)		0.90 (0.79, 1.02)

+ adjusted for age, social class, smoking, physical activity, body mass index, lung function evidence of CHD on questionnaire, diabetes and regular medication.

CHD events than occasional drinkers, even after adjustment for potential confounders (age, social class, smoking, physical activity, BMI, lung function, evidence of CHD on WHO chest pain questionnaire, diabetes and regular medication). There was little difference in all cause mortality risk between regular drinkers and occasional drinkers (Table 3.1) [20]. When examined by type of drink(s) usually consumed, the lower risk of CHD was most apparent in beer and spirit drinkers and was not observed in wine drinkers or in mixed drinking which included wine even after adjustment for confounders. For all cause mortality, there was little difference in adjusted relative risk between occasional and regular drinkers within all alcohol-type drinking categories (Table 3.1). However, all men who reported wine drinking (both occasional and regular drinkers) had lower age-adjusted absolute rates of both major CHD events and all cause mortality than non-wine drinkers (beer, spirit and mixed beer and spirits drinkers).

Wine drinking

In Table 3.2, comparison is made between the major alcoholic type categories (three groups only) using beer drinkers as the baseline category in assessment of relative risk used to determine whether wine drinking conferred any additional benefit on the risk of CHD events or on all cause mortality compared with beer and spirits. We compared the effects of

Table 3.2 Type of alcoholic drink and risk of major CHD events and of all cause and cardiovascular and non-cardiovascular mortality in occasional or regular drinkers (N=6860 men). Beer drinkers used as the reference group [20].

	Beer (N=4101)	Spirits (N=1724)	Wine (N=1035)
Major CHD events			
Age-adjusted rates/ 1000 person-years	8.3	9.2	5.8
Age-adj RR	1.00	1.12 (0.96, 1.30)	0.69 (0.56, 0.87)
Adjusted RR (+)	1.00	1.07 (0.90, 1.26)	0.82 (0.64, 1.04)
All cause mortality			
Age-adjusted rates/ 1000 person-years	12.4	11.7	7.3
Age-adj RR	1.00	0.94 (0.83, 1.07)	0.58 (0.47, 0.70)
Adjusted RR (+)	1.00	0.98 (0.85, 1.12)	0.80 (0.65, 0.98)
Cardiovascular mortality			
Age-adjusted rates/ 1000 person-years	5.4	6.0	3.0
Age-adj RR	1.00	1.04 (0.86, 1.25)	0.54 (0.40, 0.73)
Adjusted RR (+)	1.00	1.02 (0.83, 1.25)	0.71 (0.52, 0.98)
Non-cardiovascular mortality			
Age-adjusted rates/ 1000 person-years	6.8	6.0	4.2
Age-adj RR	1.00	0.86 (0.72, 1.03)	0.61 (0.47, 0.78)
Adjusted RR (+)	1.00	0.94 (0.78, 1.14)	0.87 (0.66, 1.14)

(+) adjusted for age, amount drunk, social class, smoking, physical activity, BMI, region of residence, evidence of CHD on questionnaire, diabetes, lung function and regular medication.

Table 3.3 Personal, lifestyle and biological characteristics at screening by different types of drinking [20]

Characteristics	Beer	Spirits	Wine
Age	49.7	50.5	50.0
% current smoker	45.2	42.7	24.9
% manual	66.6	48.4	28.6
% obese	19.6	20.0	15.1
% active	36.9	39.6	42.2
% inactive	8.6	8.4	6.1
% heavy drinkers	13.9	9.9	5.1
% heavy weekend	19.2	13.0	3.0
% light drinkers	33.3	34.9	41.8
% town of residence in the south	25.8	31.0	45.0
Mean lung function (FEV$_1$)	3.31	3.33	3.49
% CHD on questionnaire	9.5	11.8	9.1
% recall HBP	11.9	12.1	10.4
% diabetes	1.2	1.6	1.4
mean HDL-cholesterol (mmol/l)	1.17	1.17	1.17

the different types of drink in occasional and regular drinkers using beer drinkers (Group 1) as the reference group. All men who reported any regular wine drinking were combined (Groups 4 and 5) and similarly all men who drank spirits were combined (Groups 2 and 3) and three mutually exclusive categories were used. Men who reported wine drinking showed significantly lower absolute rates of major CHD events and all cause mortality than beer drinkers. Spirit drinkers showed similar rates to beer drinkers (Table 3.2).

Lifestyle characteristics of wine drinkers

Wine drinkers in this study had multiple advantageous characteristics (Table 3.3). They were predominantly non-manual workers, they had the lowest rates of current smoking and obesity and were more likely to be physically active and to be light drinkers. They were less likely to drink heavily when they did drink and were more likely to live in the southern part of the country which has the lowest mortality rates [24]. They also had better lung function (FEV$_1$) and a lower prevalence of CHD on WHO chest pain questionnaire. Adjustment for these baseline characteristics markedly attenuated the decreased risk of CHD associated with wine drinking compared to beer drinking and the difference was no longer significant (Table 3.2). For all cause mortality the decreased risk was markedly diminished but wine drinking remained associated with a significant reduction in risk even after adjustment, largely due to lower risk of CVD mortality.

OTHER PROSPECTIVE STUDIES

The present data from the British Regional Heart Study provide further evidence that all regular intakes of alcoholic drinks are linked with lower risk of CHD. Evidence that wine is most effective in reducing risk of CHD comes largely from ecological studies which have considerable limitations as they are based on population drinking habits and not on individuals [5,6]. In many of the cohort studies reviewed, drinks are limited to one or two alcohol-types and few prospective studies have compared the CHD and mortality risk of beer, spirits and wine drinkers *within* the same study population. Of those that have, some have found little or no difference between the effects of beer, spirits or wine on CHD [13,15], while others (The Framingham and Copenhagen Studies) have suggested wine to be most protective [14,17]. The Kaiser Permanente Study observed no difference in relationship betweeen beverage choice (beer, spirits and wine) and risk of coronary artery disease hospitalisation [15] but observed a lower risk of CHD mortality and cardio-vascular mortality in wine drinkers compared to spirit drinkers [16]. These findings are very similar to those in the British Regional Heart Study. A recent study of over 36,000 men in France showed that both moderate intake of beer and wine were associated with lower risk of cardiovascular disease compared to abstainers but only daily wine consumption was associated with lower all cause mortality than abstainers [19]. In contrast, the Honolulu Study of Japanese men living in Hawaii found beer [12] to be most protective and in the US Health Professionals Follow Up Study spirits was found to be most protective [25]. However, in these population studies no information was provided on the proportion, personal characteristics or absolute risk in the different beverage groups. The available evidence does not suggest a specific or greater benefit for wine compared with beer or spirits.

THE ROLE OF LIFESTYLE

It has been suggested that differences in findings regarding specific types of drinks, and in particular the low risk seen in wine drinkers compared to other drinkers, may be due to differences in patterns of drinking and to differences in risk traits between those choosing different beverages [11]. The Kaiser Permanente Study observed wine drinkers to have the most favourable coronary risk traits and liquor (spirit) drinkers to have the least favourable traits. Interestingly, the beneficial effect of alcohol on CHD was weakest in the liquor (spirits) drinkers [18]. In this cohort of British middle-aged men, about 15% reported wine drinking and these men had many advantageous characteristics. In particular, they were from a higher socio-economic background, they were more likely to be light drinkers and they had more favourable lifestyle patterns (less smoking, less obesity, more physical activity) than beer and spirit drinkers. These beneficial characteristics were to a considerable degree responsible for the lower relative risk of CHD and all cause mortality in wine drinkers compared to beer drinkers, although a significant reduction in all cause mortality largely due to cardiovascular causes persisted after adjustment.

Adjustment in multivariate analyses is unlikely to fully take into account the multiple advantageous lifestyle characteristics of wine drinkers. Furthermore, given that wine drinkers tend to come from a higher socio-economic background, these men are likely to have other advantages not measured in this and other studies e.g., healthier diet and better access to health care. It is a matter of conjecture as to how much more of the remaining association could be due to residual confounding. A cross sectional study conducted in Copenhagen, comprising over 23,000 men and 25,000 women aged 50–64 years showed wine drinkers to have a healthier diet than non-wine drinkers [26]. It seems likely that the significantly lower risk of all cause and cardiovascular mortality seen in wine drinkers in this and other studies is a consequence of the multiple healthier lifestyle characteristics and higher socio-economic status in wine drinkers resulting in lower fatality, rather than the result of a specific benefit of wine.

HDL-cholesterol cannot explain the lower absolute risk of wine drinking compared to other types of alcohol drinkers as the dose–response relationship between alcohol intake and HDL-cholesterol was similar in male beer, spirit and wine drinkers [27] and wine drinkers showed identical levels of HDL-cholesterol to non-wine drinkers (Table 3.2).

CONCLUSIONS

While wine has been reported to contain antioxidants and substances which have effects on thrombosis, the overall epidemiological evidence from studies in diverse populations suggests that all types of alcoholic drinks are associated with lower risk of coronary heart disease. Although wine drinkers showed a lower risk of CHD events as well as cardiovascular and all cause mortality than beer and spirit drinkers, they have lifestyle characteristics which are markedly advantageous and much if not all of the wine-drinker's advantage can be attributed to these characteristics.

REFERENCES

1 Beaglehole R, Jackson R. Alcohol, cardiovascular diseases and all causes of death: a review of the epidemiological evidence. *Drug and Alcohol Review* 1992; **11**: 275–290.
2 Marmot M, Brunner E. Alcohol and cardiovascular disease: the status of the U-shaped curve. *BMJ* 1991; **303**: 565–568.
3 Maclure M. Demonstration of deductive meta analysis: ethanol intake and risk of myocardial infarction. *Epidemiol. Rev.* 1993; **15**: 328–351.
4 Shaper AG, Wannamethee G, Walker M. Alcohol and coronary heart disease: a perspective from the British Regional Heart Study. *Int. J. Epidemiol.* 1994; **23**: 482–494.
5 St Leger AS, Cochrane AL, Moore F. Factors associated with cardiac mortality in developed countries with particular reference to the consumption of wine. *Lancet* 1979; **i**: 1017–1020.
6 Renaud S, de Logeril M. Wine, alcohol platelets and the French paradox for coronary heart disease. *Lancet* 1992; **339**: 1523–1526.
7 Frankel EN, Kanner J, German JB, Parks E, Kinsella JE. Inhibition of oxidation of human low-density lipoprotein by phenolic substances in red wine. *Lancet* 1993; **341**: 454–457.
8 Maxwell S, Cruickshank A, Thorpe G. Red wine and antioxidant activity in serum. *Lancet* 1994; **344**: 193–194.
9 Demrow HS, Slane PR, Folts JD. Administration of wine and grape juice inhibits *in vivo* platelet activity and thrombosis in stenosed canine coronary arteries. *Circulation* 1995; **91**: 1182–1188.
10 Seigneur M, Bonet J, Dorian B. Effect of the consumption of alcohol, white wine and red wine on platelet function and serum lipids. *J. Appl. Cardiol.* 1990; **5**: 215–222.
11 Rimm EB, Klatsky A, Grobbee, Stampfer MJ. Review of moderate alcohol consumption and reduced risk of coronary heart disease: is the effect due to beer, wine, or spirits? *BMJ* 1996; **312**: 731–736.
12 Yano K, Rhoads GC, Kagan A. Coffee, alcohol and risk of coronary heart disease among Japanese men living in Hawaii. *New Eng. J. Med.* 1977; **297**: 405–409.
13 Hennekens CH, Willett W, Rosner B, Cole DS, Mayrent SL. Effects of beer, wine and liquor in coronary deaths. *JAMA* 1979; **242**: 1973–1974.

14 Friedman LA, Kimball AW. Coronary heart disease mortality and alcohol consumption in Framingham. *Am. J. Cardiol.* 1986; **124**: 481–489.

15 Klatsky AL, Armstrong MA, Friedman GD. Relations of alcoholic beverage use to subsequent coronary artery disease hospitalisation. *Am. J. Cardiol.* 1986; **58**: 710–714.

16 Klatsky AL, Armstrong MA. Alcoholic beverage choice and risk of coronary heart disease mortality. Do red wine drinkers fare best? *Am. J. Cardiol.* 1993; **71**: 467–469.

17 Gronbaek M, Deis A, Sorensen TIA, Becker U, Schnohr P, Jensen G. Mortality associated with moderate intakes of wine, beer, or spirits. *BMJ* 1995; **310**: 1165–1169.

18 Klatsky AL, Armstrong MA, Friedman GD. Red wine, white wine, liquor, beer, and risk for coronary artery disease hospitalization. *Am. J. Cardiol.* 1997; **80**: 416–420.

19 Renaud SC, Gueguen R, Siest G, Salamon R. Wine, beer and mortality in middle-aged men from Eastern France. *Arch. Intern. Med.* 1999; **159**: 1865–1870.

20 Wannamethee SG, Shaper AG. Type of alcoholic drink and risk of major coronary heart disease events and all-cause mortality. *Am. J. Pub. Health* 1999; **89**: 685–690.

21 Walker M, Shaper AG. Follow-up of subjects in prospective studies in general practice. *J. R. Coll. Gen. Pract.* 1984; **34**: 365–370.

22 Wannamethee SG, Shaper AG. Men who do not drink: a report from the British Regional Heart Study. *Int. J. Epidemiology* 1988; **17**: 307–316.

23 Wannamethee SG, Shaper AG. Lifelong teetotallers, ex-drinkers and drinkers: mortality and the incidence of major coronary heart disease events in middle-aged British men. *Int. J. Epidemiol.* 1997; **26**: 523–531.

24 Pocock SJ, Shaper AG, Cook DG, Packham RF, Lacey RF, Powell P, Russell PF. British Regional Heart Study: geographic variations in cardiovascular mortality, and the role of water quality. *BMJ* 1980; **280**: 1243–1249.

25 Rimm EB, Giovannuci EL, Wilett WC, Colditz GA, Rosner B, Stampfer MJ. Prospective study of alcohol consumption and risk of coronary disease in men. *Lancet* 1991; **338**: 464–468.

26 Tjonneland A, Gronbaek M, Stripp C, Overvad K. Wine intake and diet in a random sample of 48763 Danish men an women. *Am. J. Clin. Nutr.* 1999; **69**: 49–54.

27 Brenn T. The Tromso Heart Study: alcoholic beverages and coronary risk factors. *J. Epid. Comm. Health* 1986; **40**: 249–256.

Chapter 4

Effects of gender on alcohol's heart dysfunction

Mariann R. Piano

INTRODUCTION

In both men and women, long-term heavy alcohol consumption is associated with many adverse medical consequences, including the development of a dilated cardiomyopathy (herein referred to as alcoholic heart muscle disease (AHMD)) [1]. In men, the associated clinical features of AHMD include ventricular dilation and mild hypertrophy, decreased systolic function and impaired left ventricular (LV) relaxation [2,3]. Data from recent studies indicate the female gender may be a risk factor for the development of AHMD [4,5]. This is because women who have developed AHMD report a lower total lifetime dose of alcohol compared to alcoholic men with AHMD [4,5]. The aim of this chapter is to review evidence that suggests gender differences in alcohol-related problems, specifically myocardial dysfunction and the development of AHMD.

ALCOHOLISM IN WOMEN AND INCIDENCE OF AHMD

Compared to men, women drink less and experience less alcohol-related medical problems [6]. However, one third of all alcoholics in the United States are women [6]. Over the last two decades, there is no evidence of any major increase in total alcohol consumption by women, however there has been an important change in the drinking patterns and prevalence of alcohol usage among women [7]. With regard to drinking patterns, younger women report frequent heavy drinking and frequent bouts of intoxication [8]. In addition, alcohol usage has increased among women who are employed full-time in nontraditional settings and among those who are unemployed and divorced [9]. This is of concern, because of the increase in the number of women in the work force as well as the number of women who are unemployed and divorced. Therefore, in the future, more women may experience alcohol-related medical problems.

In the United States, long-term excessive alcohol consumption (of any beverage type) in both sexes and in all races, is the leading cause of a nonischemic, dilated cardiomyopathy (DCM) [10]. AHMD represents about 3.8% of all cardiomyopathy cases and women represent approximately 14% of these cases [10]. In all races, death rates due to AHMD are greater for men compared to women. Death rates for African-American women with AHMD are two-fold greater than Caucasion women with AHMD [10].

In men, the prevalence of AHMD is variable and in selected patient populations ranges from 37% to 40% [11,12]. The prevalence of AHMD in women is lower, but is also variable depending on the setting and population sampled. For example, Fernández-Solà *et al.* found the prevalence of AHMD in women was 0.43% (3/702) in an out-patient setting [5]. Gavazzi *et al.* found that in 113 women with dilated cardiomyopathy, only one was an alcohol abuser [13]. In a larger case-control study, McKenna *et al.* found that in women with dilated cardiomyopathy, 11% of the cases were due to long-term alcohol consumption, however 10% of the randomly selected healthy control group were also alcohol abusers [12]. These latter results suggest that in some ethnic populations, alcohol may be a contributing or aggravating factor rather than a primary cause of DCM.

AHMD IN WOMEN

To date, there are only a few studies that have specifically examined sex-differences in the susceptibility and severity of alcohol-induced left ventricular (LV) dysfunction or included women in the study of AHMD. Prior to the studies of Kupari and Koskinen and Urbano-Márquez and colleagues, the prevailing notion was that the female myocardium was resistant to the adverse effects of alcohol [4,14]. In a review by Fabrizio and Regan, male gender and not female gender was listed as a risk factor for the development of AHMD [15].

In this section, studies are reviewed which have investigated abnormalities in cardiac function and structure in women with a history of alcohol abuse. In an early study, Wu *et al.* compared systolic time intervals (STI), such as left ventricular ejection time (LVET), preejection period (PEP) and the PEP/LVET ratio in healthy males/females and alcoholic males/females [16]. In brief, STIs are indexes of contractility and are measured from simultaneous fast-speed recordings of an electrocardiogram, a phonocardiogram and arterial and external carotid pulse tracings. In previous years, STIs were used as indirect measures of left ventricular performance in patients with LV dysfunction, however, these types of measurements are outdated and are infrequently used. Wu *et al.* found no differences in STIs between healthy volunteer females ($n=11$) and alcoholic females ($n=14$) with and without liver cirrhosis (Table 4.1) [16]. In this same investigation, a group of healthy volunteer males ($n=11$) and alcoholic males ($n=22$) were also studied [16]. In male alcoholics, the PEP/LVET ratio, PEP and preejection period interval values were significantly greater compared to the healthy males (Table 4.1). Based upon these data, Wu *et al.* concluded that alcoholic males had abnormal myocardial function, whereas myocardial function was preserved in alcoholic women [16]. These investigators suggested male sex might be a risk factor for the development of preclinical AHMD.

Sixteen years later, Kupari and Koskinen reported that preclinical AHMD does occur in women and occurs after a shorter period of alcohol consumption [14]. Using more reliable and sophisticated techniques (i.e., M-mode echocardiography [echo] and Doppler ultrasound) Kupari and Koskinen examined LV size, mass and systolic function in alcoholic women ($n=14$) and men ($n=22$) [14]. Kupari and Koskinen found female alcoholic patients had lower fractional shortening values and increased wall thickness-to-chamber ratio compared to healthy female subjects ($n=17$). However, there were no appreciable changes in either the end diastolic dimension (EDD) or end-systolic dimension (ESD) values between groups, indicating there was no dilation of the LV chamber. To evaluate diastolic function, Doppler indexes of LV filling, such as peak early diastolic velocity (cm/s), peak atrial velocity (cm/s), early to atrial peak velocity ratio, relaxation time (ms), acceleration of early flow velocity (cm/s^2), deceleration of early flow velocity (cm/s^2), and atrial filling fraction (%) were

Table 4.1 Summary of clinical studies of AHMD in women

Investigation	Subjects/Design	Measures	Results
Wu et al. 1976	• Non random selection of male (n = 22) and female (n = 14) alcoholics presenting to a hospital for alcohol-related diseases • Patients were excluded if signs and symptoms of other CV diseases were present, however patients did not undergo cardiac catheterization to rule out CAD • Control (n = 22) subjects were volunteers • Prospective study with a convenient sample selection	• Measures of contractility were obtained, by measuring the following systolic time intervals (STI): PEP/LVET, PEP (msec), PEPI (msec), LVETI (msec), QS$_2$I (msec)	• Female and male alcoholics were of similar age (35.7 vs. 39.4 years, respectively) • Mean duration of drinking for males was 15 ± 1.4 years compared to 14.3 ± 1.4 years for females • Estimated alcohol quantity (oz/day) for males was 16 ± 0 and for females 13.8 ± 1.9 *(see data table below)*
Kupari and Koskinen, 1992	• Non random selection of male (n = 22) and female (n = 14) patients consecutively admitted to a hospital for detoxification. Patients	• Two-dimensional and M-mode echocardiography and pulsed Doppler recordings of transmitral flow	• Female alcoholics, healthy females and alcoholic males were of similar ages (38, 37, 42 years respectively)

Data table (Wu et al. 1976):

	Females		Males	
	HC	A	HC	A
PEP/LVET	0.3 ± 0.01	0.3 ± 0.01	0.3 ± 0.01	$0.4 \pm 0.02^*$
PEP	93 ± 3	90 ± 4	92 ± 4	$107 \pm 4^*$
PEPI	120 ± 3	122 ± 4	118 ± 3	$140 \pm 4^*$
LVETI	409 ± 6	411 ± 5	401 ± 6	$397 \pm 5^*$
QS$_2$I	531 ± 7	533 ± 5	520 ± 8	$536 \pm 6^*$

- were excluded if signs and symptoms of other CV diseases were present or had cirrhosis
- Control female (n = 17) subjects were volunteers

- Healthy female subjects consumed <10 g of ethanol/day, alcoholic female patients had median duration of 5 years of heavy drinking compared to 19 years for alcoholic men
- Daily ethanol consumption for women was 200 g compared to 230 g/day for men

	HCF	AF	AM
EDD (mm)	48 ± 3†	46 ± 4	48 ± 5
ESD (mm)	32 ± 3	32 ± 4	35 ± 5
FS (%)	34 ± 3†	31 ± 6	28 ± 7
IVS (mm)	8 ± 1†	10 ± 2	11 ± 2†
PWT (mm)	9 ± 1	10 ± 2	11 ± 2
T:R ratio	0.37 ± 0.05†	0.43 ± 0.08	0.48 ± 0.09
LV Mass (g)	120 ± 22	126 ± 19	163 ± 28†‡

	HCF	AF	AM
PEDV	68 ± 7†	45 ± 11	47 ± 12
PAV	44 ± 7	40 ± 10	45 ± 10
EAPV	1.5 ± 0.25	1.2 ± 0.59	1.09 ± 0.44
RT	172 ± 18	178 ± 13	178 ± 27
AEFV	712 ± 194†	476 ± 119	548 ± 220
DEFV	−572 ± 107†	−274 ± 69	−292 ± 143
AF	27 ± 5	35 ± 12	38 ± 13

- Healthy females, alcoholic females and alcoholic males were of similar age (37, 39, 39 years, respectively)

- Skeletal muscle biopsy
- Chest x-ray
- Echocardiography

Urbano-Márquez and colleagues, 1995

- Random sample of alcoholic females (n = 50) and males (n = 100) seeking assistance for termination of their alcohol dependence

Table 4.1 (continued)

Investigation	Subjects/Design	Measures	Results
	• Patients were excluded if they had signs and symptoms of other CV diseases and underwent treadmill exercise testing to rule out other CV diseases • Control females (n = 50) were volunteers		• Mean duration of drinking for males was 17.5 years compared to 16.7 years for females, however total lifetime dose of ethanol was 14.2 kg/kg of body weight for females and 23.1 kg/kg of body weight for males

	HCF	AF	AM
EF (%)	65 ± 4	59 ± 7¶	58 ± 8
FS (%)	38 ± 6	34 ± 4¶	33 ± 6
EDD (mm/m^2)	30 ± 2	32 ± 3¶	30 ± 4
ESD (mm/m^2)	18 ± 2	21 ± 3¶	20 ± 4
LV mass (g/m^2)	78 ± 11	98 ± 21¶	121 ± 27

* Indicates male A group statistically different from male HC group
† Indicates statistically different from alcoholic females (AF)
‡ Indicates statistically different from AF and HCF
¶ Indicates significantly different from HCF group

Abbreviations used: HC – Healthy Controls, A – alcoholic, AF – alcoholic females, HCF – healthy control females, AM – alcoholic males, CV – cardiovascular, CAD – coronary artery disease, LVET – left ventricular ejection time, PEP – pre-ejection period, PEPI = PEP + 0.4 × heart rate, LVETI = LVET + 1.7 × heart rate, EDD – end diastolic dimension, ESD – end systolic dimension, IVS – interventricular thickness, PWT – posterior wall thickness, T:R – thickness to radius ratio, LV – left ventricle, PEDV – peak early diastolic velocity (cm/s), PAV – peak atrial velocity (cm/s), EAPV – early to atrial peak velocity ratio, RT – relaxation time (ms), AEFV – acceleration of early flow velocity (cm/s^2), DEFV – deceleration of early flow velocity (cm/s^2), AFF – atrial filling fraction (%).

determined. As shown in Table 4.1, significant differences in several of these Doppler parameters were found between healthy and alcoholic female subjects, indicating impaired LV filling and diastolic dysfunction in alcoholic women [14]. When echo parameters were normalized to body index, no differences were found between alcoholic men and women, suggesting no sex-differences or sex predisposition to the development of AHMD. These results suggest that after a relatively shorter duration of ethanol consumption (median 5.0 years), alcoholic women demonstrate signs of preclinical AHMD. This was exemplified by mild systolic and diastolic dysfunction (e.g., decreases in the fractional shortening values and Doppler indices of LV filling) and these changes were accompanied by a disproportionate increase in LV wall thickness relative to LV dimensions.

To date, the most comprehensive and largest study was performed by Urbano-Márquez and colleagues [4]. These investigators evaluated nutritional status, skeletal muscle and cardiac function in healthy nonalcoholic women ($n=50$), alcoholic women ($n=50$) and alcoholic men ($n=100$). Even though alcoholic women and men had the diagnosis of AHMD, they did not have overt symptoms of AHMD and therefore were designated as asymptomatic. Four percent of the asymptomatic alcoholic women had evidence of caloric malnutrition and 51% had histological criteria for skeletal muscle myopathy. In alcoholic women the ejection fraction and shortening fraction were significantly less compared to the healthy control women, while LV mass was significantly greater in the alcoholic women compared to healthy volunteers (Table 4.1). The EDD and ESD values were significantly greater in alcoholic women compared to controls (Table 4.1) [4]. Collectively, these data indicate that asymptomatic alcoholic women have evidence of both systolic dysfunction and cardio-myopathy. When compared to the alcoholic men in the same study, the mean lifetime dose of alcohol in female alcoholics with cardiac and skeletal myopathies was 40% less compared to male alcoholic subjects with a cardiac and skeletal myopathies (mean lifetime dose in women was 14.2 kg/kg of body weight compared to 23.1 kg/kg of body weight in men). These data suggest female alcoholic patients drank less, but still developed a cardiomyopathy. These data, along with those of Kupari and Koskinen indicate females are more susceptible to alcohol-induced cardiomyopathy [4,14]. However, it would be interesting to determine if men also developed AHMD at a lower level of total lifetime dose of ethanol (i.e., 14.2 kg/kg of body weight). It would be difficult to determine this, unless one conducted a large prospective study whereby cardiac structure/function were evaluated serially over time.

CLINICAL CHARACTERISTICS AND OCCURRENCE OF HEART FAILURE IN WOMEN WITH AHMD

Fernández-Solà and colleagues examined the clinical characteristics of alcoholic women with AHMD ($n=10$), who also had signs and symptoms of heart failure [5]. For comparison, alcoholic males ($n=26$) were also studied. Cardiothoracic ratios were similar between alcoholic men (0.58 ± 0.04) and women (0.58 ± 0.11) [5]. As shown in Table 4.2, women with AHMD experienced similar heart failure signs compared to men, however, some heart failure signs occurred more often in men. Interestingly, 50% of the women were New York Heart Association (NYHA) functional class II, whereas the majority of men in this sample had NYHA class III or IV heart failure [5]. The NYHA classification system is one based on the degree of physical activity required to evoke symptoms. For example, NYHA Class I indicates greater functional status and patients are able to exert themselves *without* experi-

Table 4.2 Clinical characteristics of men and women with AHMD

	Women (n = 10)	Men (n = 26)
Signs of right-sided failure	20% (2)	50 % (13)
Presence of S_3 or S_4	30% (3)	31 % (8)
Signs of pulmonary hypertension	40% (4)	85 % (22)
Abnormal electrocardiogram	80% (8)	100 % (26)
Atrial fibrillation	10% (1)	27 % (7)
Abnormal repolarization signs	50% (5)	77 % (20)

Values are expressed as percent. Values in parentheses are number of patients. Adapted and used with permission from: Fernández-Solà *et al.*, *Am. J. Cardiol.* 1997; **80**: 481–485.

encing any symptoms of heart failure, whereas NYHA Class IV heart failure patients have symptoms *at rest*. Despite differences between NYHA functional class, both alcoholic men and women had markedly reduced ejection fractions (EF) compared to their respective control groups [5]. For example, the EF in the alcoholic women was 36% compared to 65% in the control group and in alcoholic men the EF was 31% compared to 67% in the control group. In addition, Fernández-Solà *et al.* found a similar degree of LV dilation between alcoholic women and men. However LV mass was much greater in the alcoholic men compared to alcoholic women (Table 4.3) [5]. The total life time ethanol dose (kg/kg of body weight) in women was 17 ± 7 compared to 30 ± 7 for men.

These findings support those of others, which suggest women may be more sensitive to the cardiotoxic effects of ethanol. However, more alcoholic women had a better functional status as indicated by their NYHA class compared to men. It is possible that with continued drinking and a larger total lifetime dose of alcohol, women would develop more severe heart failure. In fact, Urbano-Márquez *et al.* found women with AHMD that had signs of heart failure had a much higher total lifetime ethanol dose (25.8 kg/kg of body weight) [4].

MYOCARDIAL REMODELING AND PROGRESSION OF AHMD

The specific structural remodeling events associated with AHMD in women have not been studied. Left ventricular remodeling is defined as a change in LV geometry, mass and volume

Table 4.3 Echocardiographic parameters in men and women with AHMD compared to healthy controls

	Healthy Controls		Alcoholic	
	Women (n = 20)	Men (n = 20)	Women (n = 10)	Men (n = 26)
LV shortening fraction	38 ± 6	38 ± 4	$15 \pm 8*$	$11 \pm 3\ddagger$
LV EDD (mm/m^2)	30 ± 2	27 ± 2	$36 \pm 8*$	$39 \pm 6\ddagger$
LV ESD (mm/m^2)	18 ± 2	16 ± 2	$28 \pm 10*$	$32 \pm 6\ddagger$
LV mass (g/m^2)	78 ± 11	106 ± 20	$128 \pm 28*$ †	$211 \pm 71\ddagger$

* Indicates significant differences from control healthy females † indicates significant difference from alcoholic men. ‡ Indicates significant difference from healthy men. Abbreviations used: EDD – end diastolic dimension, ESD – end systolic dimension, IVS – interventricular thickness, LV – left ventricle. Used with permission from Fernández-Solà *et al.*, *Am. J. Cardiol.* 1997; **80**: 481–485.

that occurs over a period of time [17]. The overall shape of the LV becomes more spherical with LV elongation and thinning. Over time, LV hypertrophy develops with further LV dilation and thinning and the whole heart becomes more spherically shaped. Severely abnormal LV contours are an important determinate of patient outcome and the process of LV remodeling contributes to the development of heart failure [17]. The process of LV remodeling has been extensively studied in many animal models of CV disease as well as in patients post myocardial infarction.

In terms of AHMD, Mathews *et al.* using echocardiography investigated the myocardial structural abnormalities in alcoholic men ($n = 33$) [18]. Based upon the findings of Mathews and colleagues there appears to be two stages of AHMD, asymptomatic and symptomatic, each of which is associated with different structural changes. Alcoholic patients were divided into two groups: those who were asymptomatic (i.e., symptoms of heart disease) and those who were symptomatic (i.e., symptoms of pulmonary systemic congestion, dyspnea etc.). Not surprisingly, in all symptomatic patients, there was evidence of cardiac enlargement, pulmonary congestion, left ventricular dilation and ventricular hypertrophy. Most importantly, there was a *disproportionate* increase in the radius of the left ventricular (dilation) in relationship to the increase in LV wall thickness. This leads to increases in wall tension and systolic dysfunction. These investigators also found LV dilation and increased wall thickness in the asymptomatic group of patients, however, the LV dilation was *proportionate* to the increase in wall thickness. In this situation, wall tension is usually unchanged or within normal limits.

Based upon the above findings, Mathews *et al.* proposed two models for the development of AHMD [18]. They suggested that patients who were more 'vulnerable' to further progression of AHMD had a disproportionate increase in the radius of the left ventricular (dilation) in relationship to the increase in LV wall thickness, whereas those who were less vulnerable had a more proportionate LV dilation-to-LV wall thickness change. With continued drinking, the former group remains symptomatic and develops heart failure. The progression of AHMD in terms of the progression from mild LV dilation to severe LV dilation and dysfunction has not been evaluated in women.

HOW MUCH ALCOHOL CONSUMPTION LEADS TO AHMD IN WOMEN AND DOES IT DEPEND ON BEVERAGE TYPE?

Based upon their findings, Urbano-Márquez and colleagues have suggested that a '55 kg women who drinks about 270 mL (9 oz) of 86-proof (43%) spirits or about a liter of wine a day for 20 years is a risk for the development of AHMD' [4]. These investigators also reported that, as in men, there was a positive correlation between LV mass and lifetime alcoholic intake in women. This is in contrast to Manolio *et al.*, who found alcohol use (of any beverage type) in men, but *not* women, was independently (as determined by multivariate analysis) associated with an increase in LV mass as well as an increase in internal diastolic dimension (ventricular dilation) [19]. However, when stratified by beverage type, beer and wine use in both men and women and liquor use in men were positively correlated to LV mass. This study was conducted in 4491 people (17–90 years of age), who were free of cardiac disease in the Framingham offspring and cohort study. Total weekly alcohol intake was estimated and correlated to LV mass and LV dimensions. It is important to note that the patients studied in the Framingham cohort were not alcoholics and their cardiac function was within normal limits. The findings of this study are difficult to compare to those of others, since *weekly* rather than *total lifetime* alcohol consumption was measured. Unlike many other studies reported in the literature, these investigators also used multivariate regression analysis to control for the effects of age, height, body mass index, systolic blood pressure, history of hypertension and cigarette smoking.

The results from this Framingham cohort suggest that changes in LV mass may depend on beverage type [19]. In the Urbano-Márquez *et al.* investigation women consumed alcohol predominately in the form of wine, beer, gin and anisette, rather than whisky or brandy [4]. With this limited amount of information, it is difficult to speculate whether the development of AHMD is beverage dependent.

TREATMENT OF WOMEN WITH AHMD

To the author's knowledge, there are no studies which have examined specific pharmacologic treatment modalities, other than alcohol abstinence, in the setting of AHMD. Patients with AHMD, presenting in heart failure with systolic dysfunction, should be treated according to the Agency for Health Care Policy and Research (AHCPR) and Heart Failure Consensus Recommendations [20,21]. These guidelines recommend the use of pharmacologic agents that inhibit the LV remodeling process, as well as treat the patient's symptoms. The different classes of agents include diuretics, cardiac glycosides, angiotensin-converting enzyme inhibitors and beta-adrenergic blockers.

Recently, Fauchier *et al.* examined long-term outcomes in 50 patients with alcoholic CM and 84 patients with idiopathic CM receiving ACHPR recommended pharmacologic therapies [11]. Men and women were included in this sample. Four per cent of the women had AHMD and 25% had idiopathic CM. All patients with AHMD received dietetic and alcohol abstinence counseling. Most of the patients were treated with angiotensin-converting enzyme inhibitors (81%), diuretics (70%) and digoxin (61%). Mean follow-up of patients was 47 ± 40 months. Ventricular ejection fraction improved in alcoholic patients who remained abstinent and also in those who did not remain abstinent. However, compared to patients with idiopathic CM, patients with alcoholic CM *without* abstinence had a significantly worse outcome (Figure 4.1). Furthermore, using multivariate regression, it was determined in the entire cohort that lack of abstinence, increased pulmonary capillary wedge pressure, and decreased SDNN (a time domain analysis variable of heart rate variability (standard deviation of all normal-to-normal electrocardiogram RR intervals)) were independent predicators of cardiac death. These results suggest that in the presence of recommended heart failure pharmacologic therapies, alcohol abstinence is very important.

WHAT HAVE ANIMAL MODELS TAUGHT US?

Animal models of alcoholism have revealed that long-term alcohol consumption is associated with numerous histological and cellular changes in the myocyte. Specific histological changes include myocyte loss and disarray, interstitial and perivascular fibrosis, deposition of lipids with the myocardial tissue, accumulation of fatty acid ethyl esters within intracellular organelles, and mitochondrial and sarcoplasmic reticulum disorganization [22–27]. In terms of cell function, there are reports of altered mitochondrial and sarcoplasmic reticulum function, decreased

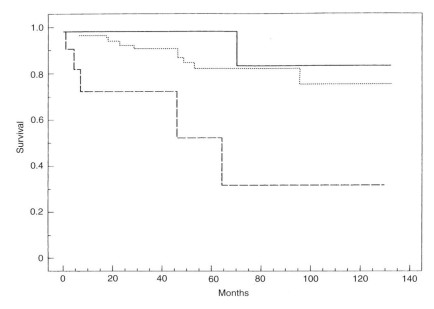

Figure 4.1 Survival curves of cardiac deaths in male patients with alcoholic dilated cardiomyopathy (DCM). Solid line indicates patients with alcoholic DCM and alcohol abstinence,
large dashed line indicates patients with alcoholic DCM without abstinence and small
dashed line indicates idiopathic DCM. Used with permission from Fauchier *et al.*
European Heart J. 2000; **21**: 306–314.

myofibrillar ATPase activity and decreased calcium sensitivity of the myofilaments [28–32].
In animal models, these changes often precede changes in cardiac structure and function.
These studies have been exclusively performed in male animal models. The only exceptions
are the studies reported by Lochner and colleagues and Brown and colleagues [33,34].
Therefore, the effects of both acute and chronic alcohol consumption on the female myo-
cardium are relatively unknown.

In the Lochner *et al.* study, female albino Wistar rats were used to study the effects of
alcohol [33]. It appears that a primary aim of this study was to contrast the effects of
acute and long-term alcohol exposure on the myocardium, rather than examine sex-
related differences. In long-term experiments, female rats received 15% ethanol in their
drinking water for 18 months. Afterwards, isolated Langendorff experiments were performed to evaluate the effects of long-term alcohol exposure as well as the effects of acute
alcohol exposure in the chronically exposed alcoholic hearts. Measures of contractility
included peak height of developed tension (PHT), tension time index (TTI), tension
time per minute (TTM), maximum rate of rise of tension (dp/dt_{max}), and time-to-and
peak height of developed tension (TPH). Except for TPH, all of the these parameters
were lower in the alcoholic hearts compared to the control hearts, however, only the
decrease in dp/dt_{max} was significantly different from the control value. In the alcohol-
exposed hearts, TPH was significantly increased compared to the control hearts. The
acute administration of ethanol (200 mM) markedly attenuated all of the aforementioned contractility parameters. However, the degree of attenuation (% reduction in

Table 4.4 Acute effects of ethanol in male and female papillary muscles

	Control	80 mg/dl	120 mg/dl	240 mg/dl	640 mg/dl
TPT (msec)					
Male	113 ± 2.3	112 ± 2.2	112 ± 1.5	108 ± 2.1	100 ± 1.5
Female	118 ± 4.2	116 ± 4.6	115 ± 4.5	$112 \pm 4.3^*$	$103 \pm 3.9^*$
RT_{90} (msec)					
Male	191 ± 15.1	192 ± 17.5	179 ± 12.5	$167 \pm 10.7^*$	$149 \pm 7.2^*$
Female	202 ± 8.7	194 ± 10.0	186 ± 9.0	$181 \pm 8.7^*$	$156 \pm 5.7^*$
+VT (g/sec)					
Male	17.9 ± 2.0	18.3 ± 2.1	17.9 ± 2.0	16.8 ± 1.9	$14.1 \pm 1.5^*$
Female	18.9 ± 2.1	18.1 ± 1.7	17.8 ± 1.6	16.9 ± 1.6	$13.1 \pm 1.2^*$
−VT (g/sec)					
Male	11.0 ± 1.9	11.1 ± 2.2	11.2 ± 1.8	10.8 ± 1.7	$8.7 \pm 1.2^*$
Female	10.3 ± 1.6	10.2 ± 1.4	10.0 ± 1.3	9.9 ± 1.2	$8.1 \pm 0.9^*$

* Indicates significant difference from same sex control value. Abbreviations used: TPT – time-to-peak tension, RT_{90} – time-to-90% relaxation, +VT – the maximum velocities of tension developed and −VT – decline in tension.

Source: Adapted and used with permission from Brown *et al. Basic Research in Cardiol.* 1996; **91**: 353–360.

tension) was similar between the alcoholic and control hearts, indicating long-term alcohol exposure had no *additional* adverse effect on contractility. These authors concluded that long-term alcohol administration had a rather modest effect on myocardial performance, because of the *lack of* statistical significance. Therefore, these authors concluded that long-term ethanol administration had no effect in the perfused female rat heart.

In a more recent study, Brown and colleagues examined the effect of acute ethanol exposure on the female and male Wistar rat myocardium [34]. Using an isolated papillary preparation, different measures of contractility such as time-to-peak tension (TPT), time-to-90% relaxation (RT_{90}), the maximum velocities of tension developed (+VT) and decline in tension (−VT) were measured after the addition of increasing concentrations of ethanol (20–640 mg/dl) to the perfusate solution. In both sexes, the addition of ethanol exerted a concentration-dependent negative inotropic effect and the magnitude of the response was similar between the sexes (Table 4.4). These data indicate that there was no sex-related difference in the negative inotropic response to acute ethanol exposure.

ONGOING RESEARCH IN FEMALE RATS

Our laboratory has been studying the effects of long-term alcohol consumption in both female and male rats. Presented below is preliminary data from our laboratory. The primary aim has been to describe in an animal model (male and female rats) the evolution of alcohol-induced changes in cardiac structure (hypertrophy and dilation) that lead to the development of a cardiomyopathy. The second aim has been to determine if these changes are associated with activation of specific peptide and neurohormonal systems.

Preliminary experiments were conducted in male ($n=5$) and female ($n=5$) Sprague-Dawley rats which received the Lieber DeCarli liquid diet for 5 months [35]. In brief and as previously described by this laboratory, control (CON) and ethanol (ETOH) groups received the nutritionally complete control or ethanol liquid Lieber-DeCarli diet [31,32]. The males received an ethanol diet (9% v/v), which provided up to 42% of their total daily caloric intake or 13.0 gm ethanol/kg/day. However, the female group received a 6.7% v/v ethanol. We were unable to titrate females up to the 9% ethanol concentration. In our laboratory and as discussed in more detail below, female rats on average drink less alcohol/day and a less concentrated (v/v ethanol) preparation of the Lieber DeCarli diet. In the control diet, maltose–dextrin was substituted isocalorically for ethanol [35]. To maintain a similar liquid diet intake between the CON and ETOH, the CON group was pair-fed to the same sex ETOH group. Liquid diet consumption was monitored daily and fresh diet was provided each day between 4 pm and 6 pm. The animals were weighed once a week. As previously reported, in male rats this ethanol consumption protocol was associated with high blood ethanol levels (BELs) [31,32] that typically ranged from 160–240 mg%.

In both groups, echocardiograms were performed by the same experienced sonographer using the Sequoia C256 Echocardiography System (Acuson Corporation, Mountain View, California) and a 7.5 MHz transducer. M-mode recordings were made by directing the ultrasound beam at the mid-papillary muscle level and echo parameters were obtained after well-defined, continuous interface of the anterior and posterior walls were visualized. For all animals, three to four beats were recorded using the same transducer position. Mean values were used for analysis. Echocardiograms were performed after 5 months of ethanol consumption.

According to the methods of the American Society of Echocardiography and other investigators in animal models, the end diastolic (EDD) and end-systolic dimensions (ESD), interventricular septum in diastole (IVSD), and posterior wall in diastole (PWD) thickness were obtained with the leading-edge method [36]. All parameters were measured with electronic calipers, and mean calculations obtained from three or more consecutive cardiac cycles. All studies were recorded on a VHS videotape recorder. Intraobserver variability for all echocardiographic parameters ranged from 0–10% (mean 7%). The LV mass (gm) was calculated based on the following echocardiogram parameters [37]: LV mass $= 1.04 \times$ [(EDD + PWD + IVSD)^3 − EDD^3].

As shown in Table 4.5, the EDD and ESD values in the male ETOH group were significantly greater than EDD and ESD values in the male CON group. No significant differences were found in IVS or PW thickness between the male ETOH and CON groups. LV mass and HW:BW ratios were greater in the ETOH group, compared to the CON group, however only the latter difference was significant (Table 4.5). In the female study, even though there was a trend for the EDD, ESD and PW thickness values to be greater in the ETOH group compared to the CON group, no significant differences were found (Table 4.5). The EDD value in the ETOH group was 42% higher than the EDD value in the female CON group, however, as noted this difference was not statistically significant, perhaps because of the small sample size. The calculated LV mass and heart-weight-to-body-weight ratios were greater in the ETOH females, however only the latter difference was significant. Representative echocardiograms are shown in Figures 4.2 and 4.3.

The female rats in this study drank a 6.7% vol/vol concentration of alcohol as compared to the males, which drank 9% vol/vol concentration. Therefore, even though the female group consumed less alcohol (gm/day), there were signs that LV dilation and hypertrophy were beginning. These results in an animal model are comparable to those of Urbano-Marquez *et al.* and of Kupari and Koskinen, who found that the mean lifetime dose of alcohol in female alcoholics with alcoholic cardiomyopathy was markedly less than male alcoholic

FEMALE

Interventricular
Septum (IVS)

Posterior
Wall

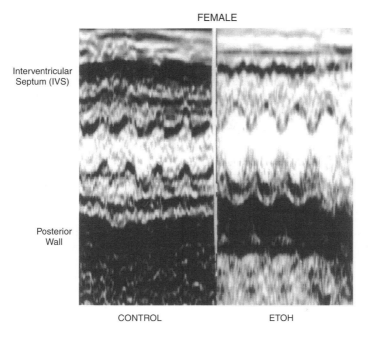

CONTROL   ETOH

Figure 4.2 Representative echocardiograms from control and ethanol-fed female rat.

MALE

Interventricular
Septum (IVS)

Posterior
Wall

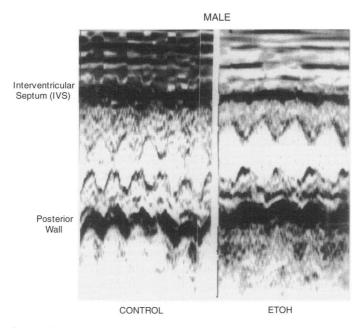

CONTROL   ETOH

Figure 4.3 Representative echocardiograms from control and ethanol-fed male rat.

Table 4.5 Echocardiographic parameters in male and female control and ethanol-fed animals

| | Dimensions | | | |
| | Males | | Females | |
	Control	Ethanol	Control	Ethanol
EDD (mm)	4.0 ± 0.05	6.3 ± 0.08*	3.9 ± 0.04	5.5 ± 0.02
ESD (mm)	1.3 ± 0.04	2.8 ± 0.05*	2.7 ± 0.04	2.8 ± 0.08
IVS thickness (mm)	2.5 ± 0.02	3.0 ± 0.02	2.5 ± 0.02	2.1 ± 0.02
PW thickness	2.2 ± 0.02	2.5 ± 0.02	2.0 ± 0.01	2.2 ± 0.01
LV mass (g)	0.76 ± 0.09	1.5 ± 0.38	0.6 ± 0.13	0.8 ± 0.17
HWBW ratio	2.4 ± 0.14	2.9 ± 0.06*	2.7 ± 0.09	3.2 ± 0.09*

All values are mean ± SEM. Within group (same sex) statistical comparisons were made and an * indicates significantly different from control value as determined by the Student's t-test. IVS and PW thickness measurements were obtained in diastole. Heart weight-to-body weight (HWBW) was calculated as follows: wet heart weight (left and right ventricles) (g)/body weight (g) × 1000. Left ventricular (LV) mass was calculated using the equation indicated in text. Abbreviations used: BW – body weight, HWBW – heart weight-to-body weight ratio, LV – left ventricle, EDD – end-diastolic left ventricular dimension, ESD – end-systolic left ventricular dimension, IVS – interventricular septal, PW – posterior wall.

subjects with alcoholic cardiomyopathy [4,14]. In addition, these preliminary findings are also supported by Capasso et al. who evaluated changes in left ventricular chamber volume in Fisher 344 rats, by measuring long and short left ventricular diameters and wall thickness of the heart [22]. The rats received 30% ethanol in their drinking water every day for 8 months. Capasso et al. found an increase in the volume of the left ventricle accompanied by a decrease in the thickness of the left ventricular free wall [22].

The preliminary studies from my laboratory were conducted following a short duration of ethanol consumption (5 months) and only included a small sample size (n = 5). Therefore, the results need to be interpreted with caution. A larger study is underway to evaluate serial changes in cardiac structure and neurohormonal levels in female rats consuming alcohol for a longer period (8 months). A serial study of this nature will allow for evaluation of cardiac structural changes with respect to body growth, age of the animal and different amounts of alcohol consumption.

ARE FEMALE ANIMAL MODELS OF ALCOHOLISM HELPFUL IN EVALUATING THE ADVERSE EFFECTS OF ALCOHOL?

Female animal models of alcoholism should be used to study the effects of long-term alcohol exposure. However, investigators need to consider variables such as the level/concentration of ethanol intake, the pattern of weight gain as well as the absolute weight gain, and hormone levels. As noted above, we have found that female rodents drink less alcohol than male rodents (Table 4.6). Our findings differ from those of others, who have reported that female rodents drink more than male rodents [38,39].

We have also found that the pattern of drinking and amount of daily Lieber DeCarli ethanol diet consumption is more variable among female rats compared to male rats (Figures 4.4 and 4.5).

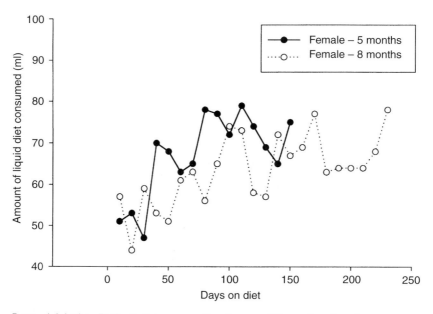

Figure 4.4 Lieber DeCarli diet consumption for two different female cohorts.

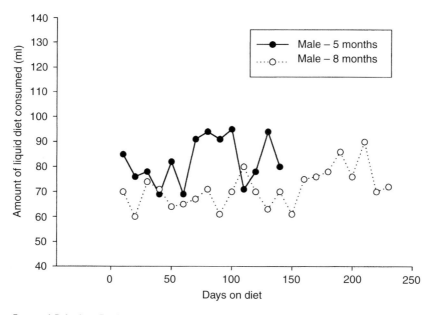

Figure 4.5 Lieber DeCarli diet consumption for two different male cohorts.

Table 4.6 Comparison of male and female body weight and Lieber DeCarli diet consumption

Sex	Drinking period	Average body weight at the end of the protocol	Ethanol Consumption		
			ml/day	gm/day	g/kg/day*
Male					
	5	526 ± 82	82 ± 2.7	5.6 ± 0.68	10.7
	8	477 ± 74	70 ± 2.1	4.9 ± 0.70	10.2
Female					
	5	393 ± 65	68 ± 2.4	3.4 ± 0.50	8.6
	8	282 ± 21	60 ± 1.6	3.1 ± 0.47	10.9

Values are mean ± SD. ml/day represents the average daily amount of diet consumed and was calculated by averaging how much animals drank every 10 days. Similarly, gm ethanol/day represents the average daily ethanol (gm/day) and was calculated by averaging how much animals drank every 10 days.
* g/kg/day was calculated by dividing the average gm/day by the ending body weight.

In addition, the pattern of drinking appears to be different between cohorts of female animals (Figure 4.4). Lieber DeCarli liquid diet intake is shown in Figure 4.4 for two different cohorts of female rats; one group drank for 5 months (preliminary data above) and another drank for 8 months (ongoing studies). Similar to others, we found that in both cohorts of female rats the average daily amount of diet consumed was variable [39]. However, the average daily ethanol intake (gm/day) in the 5-month cohort was significantly greater than in the 8-month cohort (3.4±0.50 vs. 3.1±0.47 gm ethanol/day, $p<0.05$). The end body weight of the 5-month cohort was 393±65 gm compared to the 282±21 gm body weight of the 8-month cohort. However, when ethanol intake was normalized to the end body weight, the 8-month cohort appeared to consume comparatively more ethanol (Table 4.6). These are female Sprague-Dawley rats, which are an outbred strain. Therefore, in this strain there may be more genetic variability, which may affect the ethanol preference and daily ethanol intake. Investigators should carefully consider the strain of female rat to be used in alcohol studies and choose a strain that exhibits less of a variation in daily alcohol intake.

WHY IS THE FEMALE HEART MORE SUSCEPTIBLE TO THE DEVELOPMENT OF AHMD?

There have been many reasons postulated to explain the differences between males and females, in terms of sensitivity to alcohol-related medical consequences. Several of the reasons are briefly reviewed below. A more comprehensive review is published elsewhere [40].

Female alcoholics develop a multitude of symptoms more rapidly than male alcoholics during the first few years of drinking, a phenomenon which is refered to as 'telescoping' [41,42]. Lewis *et al.* examined the effect of other co-morbidities on the rapid accrual of symptoms in women and found that this rapid accrual was independent of the number of co-morbidities [41]. Others have found that women are at greater risk for the development of alcoholic liver disease and brain damage [43–45]. These data, along with the data reviewed in this chapter, suggest that women are more vulnerable to the medical consequences of alcohol.

Putative gender-related effects may be due to sex-related differences in alcohol pharmacokinetics which allow women to achieve higher blood alcohol levels (BAL) compared to men, after consuming an equivalent amount of alcohol. Some reports suggested that higher BALs in nonalcoholic women were attributable in part to a difference in the first-pass metabolism of alcohol and the activity of gastric alcohol dehydrogenase (ADH). This is because Frezza *et al.* found no differences in BALs between nonalcoholic men and women when alcohol was administered intravenously, however after ingesting equivalent doses of alcohol orally, BALs were significantly higher in women [46]. These same investigators reported that gastric ADH activity was significantly lower in nonalcoholic women (0.025 ± 0.003 nmoles/min/mg protein) compared to nonalcoholic men (0.046 ± 0.005 nmoles/min/mg protein). A similar difference in gastric ADH activity was found between alcoholic men and women [46]. Others have also found that gastric ADH activity was lower in women compared to men, but that this effect was only found in patients (men and women) less than fifty years old and after a high concentration of ethanol was added to the gastric ADH assay (550 mM) [47]. In contrast, Yin *et al.* did not find differences in gastric ADH activity between men and women of a similar mean age [48]. Furthermore, in a recent study by Lucey *et al.* no differences in BALs were found between age-matched men and women [49]. In this investigation, BALs were compared following intravenous and oral alcohol administration in both fed and fasted states. In the fasted state, peak BALs were significantly higher in the elderly women compared to young women and young and old men. Similarly, peak BALs were significantly higher in the elderly women compared to young women and young and old men after administration of intravenous alcohol. Interestingly, this difference disappeared when peak BALs were measured in the fed state after oral alcohol consumption [49]. The results of this study suggest an age-dependent effect, rather than a sex-dependent effect on peak BALs and this in turn is influenced by the fasting or fed state of the individual.

A final parameter related to alcohol pharmacokinetics is the elimination of alcohol. Current evidence suggests that women eliminate more alcohol per unit of body mass, therefore having a faster rate in the decline in their blood alcohol level [40].

In summary, it remains controversial as to whether women achieve higher BALs after consuming similar amounts of alcohol. There appears to be more agreement among studies with regard to alcohol elimination and collectively these suggest women eliminate alcohol at a faster rate.

CONCLUSIONS

Similar to men, long-term heavy alcohol consumption in women is associated with the development of a dilated cardiomyopathy. The clinical features resemble those found in men and include a dilated LV, modest degree of hypertrophy and reduced systolic dysfunction. Most importantly, women appear to develop a preclinical, asymptomatic form of this disease with less total lifetime exposure to alcohol, suggesting female gender may be a risk factor for the development of AHMD. In terms of the amount and duration of alcohol consumption correlated with the development of AHMD, Urbano-Márquez and colleagues have suggested that a 55 kg woman who drinks about 270 mL (9 oz) of 86-proof (43%) spirits or about a liter of wine a day for 20 years is a risk for the development of AHMD [4]. In some individuals, their genetic background or environmental exposure to other toxins may also play a role in the pathogenesis of AHMD. The American Heart Association recommends that women drink no more than 1 standard drink per day (i.e., 12 fl oz regular beer, 5 fl oz wine, 1.5 fl oz 80-proof distilled spirits and each of these contains approximately 12 g of alcohol) [50]. This is because in women, the effect of alcohol on conditions other than cardiovascular disease needs to be considered. Specifically, alcohol intake between 30 and 60 g/d is associated with an increase in the relative risk of breast cancer, whereas alcohol intake of ≤10 g/d was associated with a lower relative risk [51]. Women should be advised to discuss the potential risk-to-benefit ratio of low to moderate drinking with their health care provider. Each woman, depending on their personal history (e.g., familial history of breast cancer or ischemic heart disease), will have different risk factors and should be advised accordingly.

Animal models of alcoholism have contributed a great deal to our understanding of the structural, histological, subcellular and contractile changes associated with long-term alcohol consumption. Investigators need to consider the strain of female rats. As noted above, in our laboratory, the pattern of drinking and amount consumed is variable among Sprague Dawley rats. However, Lancaster and Spiegel have found that female Long-Evans rats have a greater preference for alcohol compared to the male Long-Evans rat [38]. In fact, the female Long-Evans drank 10% beer preparations, whereas, the male Long-Evans decreased their intake at this concentration.

Clearly, there is a need for more research in women with AHMD. There is no information as yet regarding the progression of AHMD, in terms of LV structural changes and contractile performance. The effects of alcohol abstinence on AHMD is unknown. In men with AMHD, alcohol abstinence is associated with a reversal of the dilated cardiomyopathy. As with all types of cardiovascular studies, women should be well represented in the study of AHMD.

ACKNOWLEDGEMENTS

This work was supported by grant NIAAA 11112

REFERENCES

1 Piano MR, Schwertz DW. Alcoholic heart disease: A review. *Heart and Lung* 1994; **23**: 3–17.

2 Lazarević AM, Nakatani S, Nešković AN, Marinković J, Yasumura Y, Stojičić D, Muyatake K, Bojić M, Popović AD. Early changes in left ventricular function in chronic asymptomatic alcoholics: relation to the duration of heavy drinking. *J. Am. Coll. Cardiol.* 2000; **35**: 1599–1606.

3 Regan TJ. Alcohol and the cardiovascular system. *JAMA* 1990; **264**: 377–381.

4 Urbano-Márquez A, Estruch R, Fernández-Solá J, Nicloás JM, Paré JC, Rubin E. The greater risk of alcoholic cardiomyopathy and myopathy in women compared with men. *JAMA* 1995; **274**: 149–154.

5 Fernández-Solà J, Estruch R, Nicolás J-M, Paré J-C, Sacanella E, Antúnez E, Urbano-Márquez A. Comparison of alcoholic cardiomyopathy in women vs. men. *Am. J. Cardiol.* 1997; **80**: 481–485.

6 Substance Abuse and Mental Health Services Administrative Office of Applied Statistics. *Overview of the FY94 national drug and alcoholism treatment unit survey (NDATUS): Data from 1993 and 1980–1993.* 1995: **9A**: 18–19.

7 Wilsnack SC, Wilsnack RW. Epidemiology of women's drinking. *J. Subst. Abuse Treat.* 1991; **3**: 133–157.

8 Wechsler H, Davenport A, Dowdall G *et al*. Health and behavior consequences of binge drinking in college: A national survey of students at 140 campuses. *JAMA* 1994; **272**: 2939–2944.

9 Gomberg ESL. Women and Alcohol: Use and abuse. *J. Nerv. Ment. Dis.* 1993; **181**: 211–219.

10 *Vital and Health Statistics.* U.S. Department of health and human services. Centers for Disease Control and Prevention. October 1995; **13**(122).

11 Fauchier L, Babuty D, Poret P, Casset-senon D, Autret ML, Cosnay P, Faucheir JP. Comparison of long-term outcome of alcoholic and idiopathic dilated cardiomyopathy. *European Heart J.* 2000; **21**: 306–314.

12 McKenna CJ, Codd MB, McCann HA, Sugrue DD. Alcohol consumption idiopathic dilated cardiomyopathy: A case control study. *Am. Heart J.* 1998; **135**: 833–837.

13 Gavazzi A, De Maria R, Parolini M, Porcu M. On behalf of the Italian Multicenter Cardiomyopathy Study Group (SPIC). Alcohol abuse and cardiomyopathy in men. *Am. J. Cardiol.* 2000; **85**: 1114–1118.

14 Kupari M, Koskinen P. Comparison of the cardiotoxicity of ethanol in women vs. men. *Am. J. Cardiol.* 1992; **70**: 645–649.

15 Fabrizio L, Regan TJ. Alcoholic cardiomyopathy. *Cardiovasc. Drugs Ther.* 1994; **8**: 89–94.

16 Wu CF, Sudhaker M, Jaferi G, Ahmed SS, Regan TJ. Preclinical cardiomyopathy in chronic alcoholics: A sex difference. *Am. Heart J.* 1976; **91**: 281–286.

17 Piano MR, Kim SD, Jarvis C. Cellular targets linked to cardiac remodeling in heart failure: Targets for pharmacologic intervention. *J. Cardiovasc. Nursing* 2000; **14**: 1–23.

18 Mathews EC, Gradin JM, Henry WL, Del Negro AA, Fletcher RD, Snow JA, Epstein SE. Echocardiographic abnormalities in chronic alcoholics with and without overt congestive heart failure. *Am. J. Cardiol.* 1981; **47**: 570–578.

19 Manolio TA, Levy D, Garrison RJ, Castelli WP, Kannel WB. Relation of alcohol intake to left ventricular mass: The Framingham study. *JACC* 1991; **17**: 717–721.

20 Konstam M, Dracup K, Baker D *et al*. Heart failure: Evaluation and care of patients with left ventricular systolic dysfunction. *Clinical Practice guideline No. 11.* Rockville, Md: US Dept Health and Human Services, Agency for Health Care Policy and Research; 1994. ACHPR publication 94-0612.

21 Packer M, Cohn JN, Abraham WT *et al*. Consensus recommendations for the management of chronic heart failure. *Am. J. Cardiol.* 1999; **83**(2A): 1A–38A.

22 Capasso JM, Li P, Guideri G. Myocardial mechanical, biochemical and structural alterations induced by chronic ethanol ingestion in rats. *Circ. Res.* 1992; **71**: 346–356.

23 Sarma JSM *et al*. Biochemical and contractile properties of heart muscle after prolonged alcohol administration. *J. Mol. Cell Cardiol.* 1976; **8**: 951–972.

24 Weishaar RE *et al*. Reversibility of mitochondrial function and contractility changes in the myocardium after cessation of prolonged ethanol intake. *Am. J. Cardiol.* 1977; **40**: 556–562.

25 Segel LD, Rendig SV, Mason DT. Alcohol-induced hemodynamic and Ca^{2+} flux dysfunctions are reversible. *J. Mol. Cell Cardiol.* 1981; **13**: 443–455.

26 Beckemeier ME, Bora PS. Fatty acid ethyl esters potentially toxic products of myocardial ethanol metabolism. *J. Mol. Cell Cardiol.* 1998; **30**: 2487–2494.

27 Regan TJ *et al*. Myocardial function and lipid metabolism in the chronic alcoholic animal. *J. Clin. Invest.* 1974; **54**: 740–752.

28 Bing RJ, Tillmanns H, Fauvel JM, Seeler K, Mao JC. Effect of prolonged alcohol administration on calcium transport in heart muscle of the dog. *Circ. Res.* 1974; **35**: 33–38.

29 Segel LD, Rendig SV, Choquet Y, Chacko K, Amsterdam EA, Mason DT. Effects of chronic graded ethanol consumption on the metabolism, ultrastructure, and mechanical function of the rat heart. *Cardiovas. Res.* 1975; **9**: 649–663.

30 Pachinger OM, Tillmanns H, Mao C, Fauvel J-M, Bing RJ. The effect of prolonged administration of ethanol on cardiac metabolism and performance in the dog. *J. Clin. Invest.* 1973; **52**: 2690–2696.

31 Piano MR, Schwertz DW, Rosenblum C. Effect of pimobenden and isoproterenol in the alcoholic myocardium. *J. Cardiovasc. Pharmacol.* 1999; **33**: 237–242.

32 Meehan J, Piano MR, Solaro RJ, Kennedy JM. Heavy long-term ethanol consumption induces an α-MHC to β-myosin heavy chain isoforms transition in rat. *Bas. Res. Cardiol.* 1999; **94**: 481–488.

33 Lochner A, Cowley R, Brink AJ. Effect of ethanol on metabolism and function of the perfused rat heart. *Am. Heart J.* 1969; **78**: 770–780.

34 Brown RA, Filipovich P, Walsh MF, Sowers JR. Influence of sex, diabetes and ethanol on intrinsic contractile performance of isolated rat myocardium. *Basic Res. Cardiol.* 1996; **91**: 353–360.

35 Lieber C, DeCarli L. Liquid diet technique of ethanol administration: 1989 update. *Alcohol Alcohol.* 1989; **24**: 197–211.

36 Sahn DJ, DeMaria A, Kisslo J, Weyman A. The Committee on M-mode standardization of the American Society of Echocardiography Recommendations regarding quantitation in M-mode echocardiography: results of a survey of echocardiographic methods. *Circulation* 1978; **58**: 1072–1083.

37 Litwin SE, Katz SE, Morgan JP, Douglas PS. Serial echocardiography assessment of left-ventricular geometry and function after large myocardial infarction in the rat. *Circulation* 1994; **9**: 345–354.

38 Lancaster FE, Spiegel KS. Sex differences in pattern of drinking. *Alcohol* 1992; **9**: 415–420.

39 Li T-K, Lumeng L. Alcohol preference and voluntary alcohol intakes of inbred rat strains and the national institutes of health heterogenous stock of rats. *Alcohol Clin. Exp. Res.* 1984; **8**: 485–486.

40 Mumenthaler MS, Taylor JL, O'Hara R, Yesavage JA. Gender differences in moderate drinking effects. *Alcohol Research and Health* 1999; **23**: 55–64.

41 Lewis CE, Bucholz KK, Spitznagel E, Shayka JJ. Effects of gender and comorbidity on problem drinking in a community sample. *Alcohol Clin. Exp. Res.* 1996; **20**: 466–476.

42 Piazza NJ, Vrbka JL, Yeager RD. Telescoping of alcoholism in women alcoholics. *Int. J. Addict.* 1989; **24**: 19–28.

43 Norton R, Batey R, Dwyer T *et al.* Alcohol consumption and the risk of alcohol related cirrhosis in women. *Brit. Med. J.* 1987; **295**: 80–82.

44 Morgan MY, Sherlock S. Sex related differences among 100 patients with alcoholic liver disease. *Brit. Med. J.* 1977; **1**: 939–941.

45 Jacobson R. The contributions of sex and drinking history to the CT brain scan changes in alcoholics. *Psychol. Med.* 1986; **16**: 547–549.

46 Frezza M, DI Padova C, Pozzato G, Terpin M, Baraona E, Lieber CS. High blood alcohol levels in women. *NEJM* 1990; **322**: 95–99.

47 Seitz HK, Egerer G, Simanowski UA, Waldherr R, Eckey R, Agarwal DP, Goedde HW, von Wartburg J-P. Human gastric alcohol dehydrogenase activity: effect of age, sex, and alcoholism. *Gut* 1993; **34**: 1433–1437.

48 Yin S-J, Liao C-S, Wu C-W, Li T-T, Chen L-L, Lai C-L, Tsao T-Y. Human stomach alcohol and aldehyde dehydrogenases: Comparison of expression pattern and activities in alimentary tract. *Gastroenterology* 1997; **112**: 766–775.

49 Lucey MR, Hill EM, Young JP, Demo-Dannanberg L, Beresford TP. The influences of age and gender on blood ethanol concentration in healthy humans. *J. Stud. Alcohol* 1999; **60**: 103–110.

50 American Heart Association, Guide to preventive Cardiology in Women.

51 Smith-Warner SA, Spiegelman D, Yaun SS, van den Brandt PA, Folsom AR, Goldbohm RA, Grahm S, Holmberg L, Howe GR, Marshall JR, Miller AB, Potter JD, Speizer FE, Illett WC, Wolk A, Hunter DJ. Alcohol and breast cancer in women: A pooled analysis of cohort studies. *JAMA* 1998; **279**: 535–540.

Chapter 5

Alcohol and cardiac medications: interactions

Simon K.K. Cheung and Timothy J. Regan

INTRODUCTION

In the US two-thirds of the general population consume alcohol, and approximately 10% of these are considered heavy alcohol users. A majority of these also use cigarettes which, in sufficient quantity and duration, can represent a significant interaction affecting cardiac muscle function and composition [1]. About 5 million Americans have coronary artery disease and approximately 50 million have high blood pressure [2]. Treatment for these conditions may involve additive or synergistic effects when combined with ethanol and result in mild transient effects or occasional serious consequences [3]. In fact, Shinn *et al.* have reported the interaction of alcohol with about 150 medications, some of which were prescribed for the treatment of cardiovascular disease [4].

Although ingestion is the usual route of intake, ethanol can enter the circulation by cutaneous absorption or inhalation. Alcohol is also found as a solvent or an active ingredient in other commodities ranging from hair styling products and mouthwashes to cough syrups and body rubs, etc. [5].

ALCOHOL AND THE CARDIOVASCULAR SYSTEM

Ethanol has long been recognized as a toxic agent affecting different organ functions both acutely and chronically [6]. A prospective study of middle-aged Swedish males registered for alcohol addiction revealed a two-fold greater increase in the incidence of clinical cardiac events than for liver cirrhosis [7]. Several factors may be responsible for the deleterious effects of alcohol on the myocardium, including (i) a direct toxic effect of ethanol or its metabolites; (ii) associated nutritional deficiencies (i.e., thiamine); or (iii) direct toxicity of additives in the alcoholic beverage (i.e., lead or cobalt) [8].

Social drinking is often associated with a small rise of systolic blood pressure, which may have negligible effects in healthy adults. Cardiovascular events such as hypertension, stroke, arrhythmia, heart failure, and sudden death have been associated with heavy alcohol drinkers. In fact, chronic alcohol ingestion is a major cause of nonischemic cardiomyopathy in the Western world with an incidence ranging from 21–32% [9]. Most common in middle-aged individuals who have consumed large amounts of alcohol for more than 10 years resulting in heart failure [10], there is also an increased incidence of sudden death that apparently peaks about 50 years of age in the alcoholic population without heart failure.

Acute ingestion of ethanol resulting in blood levels of approximately 100 mg %, produces transient cardiac dysfunction in normal non-addictive subjects. By contrast, in chronic ethanol abusers asymptomatic but stable cardiac dysfunction has been observed for some years before evidence of heart failure appeared [11].

Early manifestations of the subclinical abnormality in chronic alcohol abusers include increased diastolic stiffness of the left ventricle, as indicated by an elevated end-diastolic pressure and diminished end-diastolic volume [12–15]. This process has been attributed to increased interstitial fibrosis. In a canine model without other risk factors, diastolic dysfunction and interstitial fibrosis were observed in studies lasting 6 months [1]. Improved basal contractility was not observed until after a period of 4 years consuming 36% of calories as ethanol [16].

In chronic studies, ethanol causes a reduction in the amount of contractile proteins, and two dimensional protein profiling implicates selective loss of individual myocardial proteins. The differential activities of lysosomal proteases may contribute to this patterned response. However, in chronic ethanol feeding, adaptive mechanisms also become important, as the synthesis of the myofibrillary proteins increases [17].

Ethanol has been shown to affect a number of molecular processes in heart muscle, including neurotransmitter receptors for amines, amino acids, and opioids and enzymes such as Na/K ATPase, acetylcholin esterase, adenylyl cyclase, as well as ion channels involved in calcium transport [18]. In a chronic canine model, increased concentrations of norepinephrine have been observed in the coronary venous effluent associated with a decrease in the ventricular fibrillatory threshold [19].

At the myocyte level, alcohol decreases the binding of calcium by the sarcoplasmic reticulum and decreases the sodium-potassium ATPase pump activity resulting in increased intracellular sodium, but these abnormalities at the levels observed are insufficient to produce systolic dysfunction [16,20,21].

MECHANISMS

Drug interactions can generally be classified as either pharmacokinetic or pharmacodynamic. Pharmacokinetic interactions result from processes that lead to a change in the disposition of one or more drugs and result in a change in clinical response. The most common form of a pharmacokinetic interaction occurs when one drug induces or inhibits the metabolism and/or elimination of another, and the steady-state concentration of a drug is lowered or raised. Alcohol can affect many medications through competition for the same microsomal oxidase system, involved in the metabolism of various drugs [22]. Pharmacodynamic interactions result when drugs have separate actions that are either augmented or antagonized when the drugs are used together. Alcohol appears to enhance aspirin-induced gastric mucosal damage and aspirin-induced prolongation of the bleeding time. Alcohol–drug interaction varies greatly in the range between social drinkers and heavy chronic drinkers. This phenomenon is also affected by the time elapsed between the alcohol ingestion and drug administration [23].

Ethanol is rapidly absorbed from the gastrointestinal tract, the main absorption occurring in the small intestine. Some absorption of ethanol, as well as 20% of its first-pass metabolism, takes place in the gastric mucosa where drug-ethanol interactions may occur [24]. Pyloric spasm caused by irritating concentrations of ethanol can slow the absorption of drugs and ethanol. During absorption, ethanol can improve the bioavailability of certain drugs which otherwise are poorly soluble or rapidly metabolized during their first pass. These interactions depend greatly on the drug concerned, but part of the inhibition of drug metabolism by ethanol results from the direct depression of the metabolic activity of hepatocytes [22].

The following discussion includes the major cardiovascular medications that can interact with ethanol.

Nitroglycerin

Nitrates induce relaxation of vascular smooth cells in both arteries and veins. At low concentration venodilation predominates, but at higher concentrations arterial vasodilation is also produced. Hypotensive reaction may result from the combination of alcohol and nitroglycerin [25]. Unless the clinician is aware of this interaction, the hypotensive episode may be attributed to coronary insufficieny or occlusion [26]. Arterial pressure and ventricular wall stress tend to be lower in subjects taking both nitroglycerin and ethanol compared to either drug alone [27].

Sympathetic antagonists (alpha-receptor blockers)

Alpha-adrenergic receptors mediate many of the important actions of endogenous catecholamines. Responses of particular relevance include alpha-1 receptor-mediated contraction of arterial and venous smooth muscle. Alpha-1 receptor antagonists effectively block the vasoconstricting effect of catecholamines and vasodilation may occur in both arteriolar resistance vessels and veins, potentially inducing postural hypotension and reflex tachycardia. They have not been as popular as many other classes of drug in treatment of essential hypertension. Recently, however interest in these antagonists has surged due to their efficacy in treating symptoms of prostatic hyperplasia has become more evident.

Alpha-2 receptors suppress central sympathetic output, increase central vagal tone, facilitate platelet aggregation, and inhibit the release of norepinephrine and acetylcholine from nerve endings. These receptors also regulate metabolic effects through suppression of insulin secretion and inhibition of lipolysis in adipose cells.

Clonidine, a centrally acting antihypertensive agent, acts primarily within the rostral ventrolateral medulla to reduce sympathetic outflow through stimulation of alpha 2 receptors thus increasing the negative feedback on norepinephrine synthesis and release [28]. On the other hand, alcohol enhances sympathetic activity [19]. In hypertensive rats, a dose of clonidine followed by intravenous alcohol in amounts similar to moderate drinking reversed the clonidine induced hypotensive effect [29]. In another animal model with moderately high ethanol blood levels, clonidine was administered intravenously. Both blood pressure and heart rate declined, indicating a dominant effect of the alpha 2 agonist [30].

Alpha-2 receptor antagonists can increase sympathetic outflow and potentiate the release of norepinephrine from the nerve endings, leading to activation of alpha 1 and beta 1 receptors in the heart and peripheral vasculature with a consequent rise in blood pressure [28].

When alcohol is fed to experimental animals, a transient alpha receptor blocking activity has been observed. A single dose of alcohol or chronic use decreased the sensitivity of adrenergic receptors [31]. In chronic alcoholism however, elevated norepinephrine levels and impaired arterial baroreceptors activity have been suggested as an underlying mechanism of ethanol-induced hypertension [32].

Guanethidine inhibits the peripheral sympathetic nervous system activity by inhibiting the release of norepinephrine vesicles from the nerve endings. Intravenous administration of acetaldehyde, a major ethanol metabolite that enhances sympathetic activity, elicits a substantial increase of blood pressure following a single dose of guanethidine. However, in animals receiving guanethidine long term, a low dose of acetaldehyde raised arterial pressure whereas a high dose of acetaldehyde diminished the blood pressure [33].

Reserpine depletes the postganglionic adrenergic neurons of norepinephrine by inhibiting its uptake into storage vesicles. Such an effect is intensified by alcohol use [34], enhancing the negative inotropic action on the heart.

Sympathetic antagonists (beta-receptors blockers)

Beta-receptor antagonist drugs have been found to be useful in a wide variety of clinical conditions and are firmly established in the treatment of hypertension, ischemic heart disease, arrhythmias, endocrinologic and neurologic disorders. Short-term studies in normal subjects indicate that ethanol increases both the elimination rate and bioavailability of propranolol [35]. The plasma clearance rate of propranolol, which is metabolized by the liver, is increased and the blood pressure-reducing effect of the drug is diminished. Ethanol and beta blockade individually affect heart rate and arterial pressure in the opposite direction. The combination of ethanol and propranolol will produce effects that are dose dependent, but both produce negative inotropic effects. Patients receiving propranolol should be dissuaded from adding more than one drink a day to their regimen [36,37]. However, subjects in alcohol withdrawal can be therapeutically affected by beta-adrenergic blockade.

Renin-angiotensin system

Angiotensin II has been shown to inhibit voluntary consumption of alcohol, an effect which is negated by ACE-inhibitor [38]. Hypothetically, angiotensin converting enzyme inhibitors (ACE-I) should exert an opposite response to the alcohol–angiotensin II effect. However, several investigators have reported that ACE-I also reduced voluntary alcohol intake [39,40]. The receptor blocker losartan administered with ethanol also blocks the intoxicating effect of ethanol in a dose dependent manner [41,42].

The renin–angiotensin system is considered to have a significant role in the development of heart failure and hypertension. The individual abusing alcohol with subclinical cardiac dysfunction responds to angiotensin with a greater rise in the left ventricular end-diastolic pressure, without a significant change of the stroke volume compared to the nonalcoholic subject [43].

Calcium channel antagonists

Phenylalkylamine (verapamil), benzothiazepine (diltiazem), diarylaminopropylamines (bepridil), the first generation dihydropyridine (nifedipine, nimodipine, nitrendipine, isradipine), and second generation dihydropyridine (amlodipine, felodipine) have different negative inotropic, vasodilatory, and A-V node conduction effects on the cardiovascular system.

Acute verapamil therapy has been found to potentiate negative inotropic and chronotropic effects of alcohol in animal models [44,45]. Consumption of ethanol following the chronic administration of verapamil results in an increased ethanol concentration in blood with the potential for an increased level of intoxication [46]. Higher blood levels are thought to be related to reduced first pass ethanol elimination in the presence of verapamil [47]. Perhaps as a consequence, rats treated with large doses of ethanol combined with verapamil have shown to have ultrastructural cardiomyocyte damage [48]. Chronic verapamil therapy diminished the negative inotropic effect of ethanol on diabetic myocardium [49]. In addition, restoration of intracellular calcium homeostasis has been reported to reverse structural, biochemical, and mechanical dysfunction in diabetic myocardium [50,51].

Chronic alcohol consumption up-regulates dihydropyridine-sensitive neuronal calcium channel binding sites. Several dihydropyridine agents are reported to have protective effects against the ethanol withdrawal syndrome. They promote the development of tolerance to alcohol and perhaps promote consumption [52,53].

Ethanol administration in healthy human volunteers resulted in a 53% increase in the nifedipine concentration-time curve but the hypotensive effect of nifedipine was not affected by ethanol [54]. Engel *et al.* reported that nifedipine antagonized the stimulant effects of ethanol on locomotion and Tuna and Eroglu found that nifedipine reversed the inhibitory effects of ethanol on locomotor activity [55,56]. In rats treated with ethanol, nifedipine did not produce cardiomyocyte damage [57].

The general anesthetic actions of ethanol have been markedly enhanced by nitrendipine while nimodipine potentiated the ataxic and hypothermic action of ethanol [58]. By contrast, pretreatment with isradipine did not significantly alter the subject-rated or performance-impairing effects of ethanol [59].

Inotropic agents

Digitalis glycosides are the most commonly used inotropic agents in patients with congestive heart failure and are also employed in patients with arrhythmias. Significant acute interaction between ethanol and this agent has not been reported. One study found that the digitalis failed to improve cardiac function in alcoholic liver disease patients [60], which may be due to the state of the cardiac tissue rather than a drug interaction.

Antiarrhythmic agents

Heavy ethanol consumption is a common cause of atrial fibrillation [61]. In general, most antiarrhythmic agents in therapeutic doses depress the automatic firing rate of spontaneously discharging ectopic sites while minimally affecting the discharge rate of the normal sinus node. Mechanisms by which different drugs suppress normal or abnormal automaticity may not be the same.

(i) **Amiodarone** as a potassium channel blocker has both alpha- and beta-adrenergic blocking properties. Filipek *et al.* reported that a low dose of ethanol did not affect the antiarrhythmic effect of amiodarone in adrenaline-induced arrhythmias but large acute doses reduced efficacy [62]. Amiodarone decreased the ethanol level in rats that received alcohol chronically but its antiarrhythmic action was impaired.

(ii) **Disopyramide** blocks sodium channels, prolongs repolarization and has negative ino-tropic effect. Concomitant disopyramide and ethanol administration had no effect on the total body clearance or half-life of disopyramide in a study of healthy volunteers [63]. The renal clearance of disopyramide significantly increased, possibly from ethanol-induced diuresis [63]. Chronic ethanol consumption may increase metabolism of disopyramide through enzyme induction.

(iii) **Phenytoin**. At therapeutic dose, this agent effectively abolishes abnormal automa-ticity caused by digitalis-induced arrhythmias. Since subjects consuming ethanol metabolize phenytoin more rapidly than control subjects [64], prolonged excessive ethanol ingestion could result in seizures in an epileptic patient controlled on pheny-toin. Whether a smaller amount of ethanol would affect phenytoin metabolism is unknown, but it is deemed unlikely [65].

(iv) **Procainamide** has electrophysiologic and hemodynamic effects similar to quinidine except for weaker anticholinergic effects and is devoid of an alpha-adrenergic blocking effect. This agent has modest negative inotropic properties that are, however, less than those of quinidine. Although acute ethanol ingestion increases the acetylation of procainamide [66], the clinical significance of this clinical interaction is unknown. However, the acetylated metabolite (N-acetylprocainamide) may mitigate the clin-ical impact of this interaction, since its clinical activity is similar to the parent drug [67]. The patient stabilized on procainamide should be monitored for an altered response following acute alcohol ingestion. Since chronic alcohol use has been reported to affect the volume of distribution of the drug and reduce the procainamide effectiveness [68], the net effect would appear to be a reduced efficacy.

(v) **Quinidine** acts to inhibit sodium channel activity, blunt the rapid upstroke of the action potential and prolong its duration, and prolong the refractory period of the myocar-dium. In addition, vagal influence on the heart is weakened. In a rat model, the com-bined effects of ethanol and quinidine decreased the papillary muscle tension. The quinidine-induced prolongation of the absolute refractory and relative refractory peri-ods were also diminished [69]. As an additional interaction a syndrome of cocktail purpura has been reported in persons drinking a cocktail with quinine water [70,71], analogous to the increased bleeding tendency in patients taking oral quinidine while simultaneously using alcohol.

Anticoagulation

Coumadin and heparin (both fractionated and unfractionated) are the two most commonly used anticoagulants. Coumadin prevents the reduction of vitamin K epoxide in liver microsomes and induces a state analogous to vitamin K deficiency by competitively inhib-iting the effects of vitamin K in the carboxylation of the vitamin K dependent plasma protein. Additionally, thrombin generation and clot formation are slowed by the biologic activity of the prothrombin complex proteins.

Ethanol-induced increases in the hypoprothrombinemic response to oral anticoagulants have been noted clinically for many years. It is clear that most patients on oral anticoagulants are not affected by moderate ethanol intake (e.g., 2 drinks per day or less) [72]. Further, daily ingestion of 592 ml (20 oz) of table wine or 296 ml (10 oz) of fortified wine (20% alcohol) had no effect on the hypoprothrombinemic response to warfarin in healthy subjects [73]. The ability of acute ethanol intoxication to enhance the hypoprothrombinemic response to oral anticoagulants may be due to inhibition of the anticoagulant metabolism. The apparent increase in warfarin metabolism in heavy drinkers when sober is presumed to be due to ethanol-induced stimulation of hepatic microsomal enzymes [74,75]. Finally, the late stages of ethanol-induced hepatic damage can be accompanied by reduced hepatic production of vitamin K-dependent clotting factors [5,76].

The interaction of heparin with ethanol is not clearly defined. The metabolite of alcohol, acetaldehyde, was shown to augment the anticoagulating activity of heparin, but only when using an unphysiological dose of acetaldehyde [77].

Antiplatelet agents

Aspirin irreversibly inactivates cyclo-oxygenase in circulating platelets, thereby interrupting the endoperoxide/thromboxane A2 pathway.

Ethanol appears to increase the gastrointestinal bleeding produced by aspirin. Both aspirin and ethanol individually damage the gastric mucosal barrier, and their combined use appears to result in additive or synergistic effects. Also, the ability of aspirin to prolong the bleeding time is enhanced by ethanol administration [77]. No effect of aspirin on the single-dose kinetics of ethanol has been found, the peak concentration of aspirin being diminished by 25% [78].

CONCLUSIONS

Ethanol is a commonly used agent that, when consumed in light to moderate amounts, may provide pleasure without undesirable side effects. However, when pharmacologic agents are used at the same time side effects may ensue. Such a response is largely dependent on the dosage of alcohol and the treatment agents. Thus, the physician prescribing treatment for cardiovascular disorders should be aware of the potential interactions and convey the appropriate message to his or her patient.

REFERENCES

1 Rajiyah G, Agarwal R, Avendano G, Lyons M, Soni B, Regan TJ. Influence of nicotine on myocardial stiffness and fibrosis during chronic ethanol use. *Alcoholism: Clinical & Experimental Research*, September 1996; **20**(6): 985–989.
2 Kannel WB. Blood pressure as a cardiovascular risk factor: Prevention and treatment. *JAMA* 1996; **275**: 1571–1576.
3 Mattila MJ. Alcohol and Drug Interactions. *Annals of Medicine* 1990; **22**: 363–369.
4 Medical safety: Avoiding Drug Interactions. *Harvard Health Letter* March 1998; **23**(5): 1–3.
5 Shinn AF, Shrewsbury RP (eds.). *Evaluations of Drug Interaction*. New York: Macmillan, 1988.
6 Bollinger O. Über die Häufigkeit und Ursachen der idiopathischen Herzhypertrophie in München. *Deutsche Med. Wchnschr.* 1884; **10**: 180–181.
7 Rosengren A *et al.* Alcoholic intemperance, coronary heart disease and mortality in middle aged Swedish men. *Acta Med. Scand.* 1987; **222**: 201–213.
8 Morin YL, Foley AR, Martineau G, Roussel J. Quebec beer-drinkers' cardiomyopathy: forty-eight cases. *Can. Med. Assoc. J.* 1967; **97**: 881–883.

9 Fuster V, Gersh BJ, Biuliani ER. The natural history of idiopathic dilated cardiomyopathy. *Am. J. Cardio.* 1981; **47**: 525.

10 Schwarz F, Mall G, Zebe H. Determinants of survival in patients with congestive cardiomyopathy: Quantitative morphologic findings and left ventricular hemodynamics. *Circulation* 1981; **70**: 923.

11 Spodick DH, Pigott VM, Chirife R. Preclinical cardiac malfunction in chronic alcoholism. Comparison with matched normal controls and with alcoholic cardiomyopathy. *N. Engl. J. Med.* 1972; **287**: 677–680.

12 Regan TJ, Levinson GE, Oldewurtel HA. Ventricular function non-cardiacs with alcoholic fattyliver: Role of ethanol in the production of cardiomyopathy *J. Clin. Invest.* 1969; **48**: 397–407.

13 Ahmed SS, Levinson GE, Fiore JJ. Spectrum of heart muscle abnormalities related to alcoholism, *Clin. Cardiol.* 1980; **3**: 335.

14 Urbano-Marquez A, Estruch R, Navarro-Lopez F, Grau JM, Mont L, Rubin E. The effects of alcoholism on skeletal and cardiac muscles. *N. Engl. J. Med.* 1989; **320**: 409–415.

15 Kupari M, Koskinen P, Suokas A, Ventila M. Left ventricular filling impairment in asymptomatic chronic alcoholic. *Am. J. Cardiol.* 1990; **66**: 1473–1477.

16 Regan TJ, Tomas G, Harder G. Progression of myocardial abnormalities in experimental alcoholism. *Am. J. Cardiol.* 1980; **46**: 233.

17 Preedy VR, Patel VB, Why HJ, Corbett JM, Dunn MJ, Richardon PJ. Alcohol and the heart: biochemical alterations. *Cardiovascular Research* January 1996; **31**(1): 139–147.

18 Habuchi Y, Furukawa T, Tanaka H, Lu LL, Morikawa J, Yoshimura M. Ethanol inhibition of Ca^{2+} and Na^+ currents in the guinea-pig heart. *European Journal of Pharmacology* January 13, 1995; **292**(2): 143–149.

19 Patel R, McArdle JJ, Regan TJ. Increased ventricular vulnerability in chronic ethanol model despite reduced electrophysiologic responses to catecholamines. *Alcohol Clin. Exp. Res.* 1991; **15**: 785–789.

20 Sarma JSM, Shigeaki I, Fischer R. Biochemical and contractile properties of heart muscle after prolonged alcohol administration. *J. Mole. Cell Cardiol.* 1976; **8**: 972.

21 Segel LD, Rendig SV, Mason DT. Alcohol-induced cardiac hemodynamic and calcium flux dysfunction are reversible. *J. Mole. Cell Cardiol.* 1981; **13**: 433.

22 Lieber. CS. Microsomal ethanol-oxidizing system. *Enzyme* 1987; **37**: 45–56.

23 Sandor P, Sellers EM, Dumbrell M, Klouw V. Effects of short- and long-term alcohol use on phenytoin kinetics in chronic alcoholics. *Clin. Pharmacol. Ther.* 1981; **30**: 390–397.

24 Caballeria J, Freaaz M, Hernandez-Munoz R, Dipadova C, Korsten MA, Baraona E, Lieber CS. Gastric origin of the first-pass metabolism of ethanol in humans: effect of gastrectomy. *Gastroenterology* 1989; **97**: 1205–1209.

25 Kupari M, Heikkila J, Ylikahri R. Does alcohol intensify the hemodynamic effects of nitroglycerin? *Clin. Cardio.* 1984; **7**: 382–386.

26 Shook TL, Kirshenbaum JM, Hundley RF, Shorey JM, Lanas GA. Ethanol intoxication complicating intravenous nitroglycerin therapy. *Ann. Intern. Med.* 1984; **101**(4): 498–499.

27 Allison RD *et al.* Effects of alcohol and nitroglycerin on vascular response in man. *Angiology* 1971; **22**: 211.

28 Goldberg MR, Robertson D. Yohimbine: a pharmacological probe of the alpha 2 adrenoreceptor. *Pharmacol. Rev.* 1983; **35**: 143–180.

29 Abdel-Rahman AA, Wooles WR. Ethanol-induced hypertension involves impairment of baroreceptors. *Hypertension* 1987; **10**: 67–73.

30 Mao L, Abdel-Rahman ARA. Ethanol counteraction of clonidine-evoked inhibition of norepinephrine release in rostral ventrolateral medulla of rats. *The Alcohol Clin. Exp. Res.* 1988; **22**(6): 1285–1291.

31 Szmigielski A, Szmigielski H, Weiman I. The effects of prolonged ethanol administration on central alpha-2 adrenoreceptors sensitivity. *Pol. J. Pharmacol. Pharm.* 1989; **41**: 263–272.

32 Russ RD, Abdel-Rahman A-RA, Wooles WR. Role of sympathetic nervous system in ethanol-induced hypertension in rats. *Alcohol* 1991; **8**: 301–307.

33 Green MA, Egle JL. The effects of acetaldehyde and acrolein on blood pressure in guanethidine-pretreated hypertensive rats. *Toxicol. Appl. Pharmacol.* 1983; **69**(1): 29–36.

34 American Society of Hospital Pharmacists. American Hospital Formulary Service Drug Information. Bethesda, MD: American Society of Hospital Pharmacists, 1984.

35 Grabowski BS *et al.* Effects of acute alcohol administration on propranolol absorption. *Int. J. Clin. Pharmacol. Ther. Toxicol.* 1980; **18**: 317.

36 Sontaniemi EA *et al.* Propranolol and sotalol metabolism after a drinking party. *Clin. Pharmacol. Ther.* 1981; **29**: 705.

37 Chakrabarti A, Grag SK, Sharma PL. A preliminary study on the interaction between ethanol and propranolol in normal human subjects. *Indian J. Physiol. Pharmacol.* 1992; **36**(3): 209–212.

38 Kulkosky PJ, Allison TG, Carr BA. Angiotensin II reduces alcohol intake and choice in water- or food-restricted rats. *Alcohol* July–August 1996; **13**(4): 359–363.

39 Spinosa G, Perlanski E, Leenen FH, Stewart RB, Grupp LA. Angiotensin converting enzyme inhibition: Animal experiments suggest a new pharmacological treatment for alcohol abuse in human. *Alcohol Clin. Exp. Res.* 1988; **12**: 65–70.

40 Lingham T, Perlanski E, Grupp LA. Angiotensin converting enzyme inhibitors reduce alcohol consumption: Some possible mechanisms and important conditions for its therapeutic use. *Alcohol Clin. Exp. Res.* 1990; **14**: 92–99.

41 Hubbell C, Chrisbacher GA, Bilski EJ, Reid LD. Manipulation of the renin–angiotensin system and intake of a sweetened alcoholic beverage among rats. *Alcohol* 1992; **9**(1): 53–61.

42 Tracy HA Jr, Wayner MJ, Armstrong DL. Losartan improves the performance of ethanol-intoxicated rats in an eight-arm radial maze. *Alcohol* September–October 1997; **14**(5): 511–517.

43 Regan TJ, Levinson GE, Oldewurtel HA. Ventricular function in non-cardiacs with alcoholic fatty liver: Role of ethanol in the production of cardiomyopathy. *J. Clin. Invest.* 1969; **48**: 397–407.

44 Posner P, Baker SP, Issacson RL. Potentiation of the negative chronotropic action of verapamil by ethanol. *J. Cardiovasc. Pharmacol.* 1986; **8**: 697–699.

45 Martinez JL, Penna M. Influence of changes in calcium concentration and verapamil on the cardiac depressant effect of ethanol in cat papillary muscle. *Gen. Pharmacol.* 1992; **23**: 1051–1056.

46 Perez-Reyes M *et al.* Interaction between ethanol and calcium channel blockers in humans. *Alcohol Clin. Exp. Res.* 1992; **16**: 769.

47 Bauer LA *et al.* Verapamil inhibits ethanol elimination and prolongs the perception of intoxication. *Clin. Pharmacol. Ther.* 1992; **52**: 6.

48 Dul B, Gajkowska B. The influence of the calcium channel antagonist, verapamil and ethanol on the myocardial ultrastructure in rat. *Exp. Toxic. Pathol.* 1997; **49**(6): 493–496.

49 Brown RA, Sundareson AM, Lee MM, Savage AO. Differential effects of chronic calcium channel blocker treatment on the inotropic response of diabetic rat myocardium to acute ethanol exposure. *Life Science* 1996; **59**(10): 835–847.

50 Pierce GN, Jutryk MJB, Dhalla NS. Alterations in calcium binding by and composition of the cardiac sacrolemmal membrane in chronic diabetes. *Proc. Natl. Acad. Sci. USA* 1983; **80**: 5412–5416.

51 Dhalla NS, Pierce GN, Innes IR, Beamish RE. Pathogenesis of cardiac dysfunction in diabetes mellitus. *Can. J. Cardiol.* 1985; **1**: 263–281.

52 Littleton JM, Little HJ, Whittington MA. Effect 1991s of dihydropyridine calcium channel antagonists in ethanol withdrawal; doses required, stereospecificity and action of Bay K 8644. *Psychopharmacology* 1990; **100**: 387–392.

53 Little HJ, Dolin SJ, Whittington MA. Calcium channel antagonists prevent adaptive responses to ethanol. *Alcohol Alcohol.* 1993; **2** (*Suppl.*): 263–267.

54 Qureshi S *et al.* Effect of an acute dose of alcohol on the pharmacokinetics of oral nifedipine in humans. *Pharm. Res.* 1992; **9**: 683.

55 Engel JA, Fahke C, Hulthe P, Hard E, Johannessen K, Snape B, Svensson L. Biochemical and behavioral evidence for an interaction between ethanol and calcium channel antagonists *J. of Neural Trans.* 1988; **74**: 181–193.

56 Tuna RK, Eroglu L. Effects of Bay K 8644 and nifedipine on locomotor activity and striatal homovanillic acid concentration in acutely ethanol-treated rats. *Alcohol Alcohol.* 1991; **26**: 465–471.

57 Dul B, Gajkowska B. The influence of ethanol and calcium channel antagonist, nifedipine on myocardial ultrastructure in the rat. *Exp. Toxic. Pathol.* 1998; **50**: 27–30.

58 Dolin SJ, Little HJ. Augmentation by calcium channel antagonists of general anesthetic potency in mice. *Br. J. Pharmacol.* 1986; **88**: 909–914.

59 Rush CR, Pazzaglia PJ. Pretreatment with isradipine, a calcium channel blocker, does not attenuate the acute behavioral effects of ethanol in human. *Alcohol Clin. Exp. Res.* 1998; **22**: 539–547.

60 Lima CJ, Guiha NH, Lekagul O, Cohn JN. Impaired left ventricular function in alcoholic cirrhosis with ascites. Ineffectiveness of ouabain. *Circulation* 1974; **49**: 755–760.

61 Rich EC, Siebold C, Campion B. Alcohol-related acute atrial fibrillation: a case-control study and review of 40 patients. *Arch. Intern. Med.* 1985; **145**: 830–833.

62 Filipek B, Krupinska J, Librowski T, Piekoszewski W. The interaction between ethanol and amiodarone, in the model of adrenaline arrhythmia in the rat. *Polish Journal of Pharmacology & Pharmacy* May–June 1989; **41**(3): 213–218.

63 Olsen H, Bredesen JE, Lunde PKU. Effect of ethanol intake on disopyramide elimination by healthy volunteers. *Eur. J. Clin. Pharmacol.* 1983; **25**: 103–105.

64 Kater RMH, Roogin G, Tobon F, Zieve P, ad Iber FL. Increased rate of clearance of drugs from the circulation of alcoholics. *Am. J. Med. Sci.* 1969; **258**: 35–39.

65 Sandor P, Seller EM, Dumbrell M, Klouw V. Effect of short- and long-term alcohol use on phenytoin kinetics in chronic alcoholics. *Clin. Pharmacol. Ther.* 1981; **30**: 390–397.

66 Olsen H, Morland J. Ethanol interaction with drug acetylation *in vivo* and *in vitro*. *Pharmacol. Biochem. Behav.* 1983; **18**(Suppl. 1): 295–300.

67 Hansten PD. Procainamide and ethanol. Drug Interactions Newsletter, Applied Therapeutics. Inc, San. Francisco. CA 1982; **2**: 23.

68 Orszulak MD, Polakowski P. Influence of ethanol on pharmacokinetic parameters of procainamide in rabbits. *Die Pharmacie* 1988; **43**(40): 260–261.

69 Guthrie SK, Wilde DW, Brown RA, Savage AO, Bleske B. Interactions of ethanol and quinidine on contractility and myocyte action potential in the rat ventricle. *Journal of Electrocardiology* January 1995; **28**(1): 39–47.

70 Belkin GA. Cocktail purpura: An unusual case of quinine sensitivity. *Ann. Intern. Med.* 1967; **66**: 583–587.

71 Siroty RR. Purpura on the rocks-with a twist. *JAMA* 1976; **235**(23): 2521–2522.

72 Udall JA. Drug interference with warfarin therapy. *Clin. Med.* 1970; **77**: 20.

73 O'Reilly RA. Lack of effect of fortified wine ingestion during fasting and anticoagulant therapy. *Arch. Intern. Med.* 1981; **141**: 458.

74 Kater RHM *et al.* Increased rate of clearance of drugs from the circulation of alcoholic. *Am. J. Med. Sci.* 1969; **258**: 35.

75 Breckenridge A. Pathophysiological factors influencing drug kinetics. *Acta Pharmacol. Toxicol.* 1971; **29**(Suppl. 3): 225.

76 Pelkonen O, Sataniemi E. Drug metabolism in alcoholics. *Pharmacol. Ther.* 1982; **16**(2): 261–268.

77 Brecher AS, Hellman K, Basista MH. Coagulation protein function VI: augmentation of anticoagulant function by acetaldehyde-treated heparin. *Digestive Diseases & Sciences.* July 1999; **44**(7): 1349–1355.

78 Deykin D *et al.* Ethanol potentiation of aspirin-induced prolongation of the bleeding time. *N. Engl. J. Med.* 1982; **306**: 852.

79 Melander O, Liden A, Melander A. Pharmacokinetic interaction of alcohol and acetylsalicylic acid. *European J. of Clin. Pharm.* 1995; **48**(2): 151–153.

Chapter 6

Alcohol abuse and hemorrhagic stroke

Seppo Juvela

INTRODUCTION

Prognosis for both spontaneous intracerebral hemorrhage (ICH) [1–4] and aneurysmal subarachnoid hemorrhage (SAH) [4–7], despite improvements in medical and neurosurgical treatment, has largely remained unaffected. Outcome of both these main hemorrhagic stroke subtypes, which together account for approximately 20% of all strokes, is still determined mainly by the severity of bleeding, and overall case-fatality still reaches 40–50% [2,3,7]. Hence, identification of modifiable risk factors for ICH and SAH as well as for impaired outcome after these strokes has been important in order to influence the incidence and outcome of these stroke subtypes as well as to understand better the pathogenesis of these hemorrhages.

Alcohol consumption has been shown to increase the risk for both ICH [4,8–14] and SAH [11,15–17]. Hypertension increases the risk for ICH [8,12,14], but its significance as a risk factor for SAH seems to be less important than for other stroke subtypes [16–18]. Cigarette smoking seems to increase the risk for SAH [16–19] but is less likely to increase the risk for ICH [8,12,14,19,20].

Other potential risk factors for hemorrhagic stroke include anticoagulant treatment [2,3,14,21], aspirin use [14,17,22], thrombolytic therapy [3,23], and use of amphetamines or cocaine [3,11,16]. These may also synergize with each other, e.g., ethanol potentiates aspirin-induced prolongation of bleeding time [24], and anticoagulant treatment increases the risk of hemorrhage associated with thrombolytic therapy [23]. In addition, alcohol consumption, cigarette smoking, hypertension, sex, and age are correlated either directly or inversely with each other so that multivariate analyses must be used to reveal independent role of each of them as a risk factor for hemorrhagic stroke subtypes [4,11].

In most risk-factor studies, ICH and SAH have been combined to form the category hemorrhagic stroke [9,11,19,22,23], which likely causes bias by either overestimation or underestimation of the significance of risk factors for different stroke subtypes. In addition, studies of hemorrhagic stroke have also included hemorrhages of different etiologies, such as non-aneurysmal SAH, arteriovenous malformation, unspecific stroke or likely also brain injuries. It is recommended that spontaneous ICH and aneurysmal SAH should not be combined in epidemiological and clinical studies because these hemorrhages have different risk factors as well as age and sex distributions [4].

This review deals with spontaneous ICH and aneurysmal SAH – the two most common and severe forms of hemorrhagic stroke – in regard to the modifiable risk factors commonly associated with hemorrhagic stroke and recovery after bleeding including alcohol consumption and other health-related habits, previous diseases, and use of antithrombotic and other medicines.

SUBARACHNOID HEMORRHAGE

Prevalence of intracranial aneurysms

Intracranial aneurysms in the general population have been studied mostly in autopsy series. Depending on whether the aneurysms were sought or merely noted as incidental findings, prevalence appears to be 2–5% (range 0.2–9%) [25–27]. More than half of these aneurysms were unruptured before death. On the other hand, aneurysm size is at least 30–60% greater before death than its size measured after death before fixation [28]. The prevalence of small aneurysms may thus be greater than reported in autopsy series.

Reported frequencies of unruptured aneurysms in angiographic series range from 1.1–6.5% [26,27,29]. The variance in prevalence has been explained by the age distributions of the different series as well as by racial differences [25,26]. Incidence of multiple aneurysms depends primarily on completeness of diagnostic procedures and can be estimated at about 30% [30,31]. Small aneurysms, which cannot be seen in angiography, may also be observed during surgery.

Aneurysms seem to be acquired degenerative lesions as a result of hemodynamic stress, but may sometimes be familial (c. 10% of cases) or associated with connective tissue diseases [25,27,32]. Many factors may increase the risk of aneurysm formation or subarachnoid hemorrhage, mainly through unknown mechanisms. These include hypertension, atherosclerosis, female sex, aging, cigarette smoking, alcohol consumption, use of oral contraceptives, arterial deficiency in collagen Type III, asymmetry of the Circle of Willis, cerebral arteriovenous malformations, viral infections, pituitary tumors, and certain HLA-associated factors [4,16,17,19,25,32,33]. Although age, sex, and hypertension may be risk factors for aneurysm formation, their association with rupture of the aneurysm itself is unlikely [34–37].

Incidence of subarachnoid hemorrhage

Incidence of SAH varies widely throughout the world, but 10/100,000/year is the generally accepted estimate for western countries [3,25,38], with the highest incidence rates (>13/100,000/year) for Finland and Japan [7,25,26,39]. During last decades, the incidence of SAH has declined somewhat [7,38,39], which is mostly explained by a greater proportion of patients investigated with computerized tomography (CT) scan. However, at least part of this decline can be explained by a well-known decrease of cigarette smoking and perhaps by improved treatment of hypertension.

Aneurysms develop during adulthood, risk for SAH increasing linearly with age [3,7,25,40]. Subarachnoid hemorrhage also is the most common form of stroke and cause of stroke mortality among young adults [40]. Although the incidence of SAH has been higher in women than in men overall [7,25,39], its incidence among young adults has been higher in men [7,17,25,40]. Proneness to SAH among young men might be partly contributed by their heavier drinking and smoking habits [17]. In recent studies, the female-to-male ratio has been approximately one also among young adults [41]. This may be due to increased smoking among young women.

Since female preponderance for SAH is not significant until the fifth decade [7,25,41], the overrepresentation of their aneurysm formation is thought to be secondary to hormonal factors [41]; it has been presumed that estrogen has an inhibitory effect on aneurysm formation; cigarette smoking also has antiestrogenic properties. The collagen content of cerebral arteries may also diminish after menopause, favoring aneurysm formation [41].

Risk factors for subarachnoid hemorrhage

Indisputable independent modifiable risk factors for SAH seems to be only cigarette smoking, alcohol consumption, and to a lesser extent, hypertension [4,16,17,19,33]. Risk factors may also differ according to race and age, with young adults having risk factors different from those of elderly people [17].

Cigarette smoking is an independent and the most important risk factor for SAH, which has already been proved in several cohort and case-control studies [4,16–19,33,42,43]. In North America and Europe, the prevalence of smoking in SAH patients ranges from 45–75%, whereas in the general adult population it is only 20–35%. Men and younger age groups smoke more than others both in SAH patients and in general populations [17,43]. Although cigarette smoking is decreasing in western countries, incidence of SAH does not necessarily change because of improved diagnostic methods and aging of populations. Of SAH cases, 38–48% can be attributed to cigarette smoking [16,17,42]. Smoking is also associated more strongly with SAH than with other forms of stroke [19].

It is also well known that heavy smokers start smoking at an earlier age, have smoked longer, and have more rarely ceased smoking than those who smoke only occasionally or less than 20 cigarettes per day [44–46]. In agreement with this, patients with SAH are more often heavy smokers [16,17], had smoked longer [17], and had ceased smoking less often [17] than controls. In addition, cigarette smoking increases the risk for SAH in a dose–response manner [16,17,19], but the mechanism by which smoking increases the risk has remained unknown.

Blood-pressure values are generally lower in smokers than in nonsmokers [19], but smoking a cigarette causes an acute increase in blood pressure for approximately three hours [16]. Transient increase in blood pressure caused by smoking may cause rupture of an aneurysm. It is also possible that long-lasting smoking can cause aneurysm formation and growth by weakening the walls of cerebral arteries. This can happen, for example, if increased amounts of proteolytic enzymes are released into the systemic circulation by smoking [4,17]. This concept is supported by some reports suggesting that former smokers also have an increased risk, which is, however, lower than that of current smokers [16,19].

Differences between SAH patients either with a single aneurysm or with multiple aneurysms can also be risk factors for aneurysm formation, since the presence of multiple aneurysms does not seem to increase the risk for rupture of an aneurysm [34,35,37]. The risk factors for aneurysm formation may only be more augmented in the patients with multiple aneurysms. Of several potential risk factors for multiple intracranial aneurysms, only two studies have used multivariate statistics to reveal independent risk factors [30,31]. Cigarette smoking [30,31], female sex [30,31], and possibly also age [31], but not hypertension, were independent risk factors for multiple intracranial aneurysms and thus possibly also for aneurysm formation. The theory that cigarette smoking causes formation of aneurysms through atherosclerosis is unlikely because atherosclerosis-promoting factors such as hypertension, and diabetes, as well as cardiovascular and ischemic cerebrovascular diseases, do not correlate with multiple aneurysms [30,31].

After diagnosis of an unruptured aneurysm, size of aneurysm [34,35,37,47], and possibly age inversely [35,36,47] and cigarette smoking [47] are independent predictors for subsequent aneurysm rupture. Cigarette smoking also seems to be the most important independent risk factor for subsequent rupture of an unruptured aneurysm, irrespective of aneurysm size, of gender, and of age of the patient at diagnosis [47]. The relative risk of cigarette smoking, tested as a time-dependent covariate in the Cox model, increased if the patient continued smoking during follow-up [47].

In a recent study, cigarette smoking and female gender were only significant independent factors affecting both aneurysm formation and growth (Juvela *et al. Stroke* 2001; **32**: 485–491). Women in particular were at high risk for aneurysm formation, and cigarette smoking hastened aneurysm growth. These findings are important since aneurysms grow before the rupture [35]. The faster the growth, the more likely is rupture.

Cigarette smokers' serum elastase/alpha-1-antitrypsin imbalance (i.e., increased elastase activity and/or decreased alpha-1-antitrypsin activity) may contribute either to aneurysm formation or to SAH [48,49]. Cigarette smoking has also been shown to increase elastase activity in the wall of the rabbit aorta [50]. Perhaps the strongest evidence is that topical application of elastase (but of neither collagenase nor papaverine) experimentally to the artery wall has caused saccular aneurysm formation, growth, and even rupture [51]. Thus, it is quite probable that regular cigarette smoking increases elastase activity in the artery wall, and this, together with hemodynamic stress, can cause aneurysm formation and even hastens aneurysm growth, leading to rupture.

The role of alcohol as a risk factor for SAH has not been as well established as smoking. Several cohort and case-control studies have shown that alcohol consumption increases – independently of cigarette smoking, age, and history of hypertension – risk for both ICH [4,8–14] and SAH [11,15–17,52], even in women [13,14,17,52]. In two studies [9,13], alcohol consumption was associated with a significantly increased risk for ICH but not with an increased risk for SAH, while in another study [15] the situation was opposite. Long-term heavy alcohol intake and problem drinking also are more infrequent in SAH patients than in ICH patients [4]. Approximately 13% of subarachnoid hemorrhages could be attributed to recent heavy drinking [17].

The risk for SAH seems to be increased when average alcohol intake is more than 150 g within a week, obtained with use of interview [11,15–17,52]. Intake of alcohol more than 40 g at a time increases the risk for SAH during subsequent 24 hours [17]. Above these limits, alcohol intake increases risk for SAH in a linear dose–response manner, and especially binge drinking is more risky than intake of corresponding amount of alcohol within a longer time period [16,17]. According to case-control studies [16,17], those with a lower alcohol intake than 150 g within a week do not seem to have an increased risk for SAH but cohort studies suggest that they have [15,52]. After adjustment for cigarette smoking, the association of heavy alcohol intake with risk for SAH has not been shown to be significant both by use of laboratory markers of alcohol intake and by interview with CAGE questionnaire which relates not merely to amount of alcohol consumed but also to abnormal drinking behavior (e.g., drinking on waking) and alcohol-induced problems [17]. Use of these parameters of alcohol intake also show that current and former heavy drinking as well as problem drinking are more common in ICH patients than in SAH patients [4,14,17]. Thus, it seems that moderate or high amount of alcohol intake has a relative short-time harmful effect on risk for SAH.

In a recent study, alcohol consumption was not an independent risk factor for aneurysm growth or formation (Juvela *et al.* Stroke 2001; **32**: 485–491). It was not even a significant risk factor in univariate analysis, except for a correlation between number of positive CAGE responses and aneurysm growth rate, although alcohol consumption is known to correlate with smoking [4,16,17]. Alcohol consumption is also not an independent risk factor for multiple aneurysms [30,31]. Thus, it is quite likely that alcohol intake does not cause aneurysm formation.

Blood pressure is raised independently by age, body mass index, pulse rate, amount of regular alcohol use, and sodium intake [53–57]. Daily drinking of alcohol results in a dose-dependent gradual elevation of blood pressure within a few days to weeks [54,55]. After cessation of drinking blood pressure is normalized. Although short-term occasional drinking may not consistently elevate blood pressure, it has been reported that, in normotensive subjects, acute consumption of alcohol can transiently raise both systolic and diastolic blood pressure [58,59]. The maximum response occurs at peak blood alcohol concentration. A reactive form of hypertension associated with increased catecholamines and vascular hyperresponsiveness is a well-known effect during alcohol withdrawal [60]. In social drinkers, binge drinking causes a transient increase in blood pressure and pulse rate only during intoxication, since blood pressure values, but not pulse rate, are even decreased after drinking and are normalized during hangover [59]. In heavy drinkers, a high variability of alcohol consumption (episodic drinking) seems to increase blood pressure values more than a low variability of alcohol intake [57].

Blood-pressure levels, which are transiently increased during alcohol intake and withdrawal, may prove to be an important mechanism for SAH [4,16,17]; such a transient increase in systemic blood pressure, together with cerebral arteriolar vasoconstriction during alcohol exposure [61], may contribute to rupture of an existing aneurysm without causing formation of an aneurysm. Use of illicit drugs amphetamines and cocaine may increase risk for SAH by this same mechanism [11,16], since presence of multiple aneurysms does not correlate with the use of such drugs [30].

History of hypertension as a risk factor for SAH seems to be less crucial than for other stroke subtypes [4,16,17,25,42]. The prevalence of hypertension among SAH patients (20–30%) has been suggested to be only slightly higher than in the general population; after adjustment for age, gender, cigarette smoking, and alcohol consumption, history of hypertension has not been shown in case-control studies to increase risk for SAH [16,17]. Smoking and alcohol consumption have thus been considered to increase risk for SAH by mechanisms other than chronic hypertension; hypertension does not even seem to increase risk for aneurysm rupture [34,35,37,47]. In a recent study, patients with hypertension did not have de novo aneurysms or aneurysm growth more often than did the non-hypertensive, nor did BP values correlate with aneurysm formation or growth (Juvela et al. Stroke 2001; **32**: 485–491).

Recently, patients of working age with hypertension also had more aneurysms than did the normotensive, although prevalence of multiple aneurysms has not been higher overall in hypertensive patients [31]. Therefore, patients with hypertension who are subject to intracranial aneurysm formation may more frequently have more than two aneurysms. The association of hypertension with SAH could be due to study populations including ICH patients been used in SAH studies [11,18,32,33]. This inclusion was possible especially in studies performed before the CT era, and occurred because ICH is the more common type of stroke in most populations [2,3,7].

Recently, family history of intracranial aneurysms has been suggested to be evidence for genetic causality of cerebral aneurysms [27,62]. However, cigarette smoking and other health-related habits should be analyzed as a confounding factor for this association since correlation of these habits between family members is higher than in the general population [62,63]. In addition, 38–48% of subarachnoid hemorrhages can be attributed to current smoking [16,17,42], whereas risk attributable to affected first-degree relatives accounts for only 5% [62]. Furthermore smoking and alcohol-intake behaviors may even to some degree be influenced by genetic factors [63], although tobacco-associated premature death from lung cancer and cardiovascular diseases does not seem to be influenced by genetic or familial predisposition [64].

Risk factors for poor outcome after subarachnoid hemorrhage

The outcome after aneurysmal SAH is determined by the severity of bleeding assessed by the clinical condition and amount of subarachnoid, intracerebral, and intraventricular blood on the CT scan, as well as by the occurrence of rebleeding or delayed cerebral ischemia (symptomatic vasospasm) [6,65–68]. Advanced age seems to impair outcome independently of factors mentioned above [67].

The risk of delayed cerebral ischemia is best predicted by the amount of subarachnoid and intraventricular blood amount [65,66,68], as well as by previous hypertension [66,68], irrespective of clinical condition on admission or hydrocephalus. Cigarette smoking has also been shown to increase the risk of symptomatic vasospasm [43] and of cerebral infarction after SAH [68].

Alcohol consumption seems not to increase the risk of death due to primary bleed although heavy drinking may increase mortality and morbidity because of severe rebleeding and delayed cerebral ischemia after SAH [6]. Poor outcome in heavy drinkers is caused mainly by an increase in mortality and morbidity due to rebleeding and delayed ischemia although frequency and time of onset of rebleeding and delayed ischemia are not affected by drinking habits [6].

There can be several mechanisms by which heavy drinking and ethanol withdrawal can predispose to a severe rebleeding or symptomatic vasospasm after SAH. These include the effects on blood pressure, platelet function, clotting factors, alcohol-induced cardiac arrhythmias, and changes in cerebral blood flow [6,10,54–60,69]. Long term severe heavy drinking can cause thrombocytopenia, reduced platelet aggregability and thromboxane formation capacity, increase in prostacyclin production in the endothelium, and defects of clotting factors [6,10]. In addition, cerebral autoregulation is impaired after SAH leading to an increase in cerebral blood flow if blood pressure is elevated [25]. Increase in blood pressure, together with cerebral arteriolar vasoconstriction during alcohol exposure [61], may increase blood pressure in large cerebral arteries. All these factors together could explain the severity of rebleeding and presence of intracerebral hematoma in heavy drinkers. Cessation of alcohol abuse results in rebound thrombocytosis and increased thromboxane formation by platelets within two weeks thus favoring thrombosis formation and severe delayed cerebral ischemia [6,69].

INTRACEREBRAL HEMORRHAGE

Incidence of intracerebral hemorrhage

Incidence of spontaneous ICH also varies widely throughout the world being most common in Asia, but 15–30/100,000/year is the generally accepted estimate for western countries

[2,3,39,70]. Although incidence of ICH is higher than that of SAH, the incidence of SAH is higher in people aged 60 or less, especially in Finland [2,7]. The incidence of SAH increases linearly by age [3,7], while that of ICH increases exponentially [2,3]. ICH also is clearly more common among men than among women.

Risk factors for intracerebral hemorrhage

Most spontaneous hematomas are attributed to chronic arterial hypertension [1–4,8,12,14]. Other risk factors for ICH include alcohol consumption [4,8–14], anticoagulant treatment [3,4,14,21], and to a lesser extent, aspirin use [14,22], thrombolytic therapy [3,23], use of amphetamines or cocaine [3,11], and possibly also diabetes mellitus [4]. These factors increase risk for ICH especially in young and middle-aged adult people, whereas amyloid angiopathy is an important cause of ICH in the older age groups. Cigarette smoking, which is the most important risk factor for SAH, seems not to increase independently of hypertension and alcohol consumption the risk for ICH, although its prevalence may be higher among ICH patients than in the general population [8,12,14,19,20]. Thus, ICH seems, contrary to SAH, to have a multifactorial pathogenesis.

History of hypertension as a risk factor for ICH is well known [1–4,8,12,14,20,70]. Its occurrence among ICH patients varies from 45–70%, whereas the prevalence of hypertension in the general adult population is about 20%. The risk is even substantially higher among those who have ceased their antihypertensive therapy [14,70]. Approximately 20% of ICH patients had not used the hypertensive medicines, which were prescribed to them before hemorrhage or these were stopped by a physician within few weeks to months before ICH [14]. The mechanism is thought to involve a hypertension-induced degeneration of the walls of small arteries (lipohyalinosis and fibrinoid necrosis or microaneurysm) that leaves them prone to rupture. Both insulin-dependent and non-insulin-dependent diabetes mellitus has been suggested, independently of chronic hypertension and other risk factors, to increase risk for ICH partly by this same mechanism: vasculopathy of perforating cerebral arteries, the walls of which are weakened by lipid and hyaline material (lipohyalinosis and fibrinoid necrosis), microaneurysm, and/or microangiopathy [4].

Several studies have shown that alcohol consumption increases the risk for ICH in a dose–response manner independent of chronic hypertension [4,8–14] – even in women [13,14]. Evidence for this has been obtained using different interview methods and laboratory markers of alcohol intake [14]. Alcohol intake seems to be more common among patients with spontaneous ICH than among those of a similar age with aneurysmal SAH [4,9,13]. The amount of alcohol used within the previous 24 hours seems to be similar in both hemorrhage types [4]. However, recent heavy drinking (>300 grams) within the previous week as well as problem drinking are more common in male ICH patients than in male SAH patients independent of their history of hypertension [4]. When the risk for SAH seems to be increased when average alcohol intake is more than 150 g within a week, risk for ICH seems to be increased already at lower levels of alcohol intake [4,11,14,17]. Average alcohol intake of <100 g within a week [71] or of less than 40 g at a time [14] seems to not increase the risk.

This alcohol-associated risk for ICH is of relative short duration. This theory is supported by the observation that recent drinking, within 24 hours of ICH, was more important as a risk factor than the amount of alcohol consumed within 1 week, and that previous drinking was not a risk factor [14]. The association of recent drinking and ICH is not influenced by sex, age, body mass index, smoking status, hypertension or other previous diseases, or by use of nonsteroidal anti-inflammatory drugs or anticoagulants [14].

The pathophysiologic mechanisms by which alcohol could contribute to ICH include hypertension [54–60], impaired hemostasis [69,72,73], decreased circulating levels of clotting factors produced by the liver [72,74], excessive fibrinolysis [75], disseminated intravascular coagulation [10], and changes in cerebral blood flow [76]. Because even anticoagulant treatment with a low- or moderate-intensity warfarin regimen seems not to increase the risk of intracranial bleeding [77], and the prevalence of thrombocytopenia as a cause of ICH seems to be uncommon [14], liver dysfunction or thrombocytopenia must be severe if bleeding or clotting disorders can be considered as the sole cause of ICH. Clotting and bleeding disorders together with alcohol-induced transient elevation of blood pressure [58–60] and plasminogen activator activity [75] could increase the risk of ICH [14].

It is unlikely that chronic hypertension is the mechanism by which alcohol consumption increases the risk for ICH, because the alcohol-associated risk has remained significant after adjustment for hypertension [8,9,12,13,14]. On the other hand, the transient increase in blood pressure during alcohol intake and withdrawal may prove to be an important mechanism [14]. Such a transient increase in systemic blood pressure [58–60] together with cerebral arteriolar vasoconstriction [61] during alcohol exposure might contribute to rupture of small cerebral arteries. Since alcohol intake is more abundant in ICH patients than in SAH patients [4,9,13], it is possible that alcohol may increase the risk of ICH also by other mechanisms than only by a transient elevation of blood pressure. Use of illicit drugs amphetamines and cocaine may increase risk for SAH by this same mechanism. During as well as after alcohol or drug intake, cerebral autoregulation, especially in patients with hypertensive cardiovascular disease, may be altered leading to arteriolar dilatation and increased cerebral blood flow even at moderately increased blood pressure levels. This may result in vascular rupture(s) [11,76,78]. Illicit drugs may also cause ICH by abrupt increase in blood pressure and by vasculitis [14].

Anticoagulant treatment has been shown to be a risk factor for ICH causing a low per cent of cases [4,14,21,77]. Intracranial bleeding caused by anticoagulant is more common in the elderly because they are treated more often by anticoagulants. Risk of hemorrhage is also directly associated with intensity of anticoagulation. Bleeding that occurs when the international normalized ratio (INR) is <3.0 is uncommon and frequently associated with an obvious underlying disease [14,77].

Use of aspirin or other nonsteroidal anti-inflammatory drugs (NSAIDs) seems to increase somewhat risk for ICH [14]. According to a meta-analysis of aspirin trials [22], although aspirin increases slightly (1.5-fold) but significantly ($p<0.05$) the risk of hemorrhagic stroke, which type of hemorrhage it increases remained unknown. It is likely that aspirin increases only the risk of ICH, since most of those SAH patients who had used NSAIDs before hemorrhage had used those agents for symptoms consistent with minor leakage, which have been suggested occurring in approximately 20–30% of SAH cases [4,5].

The risk of ICH associated with the use of thrombolytic agents has been shown to be low after myocardial infarction. This low risk may be increased somewhat by use of anticoagulants and among elderly people [23]. Thrombocytopenia as a cause of ICH also is uncommon [2,3,14]. These observations suggest that liver dysfunction or hemostatic disorders must be severe if bleeding or clotting disorders can be considered as the sole cause of ICH.

Risk factors for poor outcome after intracerebral hemorrhage

The short-term outcome (30-day mortality) after ICH is determined independently by the severity of bleeding as assessed by the initial level of consciousness, the volume of hematoma and the presence of intraventricular blood [79–84]; and the long-term functional outcome also depends on location of the hematoma, the age of patient, and the amount of alcohol consumed within one week before ICH [81,83,84]. Hematomas, which are outside the basal ganglia and brain stem are associated independently of other factors with a better prognosis than the central hematomas [84].

Patients with a subcortical or cerebellar hematoma at least 3 cm in diameter and impaired consciousness are generally considered to benefit from surgical removal of clot, which reduces both mortality and morbidity [1,84]. Patients with the most common intracerebral hematomas, which are located in the putamen are not generally accepted as candidates for surgery. Although surgery may reduce mortality of stuporous or semi-comatose patients it seems to leave these patients severely disabled [1,84,85].

Alcohol intake is not associated with case fatality due to initial bleeding but it is associated with long-term outcome [84]. Poor outcome, as well as overall outcome, are directly associated with the amount of alcohol used within the last week before ICH as well as with a laboratory marker of alcohol intake, erythrocyte mean corpuscular volume (MCV), suggesting that both recent drinking and long-term heavy alcohol intake impair outcome. At no level of alcohol intake is the outcome better in users than in abstainers [84].

Although alcohol intake and MCV were associated with variables predicting a favorable outcome (better clinical condition, younger patient age, superficial location of hematoma), they are also associated directly but non-significantly with volume of hematoma, especially MCV [84]. A possible reason for this is that patients who are long-term heavy drinkers have cerebral atrophy [86], rendering it possible that the hematoma must enlarge more in them than in those with less alcohol intake to produce similar symptoms. This might later cause more cerebral edema in heavy drinkers than expected on the basis of clinical condition owing to both the size of hematoma and the cytotoxic metabolites released from it [87].

Enlargement of the hematoma or rebleeding, which impairs clearly the outcome, occurs in 10–20% of patients when the initial CT scan is performed within 4–6 hours from the onset [84,85,88]. Enlargement of hematoma seems to be associated with initial volume of hematoma, time period between the onset of symptoms and first CT scan (inversely), heavy alcohol drinking, low level of fibrinogen, and elevated MCV [84,88].

Presence of cerebral atrophy or hematoma enlargement because of liver dysfunction could, however, not explain why patients with light or moderate recent alcohol intake have an increased risk of impaired outcome. CAGE positiveness (problem drinking), and heavy drinking were not important determinants of outcome after exclusion of amount of recent alcohol intake from the logistic models [84]. Cerebral atrophy as well as liver dysfunction seem to be reversible, which could in part explain why previous heavy drinking does not seem to impair outcome [84,86].

Pathophysiologic mechanisms by which alcohol could contribute to impaired outcome include also the same factors that increase risk for ICH: (transient) hypertension [54–60], impaired hemostasis [69,72,73], decreased circulating levels of clotting factors produced by the liver [72,74], excessive fibrinolysis [75], disseminated intravascular coagulation [10], and changes in cerebral blood flow [76]. Transient increase in blood pressure [58–60] together with cerebral arteriolar vasoconstriction during alcohol exposure [61], and/or impaired hemostasis could cause additional ruptures of small cerebral arteries causing enlargement of hematoma.

CONCLUSIONS

Cigarette smoking, alcohol consumption, and hypertension are important modifiable risk factors for hemorrhagic stroke and impaired outcome after the bleeding. Cigarette smoking and moderate to heavy alcohol consumption increase risk for SAH. Hypertension and alcohol consumption are risk factors for spontaneous ICH. Cigarette smoking may impair somewhat the outcome after SAH but alcohol consumption impairs functional recovery both after SAH and after ICH. Thus, cessation of smoking and avoiding heavy alcohol drinking, in particular binge drinking, are important factors to reduce incidence and partly also impaired outcome of these severe forms of hemorrhagic stroke.

REFERENCES

1 Juvela S, Heiskanen O, Poranen A, Valtonen S, Kuurne T, Kaste M, Troupp H. The treatment of spontaneous intracerebral hemorrhage: a prospective randomized trial of surgical and conservative treatment. *J. Neurosurg.* 1989; **70**: 755–758.

2 Fogelholm R, Nuutila M, Vuorela A-L. Primary intracerebral haemorrhage in the Jyväskylä region, Central Finland, 1985–89: incidence, case fatality rate, and functional outcome. *J. Neurol. Neurosurg. Psychiatry* 1992; **55**: 546–552.

3 Broderick JP, Brott T, Tomsick T, Miller R, Huster G. Intracerebral hemorrhage more than twice as common as subarachnoid hemorrhage. *J. Neurosurg.* 1993; **78**: 188–191.

4 Juvela S. Prevalence of risk factors in spontaneous intracerebral hemorrhage and aneurysmal subarachnoid hemorrhage. *Arch. Neurol.* 1996; **53**: 734–740.

5 Juvela S. Minor leak before rupture of an intracranial aneurysm and subarachnoid hemorrhage of unknown etiology. *Neurosurgery* 1992; **30**: 7–11.

6 Juvela S. Alcohol consumption as a risk factor for poor outcome after aneurysmal subarachnoid haemorrhage. *BMJ* 1992; **304**: 1663–1667.

7 Fogelholm R, Hernesniemi J, Vapalahti M. Impact of early surgery on outcome after aneurysmal subarachnoid hemorrhage: a population-based study. *Stroke* 1993; **24**: 1649–1654.

8 Calandre L, Arnal C, Fernandez Ortega J, Bermejo F, Felgeroso B, del Ser T, Vallejo A. Risk factors for spontaneous cerebral hematomas. Case-control study. *Stroke* 1986; **17**: 1126–1128.

9 Klatsky AL, Armstrong MA, Friedman GD. Alcohol use and subsequent cerebrovascular disease hospitalizations. *Stroke* 1989; **20**: 741–746.

10 Gorelick PB. The status of alcohol as a risk factor for stroke. *Stroke* 1989; **20**: 1607–1610.

11 Camargo CA. Moderate alcohol consumption and stroke: The epidemiologic evidence. *Stroke* 1989; **20**: 1611–1626.

12 Monforte R, Estruch R, Graus F, Nicolas JM, Urbano-Marquez A. High ethanol consumption as risk factor for intracerebral hemorrhage in young and middle-aged people. *Stroke* 1990; **21**: 1529–1532.

13 Gill JS, Shipley MJ, Tsementzis SA, Hornby RS, Gill SK, Hitchcock ER, Beevers DG. Alcohol consumption – A risk factor for hemorrhagic and non-hemorrhagic stroke. *Am. J. Med.* 1991; **90**: 489–497.

14 Juvela S, Hillbom M, Palomäki H. Risk factors for spontaneous intracerebral hemorrhage. *Stroke* 1995; **26**: 1558–1564.

15 Donahue RP, Abbott RD, Reed DM, Yano K. Alcohol and hemorrhagic stroke: The Honolulu Heart Program. *JAMA* 1986; **255**: 2311–2314.

16 Longstreth WT Jr, Nelson LM, Koepsell TD, van Belle G. Cigarette smoking, alcohol use, and subarachnoid hemorrhage. *Stroke* 1992; **23**: 1242–1249.

17 Juvela S, Hillbom M, Numminen H, Koskinen P. Cigarette smoking and alcohol consumption as risk factors for aneurysmal subarachnoid hemorrhage. *Stroke* 1993; **24**: 639–646.

18 Knekt P, Reunanen A, Aho K, Heliövaara M, Rissanen A, Aromaa A, Impivaara O. Risk factors for subarachnoid hemorrhage in a longitudinal population study. *J. Clin. Epidemiol.* 1991; **44**: 933–939.

19 Shinton R, Beevers G. Meta-analysis of relation between cigarette smoking and stroke. *BMJ* 1989; **298**: 789–794.

20 Fogelholm R, Murros K. Cigarette smoking and risk of primary intracerebral haemorrhage. A population-based case-control study. *Acta Neurol. Scand.* 1993; **87**: 367–370.

21 Fogelholm R, Eskola K, Kiminkinen T, Kunnamo I. Anticoagulant treatment as a risk factor for primary intracerebral haemorrhage. *J. Neurol. Neurosurg. Psychiatry* 1992; **55**: 1121–1124.

22 Antiplatelet Trialists' Collaboration. Collaborative overview of randomised trials of antiplatelet therapy, I: prevention of death, myocardial infarction, and stroke by prolonged antiplatelet therapy in various categories of patients. *BMJ* 1994; **308**: 81–106.

23 De Jaegere PP, Arnold AA, Balk AH, Simoons ML. Intracranial hemorrhage in association with thrombolytic therapy: incidence and clinical predictive factors. *J. Am. Coll. Cardiol.* 1992; **19**: 289–294.

24 Deykin D, Janson P, McMahon L. Ethanol potentiation of aspirin-induced prolongation of the bleeding time. *N. Engl. J. Med.* 1982; **306**: 852–854.

25 Weir B. *Aneurysms Affecting the Nervous System*. Williams & Wilkins, Baltimore, 1987.

26 Iwata K, Misu N, Terada K, Kawai S, Momose M, Nakagawa H. Screening for unruptured asymptomatic intracranial aneurysms in patients undergoing coronary angiography. *J. Neurosurg.* 1991; **75**: 52–55.

27 Ronkainen A, Miettinen H, Karkola K, Papinaho S, Vanninen R, Puranen M, Hernesniemi J. Risk of harboring an unruptured intracranial aneurysm. *Stroke* 1998; **29**: 359–362.

28 McCormick WF, Acosta-Rua GJ. The size of intracranial saccular aneurysms: an autopsy study. *J. Neurosurg.* 1970; **33**: 422–427.

29 Nakagawa T, Hashi K. The incidence and treatment of asymptomatic, unruptured cerebral aneurysms. *J. Neurosurg.* 1994; **80**: 217–223.

30 Qureshi AI, Suarez JI, Parekh PD, Sung G, Geocadin R, Bhardwaj A, Tamargo RJ, Ulatowski JA. Risk factors for multiple intracranial aneurysms. *Neurosurg.* 1998; **43**: 22–27.

31 Juvela S. Risk factors for multiple intracranial aneurysms. *Stroke* 2000; **31**: 392–397.

32 Stehbens WE. Etiology of intracranial berry aneurysms. *J. Neurosurg.* 1989; **70**: 823–831.

33 Sacco RL, Wolf PA, Bharucha NE, Meeks SL, Kannel WB, Charette LJ, McNamara PM, Palmer EP, D'Agostino R. Subarachnoid and intracerebral hemorrhage: natural history, prognosis, and precursive factors in the Framingham study. *Neurology* 1984; **34**: 847–854.

34 Wiebers DO, Whisnant JP, Sundt TM Jr, O'Fallon WM. The significance of unruptured intracranial saccular aneurysms. *J. Neurosurg.* 1987; **66**: 23–29.

35 Juvela S, Porras M, Heiskanen O. Natural history of unruptured intracranial aneurysms: a long-term follow-up study. *J. Neurosurg.* 1993; **79**: 174–182.

36 Yasui N, Suzuki A, Nishimura H, Suzuki K, Abe T. Long-term follow-up study of unruptured intracranial aneurysms. *Neurosurgery* 1997; **40**: 1155–1160.

37 The International Study of Unruptured Intracranial Aneurysms Investigators. Unruptured intracranial aneurysms – risk of rupture and risks of surgical intervention. *N. Engl. J. Med.* 1998; **339**: 1725–1733.

38 Linn FHH, Rinkel GJE, Algra A, van Gijn J. Incidence of subarachnoid hemorrhage: role of region, year, and rate of computed tomography: a meta-analysis. *Stroke* 1996; **27**: 625–629.

39 Numminen H, Kotila M, Waltimo O, Aho K, Kaste M. Declining incidence and mortality rates of stroke in Finland from 1972 to 1991: results of three population-based stroke registers. *Stroke* 1996; **27**: 1487–1491.

40 Sarti C, Tuomilehto J, Salomaa V, Sivenius J, Kaarsalo E, Narva E, Salmi K, Torppa J. Epidemiology of subarachnoid hemorrhage in Finland from 1983 to 1985. *Stroke* 1991; **22**: 848–853.

41 Kongable GL, Lanzino G, Germanson TP, Truskowski LL, Alves WM, Torner JC, Kassell NF, the Participants. Gender-related differences in aneurysmal subarachnoid hemorrhage. *J. Neurosurg.* 1996; **84**: 43–48.

42 Bonita R. Cigarette smoking, hypertension and the risk of subarachnoid hemorrhage: a population-based case-control study. *Stroke* 1986; **17**: 831–835.

43 Weir BKA, Kongable GL, Kassell NF, Schultz JR, Truskowski LL, Sigrest A, the Investigators. Cigarette smoking as a cause of aneurysmal subarachnoid hemorrhage and risk for vasospasm: a report of the Cooperative Aneurysm Study. *J. Neurosurg.* 1998; **89**: 405–411.

44 Townsend J, Wilkes H, Haines A, Jarvis M. Adolescent smokers seen in general practice: health, lifestyle, physical measurements, and response to antismoking advice. *BMJ.* 1991; **303**: 947–950.

45 Tonnesen P, Norregaard J, Simonsen K, Säwe U. A double-blind trial of a 16-hour transdermal nicotine patch in smoking cessation. *N. Engl. J. Med.* 1991; **325**: 311–315.

46 Taioli E, Wynder EL. Effect of the age at which smoking begins on frequency of smoking in adulthood [letter]. *N. Engl. J. Med.* 1991; **325**: 968–969.

47 Juvela S, Porras M, Poussa K. Natural history of unruptured intracranial aneurysms: probability and risk factors for aneurysm rupture. *J. Neurosurg.* 2000; **93**: 379–387.

48 Baker CJ, Fiore A, Connolly ES Jr, Baker KZ, Solomon RA. Serum elastase and alpha-1-antitrypsin levels in patients with ruptured and unruptured cerebral aneurysms. *Neurosurgery* 1995; **37**: 56–62.

49 Gaetani P, Tartara F, Tancioni F, Klersy C, Forlino A, Rodriguez y Baena R. Activity of alpha 1-antitrypsin and cigarette smoking in subarachnoid hemorrhage from ruptured aneurysm. *J. Neurol. Sci.* 1996; **141**: 33–38.

50 Cohen JR, Sarfati I, Wise L. The effect of cigarette smoking on rabbit aortic elastase activity. *J. Vasc. Surg.* 1989; **9**: 580–582.

51 Miskolczi L, Guterman LR, Flaherty JD, Hopkins LN. Saccular aneurysm induction by elastase digestion of the arterial wall: a new animal model. *Neurosurgery* 1998; **43**: 595–601.

52 Stampher MJ, Colditz GA, Willett WC, Speizer FE, Hennekens CH. A prospective study of moderate alcohol consumption and the risk of coronary disease and stroke in women. *N. Engl. J. Med.* 1988; **319**: 267–273.

53 Salomaa V, Tuomilehto J, Nissinen A, Korhonen HJ, Vartiainen E, Kartovaara L, Puska P. The development of hypertension care in Finland from 1982 to 1987. *J. Hypertens.* 1989; **7**: 837–844.

54 Puddey IB, Beilin LJ, Vandongen R, Rouse IL, Rogers P. Evidence for a direct effect of alcohol consumption in normotensive men: a randomized controlled trial. *Hypertension* 1985; **7**: 707–713.

55 Puddey IB, Beilin LJ, Vandongen R. Effect of regular alcohol use on blood pressure control in treated hypertensive subjects: a controlled study. *Clin. Exp. Pharmacol. Physiol.* 1986; **13**: 315–318.

56 Smith WCS, Crombie IK, Tavendale RT, Gulland SK, Tunstall-Pedoe HD. Urinary electrolyte excretion, alcohol consumption, and blood pressure in the Scottish heart health study. *BMJ* 1988; **297**: 329–330.

57 Marmot MG, Elliott P, Shipley MJ, Dyer AR, Ueshima H, Beevers DG, Stamler R, Kesteloot H, Rose G, Stamler J. Alcohol and blood pressure: the Intersalt study. *BMJ* 1994; **308**: 1263–1267.

58 Potter JF, Watson RD, Skan W, Beevers DG. The pressor and metabolic effects of alcohol in normotensive subjects. *Hypertension* 1986; **8**: 625–631.

59 Seppä K, Sillanaukee P. Binge drinking and ambulatory blood pressure. *Hypertension* 1999; **33**: 79–82.

60 Clark LT, Friedman HS. Hypertension associated with alcohol withdrawal: assessment of mechanisms and complications. *Alcohol Clin. Exp. Res.* 1985; **9**: 125–130.

61 Altura BM, Altura BT, Gebrewold A. Alcohol-induced spasms of cerebral blood vessels: relation to cerebrovascular accidents and sudden death. *Science* 1983; **220**: 331–333.

62 Wang PS, Longstreth WT Jr, Koepsell TD. Subarachnoid hemorrhage and family history: a population-based case-control study. *Arch. Neurol.* 1995; **52**: 202–204.

63 Carmelli D, Swan GE, Robinette D, Fabsitz R. Genetic influence on smoking – a study of male twins. *N. Engl. J. Med.* 1992; **327**: 829–833.

64 Carmelli D, Page WF. Twenty-four year mortality in World War II US male veteran twins discordant for cigarette smoking. *Int. J. Epidemiol.* 1996; **25**: 554–559.

65 Hijdra A, van Gijn J, Nagelkerke NJ, Vermeulen M, van Crevel H. Prediction of delayed cerebral ischemia, rebleeding, and outcome after aneurysmal subarachnoid hemorrhage. *Stroke* 1988; **19**: 1250–1256.

66 Öhman J, Servo A, Heiskanen O. Risk factors for cerebral infarction in good-grade patients after aneurysmal subarachnoid hemorrhage and surgery: a prospective study. *J. Neurosurg.* 1991; **74**: 14–20.

67 Lanzino G, Kassell NF, Germanson TP, Kongable GL, Truskowski LL, Torner JC, Jane JA, the Participants. Age and outcome after aneurysmal subarachnoid hemorrhage: why do older patients fare worse? *J. Neurosurg.* 1996; **85**: 410–418.

68 Juvela S. Plasma endothelin concentrations after aneurysmal subarachnoid hemorrhage. *J. Neurosurg.* 2000; **92**: 390–400.

69 Haselager EM, Vreeken J. Rebound thrombocytosis after alcohol abuse: A possible factor in the pathogenesis of thromboembolic disease. *Lancet* 1977; **i**: 774–775.

70 Thrift AG, McNeil JJ, Forbes A, Donnan GA. Three important subgroups of hypertensive persons at greater risk of intracerebral hemorrhage. *Hypertension* 1998; **31**: 1223–1229.

71 Berger K, Ajani UA, Kase CS, Gaziano JM, Buring JE, Glynn RJ, Hennekens CH. Light-to-moderate alcohol consumption and the risk of stroke among U.S. male physicians. *N. Engl. J. Med.* 1999; **341**: 1557–1564.

72 Ragni MV, Lewis JH, Spero JA, Hasiba U. Bleeding and coagulation abnormalities in alcoholic cirrhotic liver disease. *Alcoholism Clin. Exp. Res.* 1982; **6**: 267–274.

73 Hillbom M, Neiman J. Platelet thromboxane formation capacity after ethanol withdrawal in chronic alcoholics. *Haemostasis* 1988; **18**: 170–178.

74 Niizuma H, Suzuki J, Yonemitsu T, Otsuki T. Spontaneous intracerebral hemorrhage and liver dysfunction. *Stroke* 1988; **19**: 852–856.

75 Hendriks HFJ, Veenstra J, Velhuis-te Wierik EJM, Schaafsma G, Kluft C. Effect of moderate dose of alcohol with evening meal on fibrinolytic factors. *BMJ* 1994; **308**: 1003–1006.

76 Berglund M, Risberg J. Regional cerebral blood flow during alcohol withdrawal. *Arch. Gen. Psychiatry* 1981; **38**: 351–355.

77 Hirsh J. Oral anticoagulant drugs. *N. Engl. J. Med.* 1991; **324**: 1865–1875.

78 Kibayashi K, Mastri AR, Hirsch CS. Cocaine induced intracerebral hemorrhage: analysis of predisposing factors and mechanism causing hemorrhagic strokes. *Hum. Pathol.* 1995; **26**: 659–663.

79 Portenoy RK, Lipton RB, Berger AR, Lesser ML, Lantos G. Intracerebral haemorrhage: a model for prediction of outcome. *J. Neurol. Neurosurg. Psychiatry* 1987; **50**: 976–979.

80 Tuhrim S, Dambrosia JM, Price TR, Mohr JP, Wolf PA, Hier DB, Kase CS. Intracerebral hemorrhage: external validation and extension of a model for prediction of 30-day survival. *Ann. Neurol.* 1991; **29**: 658–663.

81 Franke CL, van Swieten JC, Algra A, van Gijn J. Prognostic factors in patients with intracerebral haematoma. *J. Neurol. Neurosurg. Psychiatry* 1992; **55**: 653–657.

82 Broderick JP, Brott TG, Duldner JE, Tomsick T, Huster G. Volume of intracerebral hemorrhage: A powerful and easy-to-use predictor of 30-day mortality. *Stroke* 1993; **24**: 987–993.

83 Daverat P, Castel JP, Dartigues JF, Orgogozo JM. Death and functional outcome after spontaneous intracerebral hemorrhage: a prospective study of 166 cases using multivariate analysis. *Stroke* 1991; **22**: 1–6.

84 Juvela S. Risk factors for impaired outcome after spontaneous intracerebral hemorrhage. *Arch. Neurol.* 1995; **52**: 1193–1200.

85 Fujitsu K, Muramoto M, Ikeda Y, Inada Y, Kim I, Kuwabara T. Indications for surgical treatment of putaminal hemorrhage. Comparative study based on serial CT and time-course analysis. *J. Neurosurg.* 1990; **73**: 518–525.

86 Charness ME, Simon RP, Greenberg DA. Ethanol and the nervous system. *N. Engl. J. Med.* 1989; **321**: 442–454.

87 Yang G-Y, Betz L, Chenevert TL, Brunberg JA, Hoff JT. Experimental intracerebral hemorrhage: relationship between brain edema, blood flow, and blood-brain barrier permeability in rats. *J. Neurosurg.* 1994; **81**: 93–102.

88 Fujii Y, Takeuchi S, Sasaki O, Minakawa T, Tanaka R. Multivariate analysis of predictors of hematoma enlargement in spontaneous intracerebral hemorrhage. *Stroke* 1998; **29**: 1160–1166.

Chapter 7

Alcohol abuse and ischemic stroke

Matti Hillbom

INTRODUCTION

Alcohol consumption has been reported to show a U-shaped [1], J-shaped [2] or linear [3] association with the incidence of total stroke, including ischemic stroke. A J-shaped association has also been observed between alcohol intake and blood pressure, the major risk factor for ischemic stroke [4]. It now seems to be generally accepted that light-to-moderate drinking does not cause any cerebrovascular harm and may even protect against athero-thrombotic stroke. However, heavy drinking clearly increases the risk of both ischemic and hemorrhagic stroke.

Alcohol abuse is known to cause both hypertension and atrial fibrillation. Alcohol abuse shows a rather high (5–30%) estimated prevalence in the western industrialized countries, but only a modest increasing effect on the risk of ischemic stroke compared to hypertension and atrial fibrillation [5]. The impact of hypertension on the incidence of stroke is much greater than that of alcohol [6,7]. The population-attributable risk for stroke caused by hypertension has been estimated to be ten-fold compared to that caused by heavy alcohol consumption [7]. However, alcohol remains among the many risk factors of ischemic stroke.

Different drinking habits certainly contribute to the diversity of observations. For example, alcohol seems to carry a much higher risk for deep cerebral infarct (lacunar stroke) in Spain than in Finland [8,9]. Regular daily drinking is much more common in the Mediterranian countries than in Scandinavia. However, the Scandinavian pattern of heavy binge drinking may be more hazardous for some other types of ischemic stroke.

The aim of the present chapter is to discuss the relationship between heavy drinking and several subtypes of ischemic stroke with particular reference to the drinking pattern. The nature of the relationship will be highlighted with case histories whenever possible. At the end of the chapter, the possible protective effect of light alcohol drinking will also be discussed.

CARDIOGENIC BRAIN EMBOLISM

Stroke admission rates have been observed to be high among heavy drinkers [10]. Some studies also suggest that alcohol abuse may associate with ischemic stroke recurrence [11,12]. A study on recent alcohol intake showed that heavy drinking is an independent risk factor for most subtypes of ischemic stroke and particularly a risk factor for cardiogenic brain embolism [13].

Table 7.1 Previously published and new case histories illustrating several different mechanisms that could link alcohol abuse to an increased risk of ischemic brain infarct

Cases [reference]	Number of cases	Type of stroke	Mechanism or underlying disease	Drinking pattern
[14]*	1	Cardioembolic	Alcoholic cardiomyopathy	Regular
[18]*	1	Cardioembolic	Atrial fibrillation	Binge
[19]*	1	Cardioembolic	Atrial flutter	Binge
Case 1	1	Cardioembolic	Atrioventricular block	Binge
Case 2	1	Cardioembolic	Myocardial infarct	Binge
Case 3	1	Cardioembolic	Left atrial thrombus	Regular
Case 4	1	Cardioembolic	Myocardial infarct	Regular
[22]*	1	Paradoxical	Atrial septal defect	Regular
Case 5	1	Paradoxical	Patent foramen ovale	Binge
Case 6	1	Paradoxical	Patent foramen ovale	Binge
[23]*	1	Undetermined	Rebound thrombocytosis	Regular
Case 7	1	Tandem embolism	Large-artery disease	Binge
Case 8	1	Lacunar infarct	Small-vessel occlusion	Regular
[37]*	1	Dissection	Hypertension	Binge
[22]*	1	Dissection	Neck trauma	Binge
[38]*	3	Dissection?	Alcoholic stupor	Binge?
[39]*	1	Dissection	Vertebral occlusion	Binge
[40]*	1	Compression	Alcoholic coma	Binge?
Case 9	1	Dissection	Neck compression	Binge
[41]*	2	Cryptogenic	Unknown	Binge
[42]*	1	Cryptogenic	Unknown	Binge

* See reference for details of the cases. In case 23 investigations to detect cardiac and vascular abnormalities were not performed.

The association between alcohol abuse with cardiogenic brain embolism suggests several mechanisms via which heavy drinking could precipitate brain infarct. First, there is the possibility of alcoholic heart muscle disease. Excessive chronic alcohol consumption leads to dilated cardiomyopathy, which often results in heart failure. In some countries, alcohol is the identifiable cause of chronic heart failure in 2–3% of cases. Embolism to the brain is a frequent complication of the disease [14]. Although case histories are infrequently reported (Table 7.1), alcoholic patients with dilated cardiomyopathy are common. In Spain, where regular daily alcohol intake is the prevailing drinking pattern of heavy drinkers, alcoholic cardiomyopathy has been observed in one-third of both male and female alcoholics [15].

Atrial fibrillation is certainly the commonest cause of cardiogenic brain embolism, and about 0.4% of the population have atrial fibrillation. The relative risk of ischemic stroke in subjects with atrial fibrillation is 5- to 7-fold compared to subjects without this condition. Alcohol abuse has been estimated to account for a substantial portion (30%) of the new-onset cases [16] and to precipitate atrial fibrillation even in healthy nonalcoholic subjects [17]. Alcohol-induced atrial fibrillation [18] and atrial flutter [19] have been reported as causes of cardiogenic brain embolism in nonalcoholic young adults. These cases were young men with neither cardiomyopathy nor coronary disease, and the strokes were precipitated by acute alcoholic intoxication. Autopsy of a patient who had two episodes of embolic stroke, both precipitated by acute alcohol drinking, did not show any cardiac abnormality [19]. These two cases illustrate that even occasional heavy drinking may precipitate cardiac arrhythmias leading to stroke. The following case history confirms that subjects prone to severe cardiac arrhythmias should avoid drinking for intoxication.

Case I

In June 1988, a 31-year-old nonsmoking man showed transient dysphasia shortly after having ingested several glasses of beer. Subsequent examinations suggested cardiogenic brain embolism. Computed tomography of the head showed a small left temporo-parietal brain infarct. His heart was in a normal position, the left ventricle was slightly enlarged (63/43 mm), and precordial echocardiography did not reveal any intracardiac thrombi, but a 17-hour Holter monitoring revealed severe bradyarrhythmias (heart rate varying from 30 to 58 beats with several asystoles >4 seconds), single ventricular extras and a third-degree atrioventricular block. The diagnosis of a congenital heart conduction defect was made. The subject was put on continuous aspirin treatment.

On the afternoon of October 4th 1991, while working, the subject suddenly developed right homonymous quadrantanopia and dysphasia. He had been taking aspirin regularly, but on the preceding evening he had ingested a large amount of alcohol (180 g ethanol). The short CAGE questionnaire [20] suggested that he was a problem drinker, and his serum gammaglutamyl transferase was clearly above normal. His total alcohol intake during the preceding week amounted to 450 grams of ethanol. He was a nonsmoker and had no other risk factors for stroke except the previously diagnosed congenital heart conduction defect and alcohol abuse. The examination revealed a new left parietal brain infarct, but transesophageal echocardiography (TEE) showed no pathological findings. The patient was put on continuous anticoagulant treatment and warned against drinking alcohol.

Other conditions, such as post-infarct abnormalities of the left ventricle and hypertensive heart disease have also been observed in subjects with alcoholic ischemic stroke. The following three case histories suggest that patients with these conditions should be warned against heavy drinking.

Case 2

In August 1992, a 57-year-old nonsmoking man, while trying to sleep after having ingested a large amount of alcohol (120 grams ethanol), suddenly became unconscious for a short moment and simultaneously developed left hemiparesis. On admission into the local hospital, a couple of hours later, his blood ethanol concentration was 40 mmol/L. Subsequent examinations revealed a large right hemispheric brain infarct (a dense media sign was visible in the first CT of the head) together with severe brain edema and herniation. The patient, who was used taking a binge once a month, died three days later. Autopsy was not performed. According to the hospital records, he had hypertension, coronary artery disease and a large anterolateral myocardial infarct resulting into infero-posterior and antero-apical hypokinetic segments. The patient had also fallen down, because of his intoxication a few hours before going to bed. Therefore, a traumatic carotid arterial dissection could not be excluded, but cardiogenic brain embolism was also possible.

Case 3

In April 1994, a 60-year-old nonsmoking man who had diabetes and untreated hypertension, but who did not use any medication, suddenly developed right hemiparesis and a visual field defect several hours after getting out of bed in the morning. He was an episodic heavy drinker and had ingested a large amount of alcohol on the preceding evening (150 g ethanol). His usual weekly alcohol intake averaged 300 g of ethanol. On admission, he had atrial fibrillation. During the preceding month, he had both an upper respiratory infection and a bacterial dental infection, and two weeks before the index stroke he experienced symptoms suggestive of a transient ischemic attack. A computed tomography head scan showed a new left temporo-occipital brain infarct and an older left deep capsular infarct. Duplex imaging of the carotid and vertebral arteries did not suggest any significant stenoses, but TEE showed an enlarged left atrium with a moving appendicular thrombus.

Case 4

In March 1990, a 42-year-old man known to be an episodic heavy drinker and regular smoker suddenly developed a right visual field defect caused by a left occipital brain infarct. A few weeks prior to the index stroke he had an anteroseptal and inferior myocardial infarct, and after discharge from hospital, he had started to drink large amounts of alcohol daily. In April 1995, he developed a right occipital brain infarct. This 'accident' was again preceded by a drinking bout of about two weeks (900 g ethanol per week). On admission, clinical examination showed tubular vision. A computed tomography head scan revealed two separate infarcts located on the left and right occipital lobes. Duplex imaging of the carotid and vertebral arteries showed neither occlusions nor significant stenoses, but transthoracic echocardiography (TTE) showed left ventricular inferior and anteroapical hypokinetic segments without any thrombi. Three days after the onset of the latter stroke, the patient's platelet count amounted to 604, suggesting rebound thrombocytosis due to the recent cessation of prolonged heavy alcohol drinking. This patient was later diagnosed for a clinically definite mitochondrial disorder, but the presumed etiology of his strokes was probable cardiogenic embolism [21].

PARADOXICAL EMBOLISM

Paradoxical embolism has also been reported as an apparent cause of a brain infarct in a heavy drinker [22]. Two further cases of possible paradoxical embolism triggered in connection with binge drinking are described below.

Case 5

In July 1990, an obese 39-year-old man who was a smoker and infrequent weekend drinker suddenly felt severe headache and developed right hemiparesis together with right hemianopia shortly after getting up from bed in the morning. He had been healthy and was not using any medication, although slightly elevated blood pressure values had been measured. He had ingested a large amount of alcohol (150 g ethanol) during the preceding evening.

On admission in the morning of the stroke onset, his blood alcohol level was still 20 mmol/L. A computed tomography head scan showed a left parietal subcortical brain infarct. An arch angiogram revealed neither any significant stenoses nor other abnormalities in his arteries. TEE showed a slightly enlarged left atrium, no thrombi, but a patent foramen ovale without any spontaneous right-to-left shunt. Venography showed a deep venous thrombosis in his right leg.

Case 6

In March 1996, a 26-year-old healthy nonsmoking man who was an infrequent weekend drinker woke up at 8 a.m., and three hours later, while jogging, suddenly developed a right visual field defect. He had been drinking alcohol during the preceding evening (alcohol intake amounted to 150 g of ethanol), and had experienced distinct signs and symptoms of hangover and vomited that morning. An arch angiogram was normal, but TEE showed a moderate-to-large patent foramen ovale, but not spontaneous right-to-left shunt. Venography was not performed, but a hematologic examination revealed resistance to protein C (APC resistance, heterozygous for the prothrombin gene).

The latter case suggests that paradoxical embolism could have been transported via a patent foramen ovale during a Valsalva manouver precipitated by vomiting, a common consequence of intoxication and hangover. Thrombocytosis and associated platelet hyperactivity have been considered as contributing factors for alcohol-induced ischemic strokes [22,23]. Case 4 and the case reported by Neiman [23] suggest a relationship between alcohol-induced rebound thrombocytosis and the onset of ischemic stroke. Although rebound thrombocytosis coincided with the onset of stroke in these cases, we still lack direct proof of a causal relation. Such factors as rebound thrombocytosis, decreased fibrinolytic activity, APC resistance, etc., could well be considered to promote the development of thrombi, but it has remained unclear whether any particular drinking pattern, such as episodic heavy drinking, precipitates thrombus formation via these mechanisms.

LARGE-ARTERY ATHEROSCLEROSIS

It is generally thought that thromboembolic strokes are mainly caused by atherosclerotic disease. Atherosclerotic disease is less prevalent among populations regularly consuming alcohol than among binge-drinking populations. The high risk of stroke in a population with a high alcohol intake does not seem to be due to large-artery atherosclerosis [24], but may be caused by other diseases promoting the onset of stroke, i.e., alcoholic cardiomyopathy. On the other hand, the age-adjusted relation between alcohol intake and carotid artery atherosclerosis has been reported to be U-shaped, with light drinkers facing a lower atherosclerosis risk than either abstainers or heavy drinkers [25].

A strong positive relation between alcohol consumption and the risk of mortality from stroke is apparent [26]. In the Scandinavian countries, binge drinking has been observed to associate with both an increased risk for ischemic stroke mortality [27] and the progression of atherosclerosis [28]. It is therefore not surprising that a weak association has been observed even between large-artery atherosclerotic stroke and recent heavy drinking [13]. An artery-to-artery embolism (tandem embolism) may easily be detached from an existing thrombus attached to an atherosclerotic vessel wall because of the abrupt increase in blood flow caused by acute alcoholic intoxication. The following case history suggests such a mechanism.

Case 7

In February 1996, a 66-year-old previously healthy, heavily smoking man suddenly developed dysphasia and right hemiparesis while getting up from a couch in the afternoon. He was an episodic drinker and had suffered from sleep apneas. He had been drinking since the preceding night, and the total amount of alcohol ingested during the index bout amounted to 150 g ethanol. On admission into hospital on the same evening, a computed tomography head scan excluded the possibility of hemorrhagic stroke, but did not show a left hemispheric infarct, either. His blood alcohol concentration was 30 mmol/L. He did not have atrial fibrillation or any other signs or symptoms of cardiac disease (normal electrocardiogram), but an arch angiogram showed a major left internal carotid arterial stenosis (80%) with a rough atheromatous plaque. A diagnosis of large-artery atherosclerotic brain infarct was made, and the patient was remitted for carotid endarterectomy.

SMALL-VESSEL OCCLUSION

Small-vessel occlusions, i.e., thrombosis of a single perforating cerebral artery, cause lacunar ischemic strokes. A lacunar infarct usually occurs in the internal capsule or thalamus and presents clinically as a pure motor stroke, pure sensory stroke, sensomotor stroke, dysarthria clumsy hand or ataxic hemiparesis. Patients with typical lacunar infarct syndromes account for approximately 20% of all ischemic strokes, and hypertensive small-vessel disease seems to be the most important etiology [29]. Because heavy drinking of alcohol is a frequent cause of arterial hypertension, it is assumed to associate with small-vessel occlusion as well. However, conflicting observations have also been reported. Some studies have not shown alcohol to be a significant risk factor [29–31], whereas others have [9,32]. The study of You et al. included a rather large series of young adults with lacunar infarcts [33]. This study suggested that long-term heavy alcohol consumption is a risk factor for ischemic brain infarct, whereas recent heavy drinking is not. The following case history suggests a relationship between alcohol drinking and the onset of lacunar brain infarct.

Case 8

In October 1994, a 55-year-old heavily smoking man with treated diabetes and hypertension suddenly developed left sensomotor hemiparesis, while sitting at home in the evening. He was a habitual heavy drinker with a regular weekly consumption of 500 g ethanol. During the afternoon preceding the onset of stroke, he had ingested 10 bottles of beer (120 g ethanol) in a pub. On admission into hospital immediately after the onset of the stroke, his blood pressure was 110/75 mmHg and blood alcohol 20 mmol/L. Duplex imaging of the carotid and vertebral arteries did not show any significant stenoses, and precordial echocardiography was unremarkable. A computed tomography head scan later confirmed the presence of a small brain infarct in the area of the right lentiform and caudate nuclei.

A few similar subjects with classical risk factors for lacunar stroke have been seen at our department during the recent years. One patient had recurrent lacunar brain infarcts during heavy binge drinking. Some recent reports of interest should be mentioned here, because they may help to orient future investigations. First, apolipoprotein E phenotype seems to significantly influence the blood-pressure-increasing effect of alcohol consumption [34] and the risk of recurrent lobar intracerebral hemorrhage [35]. Studies relating apolipoprotein E phenotype to the occurrence of strokes triggered by heavy drinking are not yet available. Second, a line of experimental studies have demonstrated alcohol-induced cerebrovascular spasms in relation to stroke-like events [36]. This mechanism of probable importance has been described in other chapters of this book. Third, it could be possible that alcohol influences cerebrovascular autoregulation in a manner that promotes the onset of lacunar stroke. Further studies are needed to demonstrate such an effect.

CERVICAL ARTERIAL DISSECTION

Cervical arterial dissection is probably one of the most common causes of ischemic stroke in young subjects. It is diagnosed by imaging with conventional or MR angiography and typically occurs after major trauma, but may also occur spontaneously or after trivial injury. Needless to say, alcoholic intoxication is a major risk factor for all types of trauma. Therefore, it is not surprising that cervical arterial dissections have also been described to have occurred in connection with alcohol abuse [22,37]. Some reports have emphasized that extracranial vessel compression due to unusual posturing during alcoholic stupor or coma could also result in a brain infarct [38–40], but it has remained unclear whether cervical arterial dissection is the underlying mechanism or not. In at least one of the reported cases dissection was excluded [40].

Surprisingly, case-control studies have not yet been able to prove alcohol as a risk factor for ischemic stroke caused by cervical arterial dissection [13]. Injury of the neck arteries may easily occur during a drunken fight or falling, but the onset of ischemic stroke is often delayed. In fact, the onset of cervical trauma may have occurred long before the onset of stroke, and the relationship is therefore difficult to establish. To show a relationship, we will need to question the subjects with dissection about their experienced trauma and violence of all kinds as well as about alcohol drinking. The following case report illustrates the problem.

Case 9

One Friday evening in May 1993, a 36-year-old man, after having been drinking heavily (180 g ethanol), started to wrestle with a drunken companion. During the fight, this man was strangled, particularly on the right hand side of his neck. The man did not feel any symptoms immediately after the fight, but later on he felt pain on his right neck and got a headache. After a fortnight, while turning his face to right, he suddenly developed a right Horner's sign and temporal hyperalgesia. After admission into hospital, an arch angiogram revealed a 3-cm-long tight stenosis with aneurysms at both ends in the extracranial part of his right internal carotid artery. A diagnosis of traumatic carotid arterial dissection was made. He was treated with anticoagulants and made good recovery without any complications.

CRYPTOGENIC STROKE

Finally, ischemic brain infarcts of unknown origin (cryptogenic stroke) have also been described in connection with heavy drinking of alcohol [41,42]. Alcohol also has complex effects on cerebral blood flow and autoregulation. Whether or not these mechanisms play a significant role is unclear. Thus far, we have not found an alcoholic binge to result in marked hypotension and watershed infarcts. We believe that many of the cryptogenic ischemic brain infarcts are due to emboli of unknown origin.

EFFECTS OF LIGHT DRINKING

Several studies have shown regular light (10–20 g of ethanol daily) or moderate (less than 300 g of ethanol per week) drinking to associate with a decreased risk for ischemic stroke of atherothrombotic origin [43–45], but the observations on the effects of light and moderate alcohol consumption on stroke mortality have been conflicting [27,46,47]. For example, one study showed light-to-moderate drinking to be associated with a 36% reduction in deaths from ischemic heart disease, but had no effect on death from stroke [47]. A recent study [48] reported that light-to-moderate alcohol consumption reduces the overall risk of stroke and the risk of ischemic stroke in men. The benefit was apparent with as little as one drink per week. More abundant consumption, up to one drink per day, did not increase the observed benefit.

Several possible mechanisms have been proposed to explain the beneficial effect of light-to-moderate alcohol consumption [49]. However, almost all of the proposed mechanisms are unable to explain a protective effect with such small amounts of alcohol as a few drinks per week. The only exception could be the increasing effect of alcohol on estrogen levels, which protects against atherogenesis. On the other hand, accurate and reliable data on alcohol consumption are hard to find in epidemiological studies, because drinking patterns have usually not been inquired.

In fact, some investigators have pointed out that there is no convincing evidence to show that light or moderate drinking is protective against stroke [50]. Nor does light-to-moderate drinking seem to protect against mortality from stroke when compared with not drinking [47]. Although many studies have taken into account several potential confounding factors, others still exist. The ones that have been poorly controlled include physical activity, psychosocial confounders and dietary factors. For example, it has been observed that moderate drinkers who do not smoke are more likely than nondrinkers to engage in regular leisure time physical activity [51]. At the moment, we cannot recommend regular drinking of small amounts of alcohol for the prevention of ischemic stroke. We know that any increase in alcohol consumption in a population is associated with a corresponding increase of heavy drinking, which has untoward consequences.

CONCLUSIONS

Heavy drinking of alcohol is a risk factor for brain infarct. This has been observed particularly in young and middle-aged men, who are frequently heavy drinkers. In many cultures, women and elderly people do not drink for intoxication and are seldom heavy drinkers.

Although in some studies, adjustment for hypertension has abolished the independent role of alcohol as a risk factor, suggesting that the risk is increased through an elevated blood pressure, other studies have shown that recent heavy drinking also increases the risk independently. The ultimate mechanisms leading to the increased risk are still unclear. Several actions of alcohol could explain why precisely recent heavy drinking increases the risk of ischemic stroke. Trauma to the neck, which frequently occurs during alcoholic intoxication, is certainly one reason. Another is alcohol-induced cardiac arrhythmias, which predispose to cardiogenic brain embolism. Some of the examples presented as case histories above may equally well suggest a coincidence as a causal relationship. Several factors have been proposed to explain the beneficial effect of light-to-moderate drinking seen in epidemiological investigations. However, direct proof of their significance is still lacking, and some counfounding factors have not yet been adequately controlled for.

REFERENCES

1 Truelsen T, Grønbæk M, Schnohr P, Boysen G. Intake of beer, wine, and spirits and risk of stroke. The Copenhagen City Heart Study. *Stroke* 1998; **29**: 2467–2472.

2 Sacco RL, Elkind M, Boden-Albala B, I-Feng Lin, Kargman DE, Hauser WA, Shea S, Paik MC. The protective effect of moderate alcohol consumption on ischemic stroke. *JAMA* 1999; **281**: 53–60.

3 Leppälä JM, Paunio M, Virtamo J, Fogelholm R, Albanes D, Taylor PR, Heinonen OP. Alcohol consumption and stroke incidence in male smokers. *Circulation* 1999; **100**: 1209–1214.

4 Gillman MW, Cook NR, Evans DA, Rosner B, Hennekens CH. Relationship of alcohol intake with blood pressure in young adults. *Hypertension* 1995; **25**: 1106–1110.

5 Sacco RL. Risk factors and outcomes for ischemic stroke. *Neurology* 1995; **45**(Suppl. 1): S10–S14.

6 Jiang He, Klag MJ, Zhenglai Wu, Whelton PK. Stroke in the People's Republic of China I. Geographic variations in incidence and risk factors. *Stroke* 1995; **26**: 2222–2227.

7 Gorelick PB. Stroke prevention, an opportunity for efficient utilization of health care resources during the coming decade. *Stroke* 1994; **25**: 220–224.

8 Caicoya M, Rodriquez T, Corrales C, Cuello R, Lasheras C. Alcohol and stroke: a community case-control study in Asturias, Spain, *J. Clin. Epidemiol.* 1999; **52**: 677–684.

9 Mäntylä R, Aronen HJ, Salonen O, Pohjasvaara T, Korpelainen M, Peltonen T, Standertskjöld-Nordenstam C-G, Kaste M, Erkinjuntti T. Magnetic resonance imaging white matter hyperintensities and mechanisms of ischemic stroke. *Stroke* 1999; **30**: 2053–2058.

10 Starr JM, Thomas B, Whalley LJ. Population risk factors for hospitalization for stroke in Scotland. *Int. J. Epidemiol.* 1996; **25**: 276–281.

11 Sacco RL, Shi T, Zamanillo MC, Kargman DE. Predictors of mortality and recurrence after hospitalized cerebral infarction in an urban community: the Northern Manhattan Stroke Study. *Neurology* 1994; **44**: 626–634.

12 Moroney JT, Bagiella E, Tatemichi TK, Paik MC, Stern Y, Desmond DW. Dementia after stroke increases the risk of long-term stroke recurrence. *Neurology* 1997; **48**: 1317–1325.

13 Hillbom M, Numminen H, Juvela S. Recent heavy drinking of alcohol and embolic stroke. *Stroke* 1999; **30**: 2307–2312.

14 Gonzales MRM, Donderis AC, Sanhauja JJ, Rieger JS. Cardiomyopathy, alcoholism and cerebral embolism. *Rev. Clin. Esp.* 1988; **182**: 79–80.

15 Urbano-Márquez A, Estruch R, Fernández-Solá J, Nicolás JM, Paré JC, Rubin E. The greater risk of alcoholic cardiomyopathy and myopathy in women compared with men. *JAMA* 1995; **274**: 149–154.

16 Lip GYH, Beevers DG, Sing SP, Watson RDS. ABC of atrial fibrillation, etiology, pathophysiology, and clinical features. *BMJ* 1995; **311**: 1425–1428.

17 Thornton JR. Atrial fibrillation in healthy non-alcoholic people after an alcoholic binge. *Lancet* 1984; **2**: 1013–1014.

18 Rosolacci T, Defaux D, Neuville V. Complete arrhythmia, caused by atrial fibrillation, causing ischemic cerebral vascular accident following acute alcoholic intoxication in a young subject. *Presse. Med.* 1995; **24**: 1911.

19 Gras P, Abdoul Karim A, Grosmaire N, Borsotti JP, Giroud M, Blettery B, Dumas R. Multiple brain embolism in acute alcohol intoxication, a clinico-pathological case. *Rev. Neurol.* 1992; **148**: 215–217.

20 Mayfield D, McLeod G, Hall P. The CAGE questionnaire: validation of a new alcoholism screening instrument. *Am. J. Psychiatry* 1974; **131**: 1121–1123.

21 Majamaa K, Turkka J, Kärppä M, Winqvist S, Hassinen IE. The common MELAS mutation A3243G in mitochondrial DNA among young patients with an occipital brain infarct. *Neurology* 1997; **49**: 1331–1334.

22 Hillbom M, Kaste M. Alcohol abuse and brain infarction. *Ann. Med.* 1990; **22**: 347–352.

23 Neiman J. Association of transient ischaemic attack in alcohol withdrawal with changes in haemostasis. *Br. J. Addiction* 1988; **83**: 1457–1459.

24 Reed DM. The paradox of high risk of stroke in populations with low risk of coronary heart disease. *Am. J. Epidemiol.* 1990; **131**: 579–588.

25 Kiechl S, Willeit J, Egger G, Oberhollenzer M, Aichner F. Alcohol consumption and carotid atherosclerosis: evidence of dose-dependent atherogenic and antiatherogenic effects. Results from the Bruneck Study. *Stroke* 1994; **25**: 1593–1598.

26 Hart CL, Smith GD, Hole DJ, Hawthorne VM. Alcohol consumption and mortality from all causes, coronary heart disease, and stroke: results from a prospective cohort study of Scottish men with 21 years of follow up. *BMJ* 1999; **318**: 1725–1729.

27 Hansagi H, Romelsjö A, Gerhardsson de Verdier M, Andréasson S, Leifman A. Alcohol consumption and stroke mortality, a 20-year follow-up of 15,077 men and women. *Stroke* 1995; **26**: 1768–1773.

28 Kauhanen J. Pattern of alcohol drinking and progression of atherosclerosis. *Arterioscler. Thromb. Vasc. Biol.* 1999; **19**: 3001–3006.

29 You R, McNeil JJ, O'Malley HM, Davis SM, Donnan GA. Risk factors for lacunar infarction syndromes. *Neurology* 1995; **45**: 1483–1487.

30 Ferro JM, Crespo M, Ferro H. Role of vascular risk factors in lacunar and unexplained strokes in young adults: a case-control study. *Cerebrovasc. Dis.* 1995; **5**: 188–193.

31 Janssens E, Mounier-Vehier F, Hamon M, Leys D. Small subcortical infarcts and primary subcortical haemorrhages may have different risk factors. *J. Neurol.* 1995; **242**: 425–429.

32 Qureshi AI, Safdar K, Patel M, Janssen RS, Frankel MR. Stroke in young black patients: risk factors, subtypes, and prognosis. *Stroke* 1995; **26**: 1995–1998.

33 You RX, McNeill JJ, O'Malley HM, Davis SM, Thrift AG, Donnan GA. Risk factors for stroke due to cerebral infarction in young adults. *Stroke* 1997; **28**: 1913–1918.

34 Kauma H, Savolainen MJ, Rantala AO, Lilja M, Kervinen K, Reunanen A, Kesäniemi YA. Apolipoprotein E phenotype determines the effect of alcohol on blood pressure in middle-aged men. *Am. J. Hypertens.* 1998; **11**: 1334–1343.

35 O'Donnell HC, Rosand J, Knudsen KA, Furie KL, Segal AZ, Chiu RI, Ikeda D, Greenberg SM. Apolipoprotein E genotype and the risk of recurrent lobar intracerebral hemorrhage. *New Engl. J. Med.* 2000; **342**: 240–245.

36 Altura BM, Altura BT. Association of alcohol in brain injury, headaches, and stroke with brain-tissue and serum levels of ionized magnesium: a review of recent findings and mechanisms of action. *Alcohol* 1999; **19**: 119–130.

37 Hess DC, Sethi KD, Nichols FT. Carotid dissection: a new false localising sign. *J. Neurol. Neurosurg. Psychiatry* 1990; **53**: 804–805.

38 Prendes JL. Cerebral infarction and alcohol. *Lancet* 1979; **1**: 219.

39 Derlon JM, Charbonneau P, Théron J, Houtteville JP, Bazin C. Edematous softening of cerebellar of the young. *Neurochirurgie* 1983; **29**: 423–428.
40 Jockers-Scherubl M, Vogel HP, Marx P. Cerebral infarct caused by compression of the carotid artery in an alcohol intoxicated patient. *Nervenarzt* 1993; **64**: 401–403.
41 Wilkins MR, Kendall MJ. Stroke affecting young men after alcoholic binges. *BMJ* 1985; **291**: 1342.
42 Sangla I, Bille-Turc F, Pouget J, Serratrice G. Ischemic cerebral vascular accident with simultaneous acute alcoholic intoxication in a young subject. *Presse. Med.* 1995; **24**: 827.
43 Palomäki H, Kaste M. Regular light-to-moderate intake of alcohol and the risk of ischemic stroke; is there a beneficial effect? *Stroke* 1993; **24**: 1828–1832.
44 Jamrozik K, Broadhurst RJ, Anderson CS, Stewart-Wynne EG. The role of lifestyle factors in the etiology of stroke, a population-based case-control study in Perth, Western Australia. *Stroke* 1994; **25**: 51–59.
45 Camargo CA, Jr. Case-control and cohort studies of moderate alcohol consumption and stroke. *Clin. Chem. Acta* 1996; **246**: 107–119.
46 Knuiman MW, Vu HTV. Risk factors for stroke mortality in men and women: the Busselton Study. *J. Cardiovascular Risk* 1996; **3**: 447–452.
47 Yuan J-M, Ross RK, Gao Y-T, Henderson BE, Yu MC. Follow up study of moderate alcohol intake and mortality among middle aged men in Shanghai, China. *BMJ* 1997; **314**: 18–23.
48 Berger K, Ajani UA, Kase CS, Gaziano M, Buring JE, Glynn RJ, Hennekens CH. Light-to-moderate alcohol consumption and the risk of stroke among U.S. male physicians. *New Engl. J. Med.* 1999; **341**: 1557–1564.
49 Hillbom M, Juvela S. Alcohol and risk for stroke. In: Zakhari S, Wassef M. (Eds.) *Alcohol and the Cardiovascular System*, Washington DC, National Institute on Alcohol Abuse and Alcoholism, NIAAA Research Monograph No. 31. 1996; 63–83.
50 Wannamethee SG, Shaper AG. Patterns of alcohol intake and risk of stroke in middle-aged British men. *Stroke* 1996; **27**: 1033–1039.
51 Barrett DH, Anda RF, Croft JB, Serdula MK, Lane MJ. The association between alcohol use and health behaviors related to the risk of cardiovascular disease: the South Carolina Cardiovascular Prevention Project. *J. Stud. Alcohol* 1995; **56**: 9–15.

Chapter 8

Alcohol consumption and the risk of stroke: the role of tobacco?

Jaana M. Leppälä

INTRODUCTION

Studies on alcohol and smoking are numerous and the epidemiologic evidence on their effects on cardiovascular diseases is overwhelming. The knowledge of their effects on different subtypes of stroke has cumulated as well, especially during the last decade, but the interaction between alcohol and tobacco with respect to the risk of stroke is mostly unexplored. This is the subject of this chapter.

ALCOHOL CONSUMPTION AND THE RISK OF STROKE

There is plenty of evidence that heavy drinking (>60 g/day) is related to increased risk of both hemorrhagic [1–9] and ischemic strokes [1,3,7,8,10–12]. In contrast, light (≤24 g/day for men and ≤12 g/day for women) and moderate (25–60 g/day for men and 13–48 g/day for women) drinking does not seem to increase and may even decrease the risk of stroke compared with non-drinking [7,13,14]. However, in order to understand the relationship between alcohol and the risk of stroke, one has to separately examine the effects of alcohol on each stroke subtype (i.e., subarachnoid and intracerebral hemorrhage, and cerebral infarction), the dose–response curve most probably differing from one subtype to another. The risk of subarachnoid hemorrhage seems to increase steeply with increasing alcohol consumption [7,15]. The relationship between alcohol and the risk of intracerebral hemorrhage is poorly known but may be U-shaped with lowest risk among light to moderate drinkers [7–9], and that of ischemic stroke appears to be J-shaped, with non-drinkers and heavy drinkers having a higher risk than light drinkers [7,8,15,16].

Alcohol causes many changes in physiological functions which may modify the risk of stroke. It increases blood pressure [17–20] and serum HDL cholesterol levels [7,18,20–26], and there is some evidence that these two factors mediate the effect of alcohol on the risk of stroke [7,15]. Alcohol seems to have a U-shaped association with fibrinogen levels [27], moderate alcohol consumption increases [28] but ethanol intoxication decreases [29] fibrinolytic activity, and immediate heavy alcohol intake decreases platelet aggregation [30] but, in binge drinkers and alcoholics, platelet aggregation is increased after alcohol withdrawal [30,31]. Cerebral blood flow is increased immediately after alcohol intake [32]. In addition, ethanol has both anti- [33] and pro-oxidant activity [34], but it has been speculated that constituents other than alcohol (e.g., flavonoids and hydroxystilbenes) might influence the development of atherosclerosis [34,35]. Alcohol also interferes with glucose metabolism, moderate alcohol consumption being associated with a decreased risk of diabetes [36]. Alcohol seems to increase insulin sensitivity and glucose tolerance [26], even though alcoholics are usually resistant to insulin [18,26].

CIGARETTE SMOKING AND THE RISK OF STROKE

Heavy smoking (>20 cigarettes/day) increases both the incidence [37–41] and mortality from stroke [40,41]. Cigarette smoking is a major modifiable risk factor for subarachnoid hemorrhage [42–48]. In contrast, evidence concerning the role of tobacco in the risk of intracerebral hemorrhage is still controversial, yet it appears that heavy, but not light-to-moderate cigarette smoking, increases the risk [9,38,49,50]. Smoking is dose-dependantly associated with the risk of ischemic stroke [38,46]. Cessation of smoking reduces stroke risk [37,39], with major reduction within 2–5 years after cessation [37,39,46], indicating that part of the effects of smoking is reversible. The risk of stroke seems to return to the level of never-smokers in light smokers, but heavy smokers seem to retain an increased risk even though also they benefit from cessation [37].

There are several mechanisms by which smoking may cause stroke. Cigarette smoking causes an immediate, yet reversible increases in blood pressure [42,51–55] and cerebral blood flow [56]. In epidemiologic studies, however, it has consistently been associated with reduced blood pressure in normotensive people [18,52,57–60], although blood pressure has been elevated in diabetic [61] and hypertensive smokers [62], and cerebral blood flow has been decreased in chronic smokers [40] compared with respective nonsmokers. It is not plausible that smoking decreases blood pressure, but smokers may initially have lower blood pressure than those who remain nonsmokers [63]. They may also have a reduced 'white coat effect', which would lead to artificially low measurements of blood pressure in clinics [59]. There is no evidence that smoking causes hypertension, but in heavy smokers the rise in blood pressure may persist during waking hours because of frequent smoking factually causing a hypertensive state [55]. Even though smoking may not be causally related to hypertension, it clearly modifies the effect of hypertension on stroke [40,51] and other cardiovascular risks [64] which are much higher in hypertensive than normotensive smokers.

Cigarette smoking is associated with reduced levels of serum HDL cholesterol [18,20,51,57, 58,60,65,66] and increased levels of serum triglycerides [18,57,65–67]. It increases platelet activity [51,53,68,69], plasma fibrinogen levels [27,51,57], hematocrit [57,65], and blood viscosity [57]. It is also associated with endothelial dysfunction [57,70,71]. Cigarette smoking increases the risks of carotid stenosis [72,73] and diabetes [36], which both are risk factors for ischemic stroke.

Tobacco smoke has over 4000 compounds, the effects of which are mostly unknown [51]. Many of the effects of smoking are attributed to nicotine, which increases systolic and diastolic blood pressure and heart rate in a dose–response manner [74,75]. Despite these hemodynamic effects, nicotine does not appear to enhance thrombosis [75,76], and the mechanism by which smoking is related to thrombogenesis is unclear. Besides nicotine, carbonmonoxide is a potential mediator of the effects of tobacco smoke on cardiovascular diseases [51,77]. It may injure the vascular endothelium [77] and thus promote atherogenesis. The causal role of smoking in the development of atherosclerosis is plausible but so far unproven.

THE EFFECT MODIFICATION OF ALCOHOL BY SMOKING

There are only two epidemiologic studies on the effect modification of alcohol by smoking and neither of them examines it in relation to the risk of stroke. In a Japanese cohort of 19,231 men, alcohol consumption and all-cause mortality had a J-shaped association in nonsmokers but not in smokers [78]. In a cross-sectional study of 5,312 German men and women, the rise in blood pressure associated with drinking was higher in smokers than in nonsmokers [79]. Some studies have instead examined the effect modification of smoking by alcohol. In a cohort of 22,071 US male physicians, alcohol attenuated the linear effect of smoking on the risk of total stroke [38]. In a Japanese cohort of 1,775 men, a dose-dependent decrease in diastolic blood pressure and serum HDL cholesterol by increasing cigarette smoking was evident in nondrinkers but not in drinkers [67].

The effects of both alcohol and tobacco are manifold, which makes them complicated to examine and understand. The effects may be additive or synergistic, or counteract each other either directly via the same mechanisms or indirectly influencing the same phenomena but through different mechanisms. Both alcohol intake and cigarette smoking increase blood pressure [17–20,42,51–55], even though the relationship between smoking and hypertension is controversial [18,52,55,57–62]. Alcohol consumption increases serum HDL cholesterol [17,18,20–26] whereas cigarette smoking has been consistently associated with reduced levels of HDL cholesterol [18,20,51,57,58,60,65,66]. Alcohol decreases platelet activity and fibrinogen levels and increases fibrinolysis [27,30], whereas smoking increases platelet aggregability and fibrinogen levels [27,51,53,57,68,69]. It is very plausible that smoking substantially modifies the effects of drinking on stroke risk, but it remains to be studied what the actual net effects of all these physiological mechanisms involved are and how smoking modifies the dose–response relationships between alcohol and each stroke subtype.

METHODOLOGICAL PROBLEMS IN STUDIES ON ALCOHOL AND TOBACCO

Studies on interactions between alcohol and tobacco are most challenging, not only because of the complexity of the effects of either factor, but also because of many inherent methodological problems. Epidemiologic studies on alcohol and tobacco are prone to imprecision in measurements and various biases, their interactions thus being even harder to evaluate in a reliable and valid manner. Alcohol consumption and smoking are usually self-reported and the measurement of either habit is susceptible to both recall and response bias. The reporting of alcohol use especially tends to be differential, heavy drinkers more likely reporting themselves as moderate-to-light drinkers than nondrinkers [24]. Differential misclassification is likely to lead to biased estimates of relative risks, and the amount and direction of such bias is hard to evaluate. Furthermore, the classification of alcohol intake and cigarette smoking, and the selection of respective reference categories (e.g., current nondrinkers vs. never-drinkers, and current nonsmokers vs. never-smokers) influence the risk ratios and, consequently, the interpretations of study results. Different category boundaries make it difficult to compare studies with each other and drawing uniform conclusions becomes unsubstantial. Alcohol and tobacco have both immediate and cumulative effects, the assessment and differentiation of which may be difficult or even impossible. This is reflected in the use of composite indices such as pack-years of smoking, such indices being appealing to use but causing considerable problems in the causal interpretation of results. There is no consensus on the most preferable way to simultaneously take into account both current use and the duration of habit.

CONCLUSIONS

Alcohol consumption and cigarette smoking are both independent risk factors for stroke, and their effects seem to vary by stroke subtype, the average daily amount of drinking and smoking, and duration of habit. It is likely that smoking modifies the effects of alcohol on the risk of stroke, depending on both stroke subtype and the relative role of each factor in the occurrence of subtype in question. However, there are no studies that have specifically examined this interaction and the risk of stroke, even though some studies have addressed this issue with respect to some other cardiovascular diseases. This multi-faceted relationship between alcohol and smoking clearly needs more research.

REFERENCES

1 Donahue RP, Abbott RD, Reed DM, Yano K. Alcohol and hemorrhagic stroke. The Honolulu Heart Program. *JAMA* 1986; **255**: 2311–2314.

2 Monforte R, Estruch R, Graus F, Nicolas JM, Urbano-Marquez A. High ethanol consumption as risk factor for intracerebral hemorrhage in young and middle-aged people. *Stroke* 1990; **21**: 1529–1532.

3 Gill JS, Shipley MJ, Tsementzis SA, Hornby RS, Gill SK, Hitchcock ER, Beevers DG. Alcohol consumption – a risk factor for hemorrhagic and non-hemorrhagic stroke. *Am. J. Med.* 1991; **90**: 489–497.

4 Longstreth WT Jr, Nelson LM, Koepsell TD, van Belle G. Cigarette smoking, alcohol use, and subarachnoid hemorrhage. *Stroke* 1992; **23**: 1242–1249.

5 Juvela S, Hillbom M, Numminen H, Koskinen P. Cigarette smoking and alcohol consumption as risk factors for aneurysmal subarachnoid hemorrhage. *Stroke* 1993; **24**: 639–646.

6 Juvela S, Hillbom M, Palomäki H. Risk factors for spontaneous intracerebral hemorrhage. *Stroke* 1995; **26**: 1558–1564.

7 Leppälä JM, Paunio M, Virtamo J, Fogelholm R, Albanes D, Taylor PR, Heinonen OP. Alcohol consumption and stroke incidence in male smokers. *Circulation* 1999; **100**: 1209–1214.

8 Caicoya M, Rodriguez T, Corrales C, Cuello R, Lasheras C. Alcohol and stroke: A community case-control study in Asturias, Spain. *J. Clin. Epidemiol.* 1999; **52**(7): 677–684.

9 Thrift AG, Donnan GA, McNeil JJ. Heavy drinking, but not moderate or intermediate drinking, increases the risk of intracerebral hemorrhage. *Epidemiology* 1999; **10**: 307–312.

10 Gorelick PB, Rodin MB, Langenberg P, Hier DB, Costigan J. Weekly alcohol consumption, cigarette smoking, and the risk of ischemic stroke: Results of a case-control study at three urban medical centers in Chicago, Illinois. *Neurology* 1989; **39**: 339–343.

11 Palomäki H, Kaste M. Regular light-to-moderate intake of alcohol and the risk of ischemic stroke. Is there a beneficial effect? *Stroke* 1993; **24**: 1828–1832.

12 Numminen H, Hillbom M, Juvela S. Platelets, alcohol consumption, and onset of brain infarction. *J. Neurol. Neurosurg. Psychiatry* 1996; **61**: 376–380.

13 Camargo CA Jr. Case-control and cohort studies of moderate alcohol consumption and stroke. *Clin. Chim. Acta* 1996; **246**: 107–119.

14 Berger K, Ajani UA, Kase CS, Gaziano JM, Buring JE, Glynn RJ, Hennekens CH. Light-to-moderate alcohol consumption and the risk of stroke among U.S. male physicians. *N. Engl. J. Med.* 1999; **341**(21): 1557–1564.

15 Camargo CA Jr. Moderate alcohol consumption and stroke. The epidemiologic evidence. *Stroke* 1989; **20**: 1611–1626.

16 Sacco RL, Elkind M, Boden-Albala B, Lin IF, Kargman DE, Hauser WA, Shea S, Paik MC. The protective effect of moderate alcohol consumption on ischemic stroke. *JAMA* 1999; **281**(1): 53–60.

17 Klatsky AL. Alcohol and hypertension. *Clin. Chim. Acta* 1996; **246**: 91–105.

18 Lee KS, Park CY, Meng KH, Bush A, Lee SH, Lee WC, Koo IW, Chung CK. The association of cigarette smoking and alcohol consumption with other cardiovascular risk factors in men from Seoul, Korea. *Ann. Epidemiol.* 1998; **8**: 31–38.

19 Beilin LJ, Puddey IB, Burke V. Alcohol and hypertension: Kill or cure? *J. Human Hyperten.* 1996; **10**(Suppl. 2): S1–S5.

20 Godsland IF, Leyva F, Walton C, Worthington M, Stevenson JC. Associations of smoking, alcohol and physical activity with risk factors for coronary heart disease and diabetes in the first follow-up cohort of the Heart Disease and Diabetes Risk Indicators in a Screened Cohort study (HDDRISC-1). *J. Intern. Med.* 1998; **244**: 33–41.

21 Suh I, Shaten BJ, Cutler JA, Kuller LH. Alcohol use and mortality from coronary heart disease: The role of high-density lipoprotein cholesterol. *Ann. Intern. Med.* 1992; **116**: 881–887.

22 Gaziano JM, Buring JE, Breslow JL, Goldhaber SZ, Rosner B, VanDenburgh M, Willett W, Hennekens CH. Moderate alcohol intake, increased levels of high-density lipoprotein and its subfractions, and decreased risk of myocardial infarction. *N. Engl. J. Med.* 1993; **329**: 1829–1834.

23 Linn S, Carroll M, Johnson C, Fulwood R, Kalsbeek W, Briefel R. High-density lipoprotein cholesterol and alcohol consumption in US white and black adults: Data from NHANES II. *Am. J. Public Health* 1993; **83**: 811–816.

24 Paunio M, Heinonen OP, Virtamo J, Klag MJ, Manninen V, Albanes D, Comstock GW. HDL cholesterol and mortality in Finnish men with special reference to alcohol intake. *Circulation* 1994; **90**: 2909–2918.

25 Kannel WB, Ellison RC. Alcohol and coronary heart disease: The evidence for a protective effect. *Clin. Chim. Acta* 1996; **246**: 59–76.

26 Eagles CJ, Martin U. Non-pharmacological modification of cardiac risk factors: Part 3: Smoking cessation and alcohol consumption. *J. Clin. Pharm. Therap.* 1998; **23**: 1–9.

27 Krobot K, Hense HW, Cremer P, Eberle E, Keil U. Determinants of plasma fibrinogen: Relation to body weight, waist-to-hip ratio, smoking, alcohol, age, and sex. *Arterioscler. Thromb.* 1992; **12**(7): 780–788.

28 Hendriks HFJ, Veenstra J, Velthuis-te Wierik EJM, Schaafsma G, Kluft C. Effect of moderate dose of alcohol with evening meal on fibrinolytic factors. *BMJ* 1994; **308**: 1003–1006.

29 Hillbom M, Kaste M, Rasi V. Can ethanol intoxication affect hemocoagulation to increase the risk of brain infarction in young adults? *Neurology* 1983; **33**: 381–384.

30 Renaud SC, Ruf JC. Effects of alcohol on platelet functions. *Clin. Chim. Acta* 1996; **246**: 77–89.

31 Hillbom M, Kangasaho M, Kaste M, Numminen H, Vapaatalo H. Acute ethanol ingestion increases platelet reactivity: Is there a relationship to stroke? *Stroke* 1985; **16**: 19–23.

32 Mathew RJ, Wilson WH. Regional cerebral blood flow changes associated with ethanol intoxication. *Stroke* 1986; **17**: 1156–1159.

33 Trevithick CC, Vinson JA, Caulfeild J, Rahman F, Derksen T, Bocksch L, Hong S, Stefan A, Teufel K, Wu N, Hirst M, Trevithick JR. Is ethanol an important antioxidant in alcoholic beverages associated with risk reduction of cataract and atherosclerosis? *Redox. Report* 1999; **4**(3): 89–93.

34 Puddey IB, Croft KD. Alcohol, stroke and coronary heart disease: Are there anti-oxidants and pro-oxidants that might influence the development of atherosclerotic cardiovascular disease? *Neuroepidemiology* 1999; **18**: 292–302.

35 Goldberg DM, Soleas GJ, Levesque M. Moderate alcohol consumption: The gentle face of Janus. *Clin. Biochem.* 1999; **32**(7): 505–518.

36 Rimm EB, Chan J, Stampfer MJ, Colditz GA, Willett WC. Prospective study of cigarette smoking, alcohol use, and the risk of diabetes in men. *BMJ* 1995; **310**: 555–559.

37 Wannamethee SG, Shaper AG, Whincup PH, Walker M. Smoking cessation and the risk of stroke in middle-aged men. *JAMA* 1995; **274**: 155–160.

38 Robbins AS, Manson JE, Lee IM, Satterfield S, Hennekens CH. Cigarette smoking and stroke in a cohort of U.S. male physicians. *Ann. Intern Med.* 1994; **120**: 458–462.

39 Kawachi I, Colditz A, Stampfer MJ, Willett WC, Manson JE, Rosner B, Speizer FE, Hennekens CH. Smoking cessation and decreased risk of stroke in women. *JAMA* 1993; **269**(2): 232–236.

40 Higa M, Davanipour Z. Smoking and stroke. *Neuroepidemiology* 1991; **10**: 211–222.

41 Lund Håheim L, Holme I, Hjermann I, Leren P. Smoking habits and risk of fatal stroke: 18 years follow up of the Oslo study. *J. Epidemiol. Comm. Health* 1996; **50**: 621–624.

42 Longstreth WT Jr, Koepsell TD, Yerby MS, van Belle G. Risk factors for subarachnoid hemorrhage. *Stroke* 1985; **16**(3): 377–385.

43 Fogelholm R, Murros K. Cigarette smoking and subarachnoid haemorrhage: A population-based case-control study. *J. Neurol. Neurosurg. Psychiatry* 1987; **50**: 78–80.

44 Knekt P, Reunanen A, Aho K, Heliövaara M, Rissanen A, Aromaa A, Impivaara O. Risk factors for subarachnoid hemorrhage in a longitudinal population study. *J. Clin. Epidemiol.* 1991; **44**(9): 933–939.

45 Teunissen LL, Rinkel GJE, Algra A, van Gijn J. Risk factors for subarachnoid hemorrhage: A systematic review. *Stroke* 1996; **27**(3): 544–549.

46 Sacco RL. Risk factors, outcomes, and stroke subtypes for ischemic stroke. *Neurology* 1997; **49** (Suppl. 4): S39–S44.

47 Weir BKA, Kongable GL, Kassell NF, Schultz JR, Truskowski LL, Sigrest A, and the Investigators. Cigarette smoking as a cause of aneurysmal subarachnoid hemorrhage and risk for vasospasm: A report of the Cooperative Aneurysm Study. *J. Neurosurg.* 1998; **89**: 405–411.

48 Morris KM, Shaw MDM, Foy PM. Smoking and subarachnoid haemorrhage: A case control study. *Br. J. Neurosurg.* 1992; **6**: 429–432.

49 Fogelholm R, Murros K. Cigarette smoking and risk of primary intracerebral haemorrhage: A population-based case-control study. *Acta Neurol. Scand.* 1993; **87**: 367–370.

50 Thrift AG, Donnan GA, McNeil JJ. Epidemiology of intracerebral hemorrhage. *Epidemiol. Rev.* 1995; **17**(2): 361–381.

51 Rigotti NA, Pasternak RC. Cigarette smoking and coronary heart disease. *Cardiol. Clin.* 1996; **14**(1): 51–68.

52 Omvik P. How smoking affects blood pressure. *Blood Pressure* 1996; **5**: 71–77.

53 Sleight P. Smoking and hypertension. *Clin. Experim. Hyperten.* 1993; **15**(6): 1181–1192.

54 Hashimoto H. Enhanced elevation of blood pressure during cigarette smoking in the elderly. *Jpn. Circ. J.* 1993; **57**: 955–959.

55 Groppelli A, Giorgi DMA, Omboni S, Parati G, Mancia G. Persistent blood pressure increase induced by heavy smoking. *J. Hyperten.* 1992; **10**: 495–499.

56 Morioka C, Kondo H, Akashi K, Matsumura K, Ochi N, Makinaga G, Furukawa T. The continuous and simultaneous blood flow velocity measurement of four cerebral vessels and a peripheral vessel during cigarette smoking. *Psychopharmacology* 1997; **131**: 220–229.

57 Price JF, Mowbray PI, Lee AJ, Rumley A, Lowe GDO, Fowkes FGR. Relationship between smoking and cardiovascular risk factors in the development of peripheral arterial disease and coronary artery disease: Edinburgh Artery Study. *Eur. Heart J.* 1999; **20**: 344–353.

58 Hughes K, Leong WP, Spothy SP, Lun KC, Yeo PPB. Relationships between cigarette smoking, blood pressure and serum lipids in the Singapore general population. *Int. J. Epidemiol.* 1993; **22**(4): 637–643.

59 Mikkelsen KL, Wiinberg N, Høegholm A, Christensen HR, Bang LE, Nielsen PE, Svendsen TL, Kampmann JP, Madsen NH, Bentzon MW. Smoking related to 24-h ambulatory blood pressure and heart rate: A study in 352 normotensive Danish subjects. Am. J. Hyperten. 1997; 10: 483–491.

60 Imamura H, Tanaka K, Hirae C, Futagami T, Yoshimura Y, Uchida K, Tanaka A, Kobata D. Relationship of cigarette smoking to blood pressure and serum lipids and lipoproteins in men. Clin. Experim. Pharmacol. Physiol. 1996; 23: 397–402.

61 Poulsen PL, Ebbehøj E, Hansen KW, Mogensen CE. Effects of smoking on 24-h ambulatory blood pressure and autonomic function in normoalbuminuric insulin-dependent diabetes mellitus patients. Am. J. Hyperten. 1998; 11: 1093–1099.

62 Verdecchia P, Schillaci G, Borgioni C, Ciucci A, Zampi I, Battistelli M, Gattobigio R, Sacchi N, Porcellati C. Cigarette smoking, ambulatory blood pressure and cardiac hypertrophy in essential hypertension. J. Hyperten. 1995; 13: 1209–1215.

63 Charlton A, While D. Blood pressure and smoking: Observations on a national cohort. Arch. Dis. Child 1995; 73: 294–297.

64 Beilin LJ. Lifestyle and hypertension: An overview. Clin. Experim. Hyperten. (New York) 1999; 21(5–6): 749–762.

65 Vriz O, Nesbitt S, Krause L, Majahalme S, Lu H, Julius S. Smoking is associated with higher cardiovascular risk in young women than in men: The Tecumseh Blood Pressure Study. J. Hyperten. 1997; 15: 127–134.

66 Connelly PW, Petrasovits A, Stachenko S, MacLean DR, Little JA, Chockalingam A. Prevalence of high plasma triglycerids combined with low HDL-C levels and its association with smoking, hypertension, obesity, diabetes, sedentariness and LDL-C levels in the Canadian population. Can. J. Cardiol. 1999; 15(4): 428–433.

67 Handa K, Tanaka H, Shindo M, Kono S, Sasaki J, Arakawa K. Relationship of cigarette smoking to blood pressure and serum lipids. Atherosclerosis 1990; 84: 189–193.

68 Rångemark C, Benthin G, Granström EF, Persson L, Winell S, Wennmalm Å. Tobacco use and urinary excretion of thromboxane A_2 and prostacyclin metabolites in women stratified by age. Circulation 1992; 86: 1495–1500.

69 Gleerup G, Winther K. Smoking further increases platelet activity in patients with mild hypertension. Eur. J. Clin. Invest. 1996; 26: 49–52.

70 Drexler H, Hornig B. Endothelial dysfunction: A novel therapeutic target: Endothelial dysfunction in human disease. J. Mol. Cell. Cardiol. 1999; 31: 51–60.

71 Pepine CJ. Clinical implications of endothelial dysfunction. Clin. Cardiol. 1998; 21(11): 795–799.

72 Mast H, Thompson JLP, Lin IF, Hofmeister C, Hartmann A, Marx P, Mohr JP, Sacco RL. Cigarette smoking as a determinant of high-grade carotid artery stenosis in Hispanic, black, and white patients with stroke or transient ischemic attack. Stroke 1998; 29: 908–912.

73 Wilson PWF, Hoeg JM, D'Agostino RB, Silbershatz H, Belanger AM, Poehlmann H, O'Leary D, Wolf PA. Cumulative effects of high cholesterol levels, high blood pressure, and cigarette smoking on carotid stenosis. New Engl. J. Med. 1997; 337: 516–522.

74 Netter P, Müller MJ, Neumann A, Kamradik B. The influence of nicotine on performance, mood, and physiological parameters as related to smoking habit, gender, and suggestibility. Clin. Investig. 1994; 72: 512–518.

75 Benowitz NL. The role of nicotine in smoking-related cardiovascular disease. Prev. Med. 1997; 26: 412–417.

76 Blann AD, Steele C, McCollum CN. The influence of smoking and of oral and transdermal nicotine on blood pressure, and haematology and coagulation indices. Thromb. Haemost. 1997; 78(3): 1093–1096.

77 Kochar MS, Bindra RS. The additive effects of smoking and hypertension: More reasons to help your patients kick the habit. Postgrad. Med. 1996; 100(5): 147–160.

78 Tsugane S, Fahey MT, Sasaki S, Baba S, for the JPHC Study Group. Alcohol consumption and all-cause and cancer mortality among middle-aged Japanese men: Seven-year follow-up of the JPHC Study Cohort I. *Am. J. Epidemiol.* 1999; **150**(11): 1201–1207.
79 Keil U, Chambless L, Filipiak B, Härtel U. Alcohol and blood pressure and its interaction with smoking and other behavioural variables: Results from the MONICA Augsburg Survey 1984–1985. *J. Hyperten.* 1991; **9**: 491–498.

Chapter 9

Alcohol, vascular cells and hemodynamic forces

Eileen M. Redmond and Paul A. Cahill

INTRODUCTION

Over the past two decades important influences of ethanol on the cardiovascular system have been recognized. Several epidemiological studies have demonstrated a consistent dose–response relationship between increasing alcohol consumption and decreasing incidence of coronary heart disease, despite an increase in mortality due to a number of other diseases [1–3]. More recently, *in vivo* animal studies have demonstrated an inhibitory effect of ethanol on neointimal formation following balloon injury [4,5]. These observations have prompted further investigation into the direct effect of ethanol on vascular endothelial and smooth muscle cell function. *In vivo*, cells of the blood vessel wall are continuously subjected to hemodynamic forces due to flowing blood that are now recognized as eliciting critical biologic responses that result in modulation of vessel function and structure [6–8]. Thus, it is important to consider these forces in any study of ethanol and vascular cells. The object of this chapter is to focus on some key functions of vascular cells that are modulated by hemodynamic forces (e.g., endothelial nitric oxide production; smooth muscle cell migration and proliferation), and how ethanol has been reported to affect these responses.

MECHANICAL FORCES AND VASCULAR CELLS

In vivo, cells of the blood vessel wall are continuously subjected to mechanical forces associated with blood flow. These hemodynamic forces can be resolved into two components; shear stress, the tangential frictional force acting at the endothelial cell surface, and pressure-stretch acting perpendicular to the vascular wall. In the arterial circulation, where blood flow is pulsatile, the endothelial cell is the recipient of most of the shear stress, whereas both the endothelial and smooth muscle cells, together with the underlying matrix, are subjected to stretch (cyclic strain) [6–8]. It is now recognized that hemodynamic forces directly influence vascular cell biology and play an important role in the acute control of vascular tone, vascular remodeling and the focal development of atherosclerotic lesions [6–8]. A large number of studies have verified the hypothesis that mechanical stresses and strains contribute to the development of vascular diseases. It has been demonstrated that increased tensile stress and strain due to hypertension may induce and/or facilitate vascular hypertrophy, whereas oscillatory low fluid shear stress and/or altered shear gradients due to eddy blood flow (typically near branches, bifurcations, regions of arterial narrowings and curvature) may initiate or promote focal atherosclerosis and intimal hyperplasia [9]. In most large-size vessels, one can estimate the magnitude of the fluid shear stress (τ), $\tau = 4\mu Q/\pi r^3$ (Hagen-Poiseuille law), as being proportional to viscosity (μ) and flow rate (Q) and inversely proportional to the third power of the internal vessel radius (r). This relation highlights the fact that relatively small decreases in vessel diameter at constant flow can markedly increase shear stress at the endothelial surface.

SHEAR STRESS AND ENDOTHELIAL CELLS

The endothelium occupies a strategic location and acts as an interface between the blood stream and the vessel wall. Because of this location, fluid shear stress is one of the most important mechanical forces acting upon vascular endothelium. Shear stress can influence a variety of endothelial cell functions including the production of vasoactive mediators, activation of transcriptional regulatory factors, and the expression of cellular adhesion molecules [6,10,11]. The molecular mechanism(s) responsible for transduction of shear stimuli and the relevant intracellular signalling pathways in endothelium are not fully defined, but likely involve the activation of integrins, guanine nucleotide-binding proteins (G-proteins) and cascades of protein kinases [10,11].

It is now well established that endothelial cells respond to increases in flow by modulating their release of vasoactive agents such as the vasorelaxants nitric oxide (NO) and prostacyclin (PGI_2), and the vasoconstrictor endothelin (Figure 9.1). Indeed, shear stress is thought to be the premiere physiological stimulus for NO [10]. Nitric oxide is synthesized

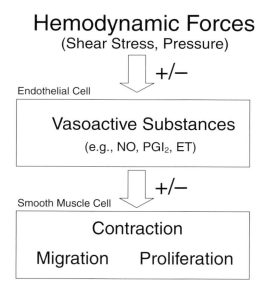

Figure 9.1 Hemodynamic forces directly influence vascular cell biology. Fluid shear stress and/or pressure (cyclic stretch) can modulate the production of vasoactive mediators such as nitric oxide (NO), prostacyclin (PGI_2) and endothelin (ET) from the endothelium, which in turn influence smooth muscle cell structure and function.

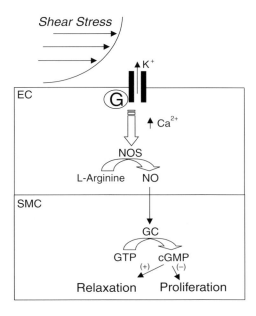

Figure 9.2 Shear stress stimulates nitric oxide (NO) production by endothelial cells. By a mechanism thought to involve a pertussis toxin-sensitive G protein (G) and a K^+ channel, shear stress stimulates nitric oxide synthase (NOS) activity in endothelial cells. The resulting NO can stimulate soluble guanylyl cyclase (GC) in adjacent smooth muscle cells, leading to increased levels of cGMP and subsequent vasorelaxation and inhibition of proliferation.

by the heme-containing enzyme nitric oxide synthase (NOS) from L-arginine in a reaction that produces stoichiometric amounts of L-citrulline [12]. Three isoforms of NOS have been identified by gene cloning. Two are constitutively expressed and one, the inducible NOS (iNOS) is produced *de novo* in response to inflammatory cytokines [12]. Activation of NOS and release of NO results in stimulation of a soluble guanylyl cyclase leading to a profound increase in intracellular cGMP levels within most target cells [12] (Figure 9.2). NO is a multifunctional molecule and plays a pivotal role in regulating blood flow by inhibiting smooth muscle contraction as well as platelet aggregation and adhesion [12]. In addition, NO has been shown to inhibit vascular smooth muscle cell proliferation [13,14]. G-proteins function as transducers of signals across the cell membrane by coupling diverse receptors to effectors and thus play a central role in signal transduction and cell biology [15,16]. Recent evidence suggests that both inhibitory G-proteins (Giα1,2,3), which are pertussis toxin sensitive, and Gαq may play a role in both agonist- and shear stress-induced activation of constitutive NOS (eNOS) in EC [17,18]. Stimulation of these G-proteins triggers a number of signal transduction cascades, including activation of K^+ channels, phospholipase C, phospholipase A_2, protein kinase C and adenylyl cyclase. Interestingly, specific interaction of ethanol with these signal transduction pathways has been reported in several cell types; in particular, ethanol-induced changes in the expression of G-proteins coupled to adenylyl cyclase [19] and phospholipase C [20].

EFFECT OF ETHANOL ON BASAL AND FLOW-INDUCED NO

Previous studies, the majority in the central nervous system looking at iNOS, have provided data to support a specific interaction between ethanol and the NOS/NO axis. Chen and LaBella demonstrated that alcohol noncompetitively inhibited rat brain NOS activity [21]. Ethanol treatment blocked LPS-mediated induction of iNOS gene expression in the lung [22] while in cultured vascular smooth muscle cells ethanol potentiated interleukin-1β-stimulated iNOS expression [23]. More recently, investigators have examined the direct effect of ethanol on eNOS in cultured endothelial cells. An ethanol enhancement of the NOS response to agonists such as bradykinin has been reported in bovine pulmonary artery endothelial cells [24]. In another study, the ethanol augmentation of NO production was associated with increased eNOS protein and mRNA expression [25].

Because fluid shear stress is such an extremely important physiological pathway for eNOS activation [6], the effect of ethanol on flow-stimulated NOS has been investigated. In a series of *in vitro* experiments, Hendrickson *et al.* demonstrated that cultured endothelial cells exposed to either steady laminar flow or pulsatile flow exhibited a flow- and time-dependent increase in eNOS activity [26]. Ethanol significantly enhanced basal and flow-induced eNOS activity. The enhanced eNOS activity was independent of a change in eNOS or iNOS protein expression but was dependent on activation of an inhibitory guanine nucleotide binding protein (Gi protein) inasmuch as ethanol treatment increased pertussis-catalyzed ribosylation of Giα substrates and pertussis toxin pretreatment inhibited eNOS activity in static and flow-stimulated cells after ethanol treatment [26]. However, ethanol did not alter G protein (Giα3, Giα1–2, Gαq) expression in these cells [26]. These data suggest an important role for ethanol-induced potentiation of shear stress-stimulated eNOS activity *in vitro*. They further invite speculation that the beneficial effects of ethanol consumption on vascular function are mediated, at least in part, by ethanol-induced stimulation of eNOS activity. Moreover, the augmentation of shear stress-induced eNOS activity by ethanol represents a potential mechanism whereby the protective effects of NO-mediated inhibition of vascular smooth muscle cell proliferation [27] and migration [28] are potentiated. Further *in vivo* experiments using specific eNOS inhibitors will be required to elucidate the importance of these mechanisms.

EFFECT OF ETHANOL ON PROSTACYCLIN

The effects of ethanol on PGI_2, another endothelium-derived vasodilator and potent inhibitor of platelet aggregation, have also been investigated. Ethanol increased PGI_2 production in cultured human umbilical vein endothelial cells and elevated plasma levels of PGI_2 in volunteers administered ethanol [29]. Guivernau *et al.* found that while ethanol did not affect vascular PGI_2 release in control rats, in aortas from alcohol-fed animals ethanol stimulated PGI_2 production [30]. These data imply that this response to ethanol may be altered by chronic alcohol consumption. In any case, ethanol's modulatory effect on endothelial PGI_2 production could also contribute to its cardiovascular protective effects *in vivo*. As in the case of NO, fluid shear stress is an important physiological stimulus for enhanced cyclooxygenase activity and subsequent PGI_2 release by endothelial cells [10]. Moreover, agonist and shear stress induced PGI_2 release is dependent on activation of an inhibitory guanine nucleotide binding protein (Giα protein) inasmuch as pertussis-catalyzed ribosylation of Giα substrates inhibits PGI_2 release in static and flow-stimulated cells [31]. Since ethanol increases endothelial Giα functionality in cultured endothelial cells [26], and since PGI_2 release is shear stress-dependent, it is tempting to speculate that ethanol may modulate shear stress induced activation of endothelial PGI_2 release via activation of a pertussis toxin sensitive Giα protein. It would therefore be of interest to determine the specific effect of ethanol on flow-induced cyclooxygenase activity and PGI_2 production in endothelial cells. Of note, ethanol has been shown to increase cyclo-oxygenase-2 expression in both brain and uterine tissues [32].

VASCULAR SMOOTH MUSCLE CELL (SMC) PROLIFERATION AND MIGRATION

Arterial SMC migration and proliferation are two distinct processes that play an important role in the pathogenesis of atherosclerosis as well as in the normal development of blood vessels and the arterial response to injury (for review see [13,14]). In addition, accelerated SMC proliferation and migration leading to neointimal formation is a characteristic feature in arteries of hypertensive patients and animals [33,34]. An ethanol-induced reduction in neointimal formation following balloon injury has been reported in both rabbit and pig models [4,5]. This inhibition of intimal hyperplasia was observed following either local delivery of ethanol or alcohol feeding [4,5]. The preservation of arterial lumen diameter was achieved by decreasing neointimal proliferation in part by decreasing LDL oxidation in these animals [4]. However, the primary pathogenesis of neointimal formation is SMC migration, proliferation and extracellular matrix production and these are therefore likely targets for ethanol in inhibiting neo-intimal formation.

ETHANOL AND VASCULAR SMOOTH MUSCLE CELL MIGRATION

The accumulation of SMC in the intima of arteries is one of the most prominent features of the atherosclerotic plaque and of the intimal hyperplastic lesions which cause restenosis following angioplasty [35,36]. It is increasingly recognized that migration of SMC from the media is a key event in progressive intimal thickening leading to atherosclerosis and restenosis [35–37]. Consequently, there has been extensive interest in defining both positive and negative regulators of this process and many factors have been identified that may play a role. While ethanol has been shown *in vitro* to differentially influence the migration of neuronal cells [38] and melanoma cells [39], its effect on SMC migration has not been defined until recently.

The fibrinolytic plasminogen activator system (Figure 9.3) has been hypothesized to play an important role in intimal thickening after various types of vascular injury [40]. The inactive proenzyme plasminogen is activated to the proteolytic enzyme plasmin by two plasminogen activators, tissue-type plasminogen activator (tPA) and urokinase-type plasminogen activator (uPA). The system is regulated by a series of plasminogen activator inhibitors, the most import-ant of which is thought to be plasminogen activator inhibitor type-1 (PAI-1). Several groups have reported the involvement of the fibrinolytic plasminogen system in SMC migration.

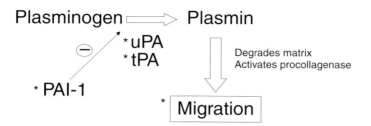

Figure 9.3 The fibrinolytic plasminogen activator system. The inactive proenzyme plasminogen is converted to the proteolytic enzyme plasmin by urokinase-type plasminogen activator (uPA) or tissue-type plasminogen activator (tPA). The system is regulated by a series of plasminogen activator inhibitors (PAI), of which PAI-1 is believed to be the most physiologically important. (* modulated by hemodynamic forces).

Clowes *et al.* have demonstrated that neointimal thickening post-vascular injury is associated with upregulation of both uPA and tPA [40]. Carmeliet *et al.* demonstrated that uPA null mice do not exhibit exuberant thickening of the intima after vascular injury [41]. PAI-1 has been shown to inhibit SMC migration [42] and inactivation of the PAI-1 gene results in abundant neointimal thickening [43]. Recently, it has been demonstrated that pulse pressure due to pulsatile flow increases SMC migration *in vitro* via uPA- and metalloproteinase (MMP)-dependent mechanisms [44]. Indeed, uPA gene deletion resulted in blunting of pressure-induced SMC migration despite the endogenous upregulation of MMP [44]. A role for the endothelium in protecting the underlying smooth muscle from hemodynamic forces and in playing a pivotal role in hemodynamic force-induced remodelling is underscored by the finding that endothelial cells prevented flow-induced SMC migration [44,45]. It appears that, at least *in vitro*, fluid shear stress induces endothelial cell PAI-1 gene expression and activity and that this in turn inhibits the flow-induced SMC migratory response [45]. Modulation of vascular cell uPA and PAI-1 expression by pulse pressure and shear stress may thus represent an important mechanism whereby hemodynamic forces regulate SMC migration and represent potential targets for ethanol to mediate its vascular effects.

With this in mind, the direct effect of ethanol on SMC migration *in vitro* has been investigated. Hendrickson *et al.* pretreated cultures of human smooth muscle cells (HuSMC) under static (no flow) or pulsatile flow conditions in the absence or presence of ethanol and then assessed their migration by Transwell assay. Ethanol dose-dependently inhibited migration of SMC from static cultures. Furthermore, ethanol inhibited the flow-induced increase in SMC migration (Figure 9.4) in the absence of any effect on uPA mRNA expression [46]. Other mechanisms that are involved in the smooth muscle cell migratory response under basal and flow conditions that ethanol may modulate include the matrix metalloproteinases (MMPs), tissue inhibitors of metalloproteinases (TIMPs), mitogen activated protein kinase (MAPK), and calcium/calmodulin kinase (CaM kinase II). The possible role of these signaling pathways in pulse pressure-induced SMC migration and the effect, if any, of ethanol on their function and activity merits further investigation.

There have been a number of *in vitro* studies, using cells cultured under static (no flow) conditions, on the molecular regulatory effects of ethanol on endothelial cell-mediated fibrinolysis. Laug demonstrated an ethanol-induced increase in tPA secretion in cultured bovine

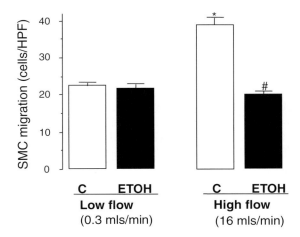

Figure 9.4 The effect of ethanol on pulse pressure-induced smooth muscle cell migration. Human smooth muscle cells (HuSMC) in perfused transcapillary cultures were exposed to low or high pulsatile flow conditions, in the absence or presence of ethanol (20 mM). Cells were then harvested and their migration assessed by Transwell assay. Ethanol inhibited the flow-induced increase in HuSMC migration. (Reproduced by permission of Academic Press from Hendrickson *et al.* (1999), [46].)

aortic endothelial cells [47]. An increase in tPA and uPA mRNA and a simultaneous decrease in PAI-1 mRNA in cultured human endothelial cells, concomitant with increased surface-localized EC fibrinolytic activity have been shown [48,49]. Miyamoto *et al.* reported that ethanol enhances agonist-stimulated cAMP-dependent tPA gene transcription in human and bovine EC through differential modulation of a G-protein [50]. These *in vitro* studies may explain the increased fibrinolytic activity found in the plasma of persons consuming moderate amounts of alcohol. As the fibrinolytic plasminogen system is modulated by hemodynamic forces it may be more physiologically relevant to study the effect of ethanol on endothelial fibrinolytic activity in cells exposed to fluid shear stress.

ETHANOL AND SMOOTH MUSCLE CELL PROLIFERATION

Excessive proliferation of arterial SMC plays an important role in the process of atherogenesis and hypertension [14]. Therefore, inhibition and stimulation of VSMC proliferation may be crucial for preventing and exacerbating, respectively, the development of cardiovascular disease. One key regulatory enzyme pathway for control points within the cell cycle has been identified as mitogen-activated protein kinases (MAPKs) [51]. They are serine/threonine protein kinases that are activated by dual phosphorylation of both tyrosine and threonine residues. Highly conserved during eukaryotic evolution, they are rapidly activated in response to ligand binding by both growth factor receptors with intrinsic tyrosine kinase activity, such as the platelet derived growth factor (PDGF) receptor, and receptors that are coupled to G-proteins such as the thrombin receptor [51–53]. They are also activated by hemodynamic stimuli [11]. Members of the MAPK family include the ERKs (ERK-1 and

ERK-2) which are activated by MEK (also referred to as MAPK kinase). MEK itself is activated by phosphorylation on two conserved serine residues by Ser/Thr kinases such as Raf, Mos and Mek kinase (MEKK) [54]. ERKs are dephosphorylated and inactivated by MAPK phosphatase-1 (MKP-1). Several studies have provided compelling evidence for a role of MAPKs in regulating SMC growth [55]. MAPK signaling, in particular ERK activity, is increased in rat carotid arteries following balloon injury concomitant with enhanced medial cell proliferation [56]. Furthermore, inhibition of MAPK signaling with PD 098059, a MEK inhibitor, reduced medial cell replication following injury [56]. MKP-1 expression is high in normal arterial tissue, whereas ERK expression is low [55,57]. However, following balloon injury the expression of MKP-1 decreases dramatically, whereas that of ERK is increased [57]. In proliferating cells it has been postulated that activated ERK-MAPKs phosphorylate specific cytoplasmic and nuclear proteins needed for passage through certain checkpoints in the cell cycle (e.g., G1/S and G2/M) [58].

The effect of ethanol on MAPK in VSMC *in vitro* has been investigated and divergent effects reported. Hendrickson *et al.* demonstrated that ethanol treatment (24 h), at physiologically relevant concentrations, inhibited serum-stimulated growth and MAPK activity in cultured SMC in the absence of any effect on cell viability (Figure 9.5) [59]. The mechanism of ethanol's induced changes in smooth muscle MAPK signaling and growth remain unclear. The decreased phosphorylation of ERK-1 and ERK-2 by MEK in cells exposed to ethanol suggests that MEK inhibition determines ERK inhibition by ethanol in these cells. Several studies have demonstrated that ethanol can inhibit the proliferation of cells at the level of growth factor receptor expression [60]. Ethanol inhibited basic fibroblast growth factor (bFGF)-induced proliferation of C6 astrocytoma cells [61]. In addition, ethanol markedly inhibited cell growth stimulation in response to insulin like growth factor-1 (IGF-1) and depressed tyrosine phosphorylation of the IGF-1 receptor [60]. Since ethanol induces G1 phase arrest in SMC *in vitro*, it is possible that inhibition of specific growth factor receptor autophosphorylation may in part account for the antiproliferative effects of ethanol in SMC. However, Sachinidis *et al.* demonstrated that ethanol had a different effect on SMC depending on the exposure time used. In their hands, acute treatment of VSMC with ethanol (3–5 min) led to a substantial increase in DNA synthesis and stimulated the same intracellular signalling events (including PIP_2 hydrolysis, MAPK activation, and stimulation of c-fos mRNA expression) associated with the potent growth factors PDGF-BB and Angiotensin II, whereas more chronic treatment (>30 min) resulted in cell necrosis [62].

Changes in intravascular hemodynamic forces that occur in disease states such as hypertension are profoundly associated with remodeling of the vascular media. Several studies have confirmed that subjecting SMC to increased pressure and/or stretch, in the absence of a functional endothelium, can result in increased wall thickness *in vivo* and proliferation of SMC *in vitro* [63,64]. Under normal circumstances in adult organisms, the vascular system functions in a relatively quiescent state despite these forces impacting on the vascular smooth muscle [8]. In contrast, following vascular injury due to endothelial dysfunction or denudation, SMC abandon their quiescent state and actively proliferate under the influence of mitogenic and other factors [65].

Several studies have demonstrated a marked heterogeneity of SMC phenotypes in rodents and humans [66,67]. Intimal SMC associated with vascular remodeling following injury are phenotypically distinct from their medial counterparts [66,67]. Characteristically, intimal cells resemble immature, dedifferentiated SMC and have lower levels of contractile proteins, fewer

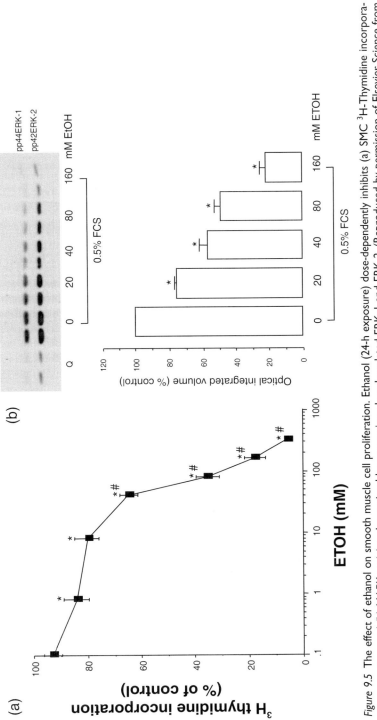

Figure 9.5 The effect of ethanol on smooth muscle cell proliferation. Ethanol (24-h exposure) dose-dependently inhibits (a) SMC ^{3}H-Thymidine incorporation, and (b) MAPK activity, determined by measuring phosphorylated ERK-I and ERK-2. (Reproduced by permission of Elsevier Science from Hendrickson et al. (1998), [59]).

myofilaments and express a large number of proteins involved in lesion development [66,67]. In contrast, medial SMC express differentiated cell markers associated with contractile function (α-actin, myosin, calponin and phospholamban) and the synthesis and maintenance of extracellular components of the vessel wall (e.g., osteopontin, elastin). Cappadona *et al.* demonstrated that SMC phenotype is a critical determinant of the proliferative response of SMC to hemodynamic forces [68], in that phenotypically distinct cells respond negatively to pulse pressure in a MAPK-dependent manner. Interestingly, in a recent study using rabbit iliac arteries following balloon angioplasty, significant inhibition of SMC phenotype conversion from contractile to synthetic was observed following ethanol treatment that was indicative of an inhibition of SMC proliferation [69]. Moreover, ethanol treatment at low concentrations results in inhibition of SMC growth in a MAPK-dependent manner [59]. Further investigation of the effect of ethanol on SMC phenotype and how the differentiation state of these cells affect hemodynamic force-induced signaling and growth in SMC is warranted.

CONCLUSIONS

The regular consumption of alcohol in moderate amounts has been recognized as a negative risk factor for atherosclerosis and its clinical sequelae: coronary heart disease, ischemic stroke and peripheral vascular disease. Mortality and morbidity attributable to CHD are 40–60% lower in moderate drinkers than among abstainers. Among the mechanisms accounting for these reductions, increased circulating concentrations of HDL-cholesterol and inhibition of blood coagulation appear to be paramount. However, additional benefits may be attributable to the direct effects of alcohol on vascular function and structure.

Mechanical forces that impact on vascular cells (shear stress and pulse pressure) are known to play a critical role in determining vascular structure following endothelial dysfunction or denudation following injury by modulating vascular smooth muscle cell proliferation and migration. Ethanol, at physiologically relevant concentrations, inhibits these processes *in vitro* and *in vivo* and thus may account, in part, for the protective effect of ethanol under both normal conditions and following vascular injury. The mechanisms involved in mediating ethanol-induced inhibition of pressure-induced SMC proliferation and migration are currently under investigation and include the effects of ethanol on SMC signaling (MAPK, Cam Kinases, MMP's and TIMP's). Ethanol may also be protective against neointimal formation and vascular remodeling in intact vessels by potentiating the release of the anti-migratory and anti-proliferative substances, NO and PGI_2, both of which are released from the endothelium in response to mechanical stimuli (shear stress and cyclic strain). The ability of moderate ethanol consumption to inhibit key steps in mechanical force-induced changes in the atherogenic process, at least *in vitro*, warrants further investigation into whether these effects contribute to the beneficial effects of moderate alcohol consumption on coronary artery disease.

REFERENCES

1 Friedman LA, Kimball AW. Coronary heart disease mortality and alcohol consumption in Framingham. *Am. J. Epidemiol.* 1986; **124**: 481–489.
2 Doll R, Peto R, Hall E, Wheatly K, Gray R. Mortality in relation to consumption of alcohol: 13 years observations on male British doctors. *BMJ* 1994; **309**: 911–918.

3 Klatsky AL, Armstrong MA, Friedman GD. Alcohol and mortality. *Ann. Int. Med.* 1992; **117**: 646–654.

4 Merritt R, Guruge BL, Miller DD, Chaitman BR, Bora PS. Moderate alcohol feeding attenuates post-injury vascular cell proliferation in rabbit angioplasty model. *J. Cardiovasc. Pharm.* 1997; **30**: 19–25.

5 Liu MW, Anderson PG, Luo JF, Roubin GS. Local delivery of ethanol inhibits intimal hyperplasia in pig coronary arteries after balloon injury. *Circulation* 1997; **96**: 2295–2301.

6 Davies P. Flow mediated endothelial mechanotransduction. *Physiol. Rev.* 1995; **75**: 519–560.

7 Skalak TC, Price RJ. The role of mechanical stresses in microvascular remodelling. *Microcirculation* 1996; **3**: 143–165.

8 Osol G. Mechanotransduction by vascular smooth muscle. *J. Vasc. Res.* 1995; **32**: 275–292.

9 Ku DN, Giddens DP, Zarins CK, Glagov S. Pulsatile flow and atherosclerosis in the human carotid bifurcation. Positive correlation between plaque location and low and oscillating shear stress. *Arteriosclerosis* 1985; **5**: 293–301.

10 Busse R, Fleming I. Pulsatile stretch and shear stress: Physical stimuli determining the production of endothelium-derived relaxing factors. *J. Vasc. Res.* 1998; **35**: 73–84.

11 Takahashi M, Ishida T, Traub O, Corson MA, Berk BC. Mechanotransduction in endothelial cells: Temporal signaling events in response to shear stress. *J. Vasc. Res.* 1997; **34**: 212–219.

12 Moncada SR, Palmer M, Higgs EA. Nitric oxide: Physiology, pathophysiology and pharmacology. *Pharmacol. Rev.* 1991; **43**: 109–129.

13 Schwartz SM, Liaw L. Growth control and morphogenesis in the development and pathology of arteries. *J. Cardiovasc. Pharm.* 1993; **21**(Suppl. 1): S31–S49.

14 Schwartz SM, DeBlois D, O'Brien ERM. The intima: Soil for atherosclerosis and restenosis. *Circ. Res.* 1995; **77**: 445–465.

15 Levitzki A, Bar-Sinai A. The regulation of adenylyl cyclase by receptor G proteins. *Pharmacol. Ther.* 1991; **50**: 271–283.

16 Helmreich EJ, Hofmann KP. Structure and function of proteins in G-protein-coupled signal transfer. *Biochim. Biophys. Acta* 1996; **1286**: 285–322.

17 Ohno M, Gibbons GH, Dzau VJ, Cooke JP. Shear stress elevated endothelial cGMP. Role of a potassium channel and G-protein coupling. *Circulation* 1993; **88**: 193–197.

18 Cooke JP, Rossitch E, Ardon NA, Loscalzo J, Dzau VJ. Flow activates an endothelial potassium channel to release an endogenous nitrovasodilator. *J. Clin. Invest.* 1991; **88**: 1663–1671.

19 Wand GS, Diehl AM, Levine MA, Wolfgang D, Samy S. Chronic ethanol treatment increases expression of inhibitory G-proteins and reduces adenylyl cyclase activity in the central nervous system of two lines of ethanol-sensitive mice. *J. Biol. Chem.* 1993; **268**(4): 2595–2601.

20 Thurston AW, Shukla S. Ethanol modulates epidermal growth factor-stimulated tyrosine kinase and phosphorylation of PLC-gamma 1. *Biochem. Biophys. Res. Commun.* 1992; **185**: 1062–1068.

21 Chen QM, LaBella FS. Inhibition of nitric oxide synthase by straight chain and cyclic alcohols. *Eur. J. Pharm.* 1997; **321**: 355–360.

22 Kolls JK, Xie J, Lei D, Greenberg S, Summer WR, Nelson S. Differential effects of *in vivo* ethanol on LPS-induced TNF and nitric oxide production in the lung. *Am. J. Physiol.* 1995; **268**: L991–L998.

23 Durante W, Cheng K, Sunahara RK, Schafer AI. Ethanol potentiates interleukin-1β-stimulated inducible nitric oxide synthase expression in cultured vascular smooth muscle cells. *Biochem. J.* 1995; **308**: 231–236.

24 Davda RK, Chandler J, Crews FT, Guzman NJ. Ethanol enhances the endothelial nitric oxide synthase response to agonists. *Hypertension* 1993; **21**: 939–943.

25 Venkov CD, Myers PR, Tanner MA, Su M, Vaughan DE. Ethanol increases endothelial nitric oxide production through modulation of nitric oxide synthase expression. *Thromb. Haemost.* 1999; **81**: 638–642.

26 Hendrickson RJ, Cahill PA, Sitzmann JV, Redmond EM. Ethanol enhances basal and flow-stimulated nitric oxide synthase activity *in vitro* by activating an inhibitory guanine nucleotide binding protein. *J. Pharm. Exp. Ther.* 1999; **289**: 1293–1300.

27 Garg UC, Hassid A. Nitric oxide-generating vasodilators and 8-bromo-cyclic guanosine mono-phosphate inhibit mitogenesis and proliferation of cultured rat vascular smooth muscle cells. *J. Clin. Invest.* 1989; **83**: 1774–1777.

28 Gorog P, Kovacs IB. Inhibition of vascular smooth muscle cell migration by intact endothelium is nitric oxide-mediated: interference by oxidised low density lipoproteins. *J. Vasc. Res.* 1998; **35**: 165–169.

29 Landolfi R, Steiner M. Ethanol raises prostacyclin *in vivo* and *in vitro*. *Blood* 1984; **64**: 679–682.

30 Guivernau M, Baraona E, Lieber CS. Acute and chronic effects of ethanol and its metabolites on vascular production of prostacyclin in rats. *J. Pharmacol. Exp. Ther.* 1987; **240**: 59–64.

31 Redmond EM, Cahill PA, Sitzmann JV. Flow-mediated regulation of G-protein expression in co-cultured vascular smooth muscle and endothelial cells. *Arterioscler. Thromb. Vasc. Biol.* 1998; **18**: 75–83.

32 Knapp DJ, Crews FT. Induction of cyclooxygenase-2 in brain during acute and chronic ethanol treatment and ethanol withdrawal. *Alcohol Clin. Exp. Res.* 1999; **23**: 633–643.

33 Dzau VJ, Gibbons GH. Vascular remodelling: Mechanisms and implications. *J. Cardiovasc. Pharm.* 1993; **21**: S1–S5.

34 Cho A, Mitchell L, Koopmans D, Langille BL. Effects of changes in blood flow rate on cell death and cell proliferation in carotid arteries of immature rabbits. *Circ. Res.* 1997; **81**: 328–337.

35 Ross R. The pathogenesis of atherosclerosis: a perspective for the 1990's. *Nature* 1993; **362**: 801–809.

36 Raines EW, Ross R. Smooth muscle cells and the pathogenesis of the lesions of atherosclerosis. *Br. Heart J.* 1993; **69**: S30–S37.

37 Abedi A, Zachary I. Signalling mechanisms in the regulation of vascular cell migration. *Cardiovasc. Res.* 1995; **30**: 544–556.

38 Miller MW. Migration of cortical neurons is altered by gestational exposure to ethanol. *Alcohol Clin. Exp. Res.* 1993; **17**(2): 304–314.

39 Silberman S, McGarvey TW, Comrie E, Persky B. The influence of ethanol on cell membrane fluidity, migration and invasion of murine melanoma cells. *Exp. Cell Res.* 1990; **189**(1): 64–68.

40 Clowes AW, Clowes MM, Au YP, Reidy MA, Belin D. Smooth muscle cells express urokinase during mitogenesis and tissue-type plasminogen activator during migration in injured rat carotid artery. *Circ. Res.* 1990; **67**: 61–67.

41 Carmeliet P, Moons L, Herbert J-M *et al.* Urokinase but not tissue plasminogen activator mediates arterial neointima formation in mice. *Circ. Res.* 1997; **81**: 829–839.

42 Stefansson S, Lawrence DA. The serpin PAI-1 inhibits cell migration by blocking integrin αvb3 binding to vitronectin. *Nature* 1996; **383**: 441–443.

43 Carmeliet P, Stassen JM, De Mol M, Bouche A, Collen D. Arterial neointima formation after trauma in mice with inactivation of the tPA, uPA or PAI-1 genes. *Circulation* 1994; **90**: 1–144.

44 Redmond EM, Cahill PA, Hirsch M, Wang YN, Sitzmann JV, Okada SO. Effect of pulse pressure on vascular smooth muscle cell migration: The role of urokinase and matrix metalloproteinase. *Thromb. Haemost.* 1999; **81**: 293–300.

45 Redmond EM, Cullen JP, Cahill PA, Sitzmann JV, Stefansson S, Lawrence DA, Okada SS. Endothelial cells inhibit flow-induced smooth muscle cell migration. Role of plasminogen activator inhibitor-1. *Circulation* 2001; **103**: 597–603.

46 Hendrickson RJ, Okada SS, Cahill PA, Yankah EN, Sitzmann JV, Redmond EM. Ethanol inhibits basal and flow-induced vascular smooth muscle cell migration *in vitro*. *J. Surg. Res.* 1999; **84**: 64–70.

47 Laug WE. Ethyl alcohol enhances plasminogen activator secretion by endothelial cells. *JAMA* 1983; **250**: 772–776.

48 Venkov CD, Su M, Shry Y, Vaughan DE. Ethanol-induced alterations in the expression of endothelial-derived fibrinolytic components. *Fibrinol. Proteol.* 1997; **11**: 115–118.

49 Aikens ML, Grenett HE, Benza RL, Tabengwa EM, Davis GC, Booyse FM. Alcohol-induced upregulation of plasminogen activators and fibrinolytic activity in cultured human endothelial cells. *Alcohol Clin. Exp. Res.* 1998; **22**: 375–381.

50 Miyamoto A, Yang SX, Laufs U, Ruan XL, Liao JK. Activation of guanine nucleotide binding proteins and induction of endothelial tissue-type plasminogen activator transcription by alcohol. *J. Biol. Chem.* 1999; **274**: 12055–12060.

51 Pelech SL, Sanghera JS. Mitogen-activated protein kinases: versatile transducers for cell signaling. *Trends. Biochem. Sci.* 1992; **17**; 233–238.

52 Boulton TJ, Nye SH, Robbins DJ, Ip NY, Radziejewska E, Morgenbesser SD, DePinho RA, Panayotatos HN, Cobb MH, Yancopoulos GD. ERKs: a family of protein-serine/threonine kinases that are activated and tyrosine phosphorylated in response to insulin. *Cell* 1991; **65**: 663–675.

53 L'Allemain G, Pouyssegar J, Weber MJ. p42/mitogen-activated protein kinase as a converging target for different growth factor signaling pathways: use of pertussis toxin as a discrimination factor. *Cell Regul.* 1991; **2**: 675–684.

54 Gardner AM, Vaillancourt RR, Lange-Carter CA, Johnson GL. MEK-phosphorylation by MEK kinase, Raf, and mitogen-activated protein kinase: analysis of phosphopeptides and regulation of activity. *Mol. Biol. Cell* 1994; **5**: 193–201.

55 Mii S, Khalil RA, Morgan KG, Ware JA, Kent KC. Mitogen-activated protein kinase and proliferation of human vascular smooth muscle cells. *Am. J. Physiol.* 1996; **270**: H142–H150.

56 Koyama H, Olson NE, Dastvan F, Reidy MA. Cell replication in the arterial wall: Activation of signaling pathway following *in vivo* injury. *Circ. Res.* 1998; **82**: 713–721.

57 Lai K, Wang H, Lee W-S, Jain M, Lee M-E, Haber. Mitogen activated protein kinase phophatase-1 in rat arterial smooth muscle cell proliferation. *J. Clin. Invest.* 1996; **98**: 1560–1567.

58 Tamemoto H, Kadowaki T, Tobe K, Ueki K, Izumi T, Chatani Y, Kohno M, Kasuga M, Yawaki Y, Akanuma Y. Biphasic activation of two mitogen-activated protein kinases during the cell cycle in mammalian cells. *J. Biol. Chem.* 1992; **267**: 20293–20297.

59 Hendrickson RJ, Cahill PA, McKillop IH, Sitzmann JV, Redmond EM. Ethanol inhibits mitogen activated protein kinase activity and growth of vascular smooth muscle cells *in vitro. Eur. J. Pharmacol.* 1998; **362**: 251–259.

60 Resnicoff M, Sell C, Ambrose D, Baserga R, Rubin R. Ethanol inhibits the autophosphorylation of the insulin-like growth factor 1 (IGF-1) receptor and IGF-1 mediated proliferation of 3T3 cells. *J. Biol. Chem.* 1993; **268:** 21777–21782.

61 Luo J, Miller MW. Ethanol inhibits basic fibroblast growth factor-mediated proliferation of C6 astrocytoma cells. *J. Neurochem.* 1996; **67**: 1448–1456.

62 Sachinidis A, Gouni-Berthold I, Seul C, Seewald S, Ko Y, Schmitz U, Vetter H. Early intracellular signalling pathway of ethanol in vascular smooth muscle cells. *Br. J. Pharmacol.* 1999; **128**: 1761–1771.

63 Miyashiro JK, Poppa V, Berk BC. Flow-induced vascular remodelling in the rat carotid artery diminishes with age. *Circ. Res.* 1997; **81**: 311–319.

64 Watase M, Awolesi MA, Ricotta J, Sumpio BE. Effect of pressure on cultured smooth muscle cells. *Life Sci.* 1997; **61**: 987–996.

65 Allaire E, Clowes A. Endothelial cell injury in cardiovascular surgery: the intimal hyperplastic response. *Ann. Thorac. Surg.* 1997; **63**: 582–591.

66 Bochaton-Piallat M-L, Ropraz P, Gabbiani F, Gabbiani G. Phenotypic heterogeneity of rat arterial smooth muscle cell clones. Implications for the development of experimental intimal thickening. *Arterioscl. Thromb. Vasc. Biol.* 1996; **16**: 815–820.

67 Shanahan CM, Weisberg PL, Metcalfe JC. Isolation of gene markers of differentiated and proliferating smooth muscle cells. *Circ. Res.* 1993; **73**: 193–204.

68 Cappadona C, Redmond EM, Theodorakis NG, McKillop IH, Hendrickson R, Chhabra A, Sitzmann JV, Cahill PA. Phenotype dictates the growth response of vascular smooth muscle cells to pulse pressure *in vitro. Exp. Cell Res.* 1999; **250**: 174–186.

69 Liu MW, Lin SJ, Chen YL. Local alcohol delivery may reduce phenotype conversion of smooth muscle cells and neointimal formation in rabbit iliac arteries after balloon injury. *Atherosclerosis* 1996; **27**: 221–227.

Chapter 10

Moderate alcohol exposure protects cardiac myocytes from ischemia-reperfusion injury

Mary O. Gray and Daria Mochly-Rosen

INTRODUCTION

The effects of ethanol on the cardiovascular system have long been of interest to physicians, scientists, and the public. Although certain genetic backgrounds or pre-existing cardiac disease may leave individuals more vulnerable to ethanol toxicity, in general the detrimental effects of alcohol on cardiac function are linked to heavy consumption and the cardioprotective effects to moderate consumption [1]. Moderate alcohol intake, defined as one drink or less per day for women and two drinks or less per day for men [2], has been shown to reduce coronary heart disease (CHD) in a large number of observational studies [3–5]. The relationship between alcohol intake and total mortality is usually reported as U- or J-shaped and represents the sum of the protective effect of moderate consumption on CHD mortality and the detrimental effect of heavy drinking on other causes of death [2].

EPIDEMIOLOGICAL STUDIES

Recently, the South Bay Heart Watch (Torrance, CA) reported a study of 1,196 asymptomatic subjects with coronary risk factors who were assessed for alcohol consumption history and for the presence of calcium deposits in coronary atherosclerotic lesions as measured by electron beam computed tomography (EBCT). Participants were followed prospectively for 41 months for coronary events, defined as the occurrence of myocardial infarction or CHD death [6]. Subjects who drank alcohol had a relative risk of 0.3 of having a coronary event compared with abstainers. The diminished risk of myocardial infarction or CHD death associated with moderate alcohol consumption was independent of serum HDL cholesterol levels, EBCT coronary calcium scores, and all other coronary risk factors. Abstention from alcohol in this study was as strong a predictor of coronary events as diabetes, smoking, hypertension, and coronary calcification [6].

Also reported recently was an analysis of the relationship between light-to-moderate alcohol consumption and cause-specific mortality in the Physicians' Health Study enrollment cohort [7]. Participants in the study (89,299 asymptomatic male physicians) were assessed for alcohol consumption history and other baseline characteristics and then followed prospectively for 5.5 years. Investigators observed significant reductions in mortality from myocardial infarction of 32% to 47% among participants who consumed one drink or more per week [7]. Also observed in this cohort was a significant decrease in total mortality among light-to-moderate drinkers (<2 drinks per day) after adjustment for age. Similar reductions in mortality were found for alcohol consumption between one and seven drinks per week, with a slightly greater reduction in all-cause mortality at one drink per week. Therefore, current studies of risk factors for coronary artery disease continue to support a beneficial effect of moderate consumption in decreasing the risk of myocardial infarction and death.

MEDIATORS OF CARDIAC PROTECTION INDUCED BY CHRONIC EXPOSURE TO ETHANOL

Because no clinical trials actually test prospectively the relationship between alcohol consumption and coronary heart disease, efforts to identify the mediators of ethanol-induced cardiac protection in humans focus on statistical modeling of observational data. These analyses have identified increased HDL cholesterol levels [8,9], decreased platelet aggregation [10], and increased expression of tissue-type plasminogen activator [11] as potential mechanisms underlying ethanol-induced cardiac protection. Moderate ethanol exposure may also protect against CHD through direct effects on heart muscle. For example, Auffermann et al. reported that ethanol significantly reduces the functional and structural damage caused by one component of ischemia-reperfusion injury, the pathological influx of Ca^{2+} into myocardial cells termed the calcium paradox injury [12]. Using isolated Langendorff-perfused rat hearts, these investigators found that addition of 2.5% (vol/vol) ethanol to the perfusate protected against massive calcium overload in cardiac myocytes and greatly enhanced hemodynamic recovery as measured by left ventricular developed pressure and end-diastolic pressure [12].

PROTEIN KINASE C IN CARDIOPROTECTION INDUCED BY CHRONIC EXPOSURE TO ETHANOL

The cellular mechanisms by which moderate alcohol exposure directly protects, or preconditions, cardiac myocytes from ischemia-reperfusion injury are unknown. However, substantial experimental evidence suggests that an intracellular signal transduction pathway common to several important forms of cardiac preconditioning involves activation of protein kinase C [13]. Ischemic preconditioning, a protective mechanism induced when the heart is exposed to brief sublethal episodes of ischemia, is the most potent experimental means of reducing cardiac myocyte damage during subsequent prolonged ischemia. Data from clinical studies suggest that ischemic preconditioning occurs in humans [14–16]. Speechly-Dick et al. have reported an in vitro model in which isolated human right atrial trabeculae were subjected to a preconditioning stimulus consisting of 3 minutes of simulated ischemia (hypoxic substrate-free superfusion combined with pacing at 3 Hz) followed sequentially by 7 minutes of reperfusion, 90 minutes of simulated ischemia, and 120 minutes of reperfusion [17]. They found that ischemic preconditioning significantly improved contractile recovery compared with the non-preconditioned group ($63.5 \pm 5.4\%$ of baseline developed force vs. $29.5 \pm 3.6\%$ of baseline for controls, $p < 0.01$). Furthermore, exposure of trabeculae to the protein kinase C (PKC) activator 1,2-dioctanoyl glycerol mimicked ischemic preconditioning, and treatment with the PKC antagonist chelerythrine blocked the protective effect of brief simulated ischemia [17].

In studies of rodent heart, PKC activation by transient ischemia or by pharmacological agonists also induces protection against myocardial dysfunction and infarction, and PKC antagonists inhibit cardiac preconditioning [13]. Several laboratories have further demonstrated a critical role for selective activation and translocation of the epsilon PKC isozyme in cardiac preconditioning. For example, in a conscious rabbit model, one to six cycles of 5 minute coronary occlusion induced protection from myocardial infarction and caused dose-dependent and selective translocation of εPKC from the cytosolic to the particulate fractions of cardiac myocyte preparations [18]. Our laboratory previously reported a neonatal rat cardiac myocyte culture model in which hypoxic preconditioning produced resistance to subsequent prolonged hypoxia and glucose deprivation as well as activation and translocation of εPKC [19]. In this model, introduction into cardiac myocytes of a novel isozyme-selective peptide antagonist of εPKC inhibited both εPKC translocation and the protection from cellular injury during prolonged hypoxia [19]. More recently, we reported development of a rationally designed peptide that causes selective ε protein kinase C translocation in both neonatal and adult cardiac myocytes [20]. Acute introduction of the εPKC agonist into isolated cardiac myocytes protected against cell death induced by simulated ischemia, measured by abnormal uptake of trypan blue or ethidium homodimer. Furthermore, chronic postnatal expression of the εPKC agonist in the hearts of transgenic mice improved left ventricular contractile recovery after 30 minutes of global ischemia by 43% compared with nontransgenic sibling controls and reduced by 61% the release of creatine kinase into coronary effluent during 15 minutes of reperfusion [20]. Therefore, activation of epsilon protein kinase C appears to be both necessary and sufficient for the induction of powerful protective mechanisms against ischemia-reperfusion injury in rodent heart models.

In collaboration with Vincent Figueredo, we developed a guinea pig model of chronic ethanol consumption to test the hypothesis that moderate alcohol exposure also protects against ischemia-reperfusion injury via selective activation of εPKC in cardiac myocytes [21]. In this study, Hartley guinea pigs were fed a nutritionally supplemented liquid diet containing 15% or 0% ethanol-derived calories for 8 weeks. Hearts from control and treated animals were isolated and perfused using a modified Langendorff method. After a 20 minute equilibration period, hearts were subjected to 45 minutes of no-flow ischemia and 48 minutes of reperfusion. Serum ethanol levels were 10 ± 2 mg/dL (2 mM) after 8 weeks of feeding with 15% ethanol-derived calories. Body weight, dry heart weight to body weight ratio, baseline left ventricular (LV) developed pressure, coronary flow, and perfusion pressure were the same in control and ethanol-fed animals. However, hearts from control and ethanol-treated guinea pigs differed significantly in their resistance to ischemia-reperfusion injury. LV developed pressure recovered to 42% of pre-ischemic levels in hearts from ethanol-fed animals compared to only 22% in controls ($p < 0.05$). LV end-diastolic pressure (LVEDP), an index of myocyte contracture and injury, was lower during reperfusion in hearts from ethanol-fed animals compared with controls. Creatine kinase release was also lower from hearts of ethanol-fed animals compared with controls (260 ± 40 vs. 469 ± 74 units/mL/gdw, $p < 0.05$). Importantly, protection obtained by chronic moderate ethanol exposure *in vivo* was unchanged by termination of ethanol exposure 16 hours prior to heart isolation compared with termination immediately prior to isolation. These data suggested a sustained cardioprotective effect due to ethanol exposure *in vivo* [21].

Additional experiments were performed using chelerythrine chloride, a potent selective inhibitor of the catalytic domain of PKC [22], added to the perfusate 10 minutes prior to ischemia. Chelerythrine treatment abolished resistance to ischemia-reperfusion injury in hearts from ethanol-fed guinea pigs, supporting a critical role for PKC activation in ethanol-induced protection [21]. Furthermore, selective activation of the εPKC isozyme correlated with ethanol-mediated preconditioning. Cardiac myocytes were isolated by perfusing hearts from control and ethanol-fed animals with buffer containing collagenase B. Western analysis and immunofluorescence staining were used to determine the subcellular distribution of αPKC, δPKC, and εPKC in control and ethanol-exposed cardiac myocytes. The subcellular distribution of αPKC and δPKC did not differ in cardiac myocytes isolated from control and ethanol-fed animals. In contrast, the ratio of particulate to cytosolic εPKC was greater in myocytes from hearts of ethanol-fed guinea pigs (2.7 ± 0.1 vs. 1.5 ± 0.4 for controls, $p < 0.05$) as measured by western analysis [21]. The percentage of myocytes exhibiting activated εPKC in an activated, cross-striated pattern of immunofluorescence was also greater in hearts from ethanol-fed animals ($61 \pm 3\%$ vs. $22 \pm 5\%$ for controls, $p < 0.05$). These data support the hypothesis that moderate alcohol intake protects myocardium against ischemia-reperfusion injury via chronic activation and translocation of εPKC in guinea pig cardiac myocytes [21].

We have subsequently developed an isolated mouse heart model that allows us to make detailed hemodynamic measurements in wild-type and genetically altered mice [23]. C57BL/6 mice (34–$40\,g$) were preconditioned by feeding with 18% ethanol (vol/vol) in their drinking water for 12 weeks. At the end of the treatment period, there were no differences in body weight, heart weight, baseline LV developed pressure (LVDP), or coronary flow between ethanol-fed mice and age-matched controls. Serum ethanol levels were measured prior to each experiment and averaged $31 \pm 4\,mg/dL$ ($6\,mM$). Hearts from control and treated mice were isolated and perfused using a modified Langendorff method. After a 20 minute equilibration period, hearts were subjected to 20 minutes of no-flow ischemia and 30 minutes of reperfusion. Ethanol preconditioning increased recovery of LVDP during postischemic reperfusion ($64.8 \pm 7.3\%$ of baseline vs. $36.9 \pm 9.4\%$ for control, $p < 0.05$) and lowered LVEDP ($19 \pm 3.4\,mmHg$ vs. $34 \pm 4.3\,mmHg$ for control, $p < 0.05$). Creatine kinase release was also lower from the hearts of ethanol-fed animals compared with controls (0.28 ± 0.04 vs. $0.51 \pm 0.08\,U/min/gww$, $p < 0.05$). Withdrawal of alcohol from drinking water 16 hours prior to sacrifice lowered the mean serum ethanol level to $3.2 \pm 1.3\,mg/dL$ ($0.6\,mM$) but had no effect on preservation of LVDP, again supporting a sustained cardio-protective effective due to moderate alcohol exposure *in vivo* [23].

In our mouse model of chronic moderate ethanol exposure, western analysis of LV homogenates demonstrated a 2.4-fold increase in total εPKC expression in hearts from ethanol-fed animals (96.3 ± 13.3 vs. 39.5 ± 2.2 density units for control, $p < 0.05$) and an absolute increase in active εPKC localized to particulate fractions [23]. There was no change in the relative or absolute subcellular distribution of αPKC, βPKC, δPKC, or λPKC, the other isozymes present in mouse heart [24]. These data suggest a role for upregulation and activation of εPKC in the protective effect of chronic moderate alcohol exposure in the mouse. Studies to determine whether εPKC knockout mice [25] or transgenic mice with chronic postnatal expression of εPKC antagonist [26] develop cardiac protection in response to moderate alcohol exposure are currently underway in our laboratories.

Guinea pig [21], rat [27], and mouse [23] models of chronic ethanol feeding are important because they validate the beneficial effects of moderate consumption observed in human epidemiological studies and because they confirm the greater contribution of ethanol content over that of nonalcoholic components of alcoholic beverages to the induction of cardiac protection. However, the utility of chronic feeding strategies in the identification of cellular preconditioning mechanisms is limited by several considerations. First, increased resistance to ischemia-reperfusion injury in hearts isolated from ethanol-fed animals strongly suggests but does not prove a direct preconditioning effect of ethanol on cardiac myocytes. Ethanol-mediated protection might instead proceed via paracrine stimulation of endothelial cells, fibroblasts, or other nonmyocyte cells present in cardiac tissue. For example, we recently reported a neonatal rat cell culture model in which angiotensin II stimulated myocyte hypertrophy via paracrine release of transforming growth factor-β1 and endothelin-1 from fibroblasts [28]. Second, although εPKC activation was detected in the guinea pig model of chronic ethanol consumption [21], biochemical and histological analysis of hearts isolated from chronically fed animals may fail to identify the earliest signal transduction events required for ethanol-induced cardiac protection. Finally, some of the most powerful experimental tools available for modulation of protein–protein interactions in intracellular signaling [29], including isozyme-selective agonists and antagonists of protein kinase C [19,20,30], are currently active in isolated or cultured cells but not in intact heart.

PKC IN CARDIOPROTECTION INDUCED BY ACUTE EXPOSURE TO ETHANOL

We addressed these concerns by adapting an isolated adult myocyte model originally designed to assess ischemic and pharmacological preconditioning in rabbit cardiac myocytes [31] for our study of ethanol-mediated cardiac protection [32]. Isolated adult rat hearts were perfused with collagenase on a Langendorff apparatus. Ventricular myocytes were isolated by maceration of collagenase-digested tissue and gentle centrifugation of the resultant cellular suspension. Cardiac ischemia was simulated by pelleting of freshly-isolated cells in microcentrifuge tubes, removal of supernatant, and layering of mineral oil or microballoons over the packed myocytes to create an air-tight environment [32]. Samples were drawn from the myocyte pellet at given time intervals and assayed for viability. We assessed ischemia-induced cell damage using an osmotic fragility test in which myocytes were incubated in a hypotonic (85 milliosmolar) trypan blue solution. Cells that did not exclude trypan blue dye were considered nonviable because of membrane fragility [31]. During simulated ischemia, myocytes became progressively more fragile as evidenced by an increasing percentage of myocytes stained with trypan blue [32]. This *in vitro* model of cardiac ischemia is a useful approach to identification of cellular mediators of preconditioning because it permits direct comparison of control and acutely treated myocytes obtained from the same animal without the complications of other organ effects.

We found that acute moderate alcohol exposure directly protected cardiac myocytes from ischemia-induced damage [32]. Under normoxic conditions over 3 hours of incubation, 10% of cells demonstrated osmotic fragility, indicating that isolated myocytes remained healthy. Under simulated ischemic conditions over 3 hours of incubation, 75% of myocytes demonstrated osmotic fragility. Ten minute exposure of myocytes to 50 mM ethanol before, but not during, simulated ischemia reduced cell damage by 35%. Exposure of cardiac myocytes to just 10 mM ethanol throughout simulated ischemia reduced cell damage by 56%. Furthermore, 20 minute Langendorff perfusion of isolated rat heart with 10 mM ethanol reduced creatine kinase release after 45 minutes of ischemia and 30 minutes of reperfusion by 70%. Therefore, brief exposure to physiological levels of ethanol induced powerful protective mechanisms against ischemia-reperfusion injury in both isolated cardiac myocytes and intact rat myocardium [32].

Three lines of evidence support a critical role for εPKC activation and translocation in acute ethanol-mediated preconditioning in this model. First, the presence of the general PKC inhibitors chelerythrine or GF109203X during ethanol pretreatment of myocytes abolished protection during subsequent ischemia [32]. Second, treatment of cardiac myocytes with 10–50 mM ethanol doubled the amount of εPKC translocated from the cell soluble to the cell particulate fraction compared with controls [32]. Finally, the presence of the εPKC-selective inhibitor peptide, εV1–2 [19], during ethanol pretreatment of myocytes selectively abolished protection during subsequent ischemia. In contrast, a peptide inhibitor of the classical PKC isozymes, βC2–4 [30], had no effect [32]. Therefore, cardiac protection from ischemic injury following acute exposure to 10 mM ethanol not only correlated with activation of specific PKC isozymes but would not have occurred without activation of εPKC [32].

DOWNSTREAM MEDIATORS OF ETHANOL-INDUCED CARDIOPROTECTION

Because activation of epsilon protein kinase C is a critical event in several important forms of cardiac preconditioning, interest in the field is now focused on uncovering the downstream mediators of protection. Exhaustive examination of ischemic preconditioning in a conscious rabbit model by Ping *et al.* has identified p44/p42 mitogen-activated protein kinases [33], p46/p54 c-Jun NH2-terminal kinases [34], and Src and Lck tyrosine kinases [35] as downstream elements of εPKC-mediated signal transduction. Studies to determine the precise mechanisms linking εPKC to these signaling molecules, the requirement for their activation in other forms of preconditioning, and their own downstream cellular targets, are ongoing. Our laboratory has cloned the anchoring protein or RACK (receptor for activated C-kinase) for activated εPKC, that was identified as the COPI coatomer protein β'-COP [36]. The εPKC inhibitor peptide, εV1–2 [19], acts by competing for binding of activated εPKC to β'-COP [36] and selectively abolishes protection of adult rat cardiac myocytes from ischemic injury following acute exposure to ethanol [32]. Studies to determine the εPKC substrates responsible for cardiac protection and the mechanisms by which RACKs facilitate their activation in response to acute and chronic moderate alcohol exposure are currently underway in our laboratories.

One intriguing possibility is that moderate alcohol consumption protects cardiac myocytes from ischemia-reperfusion injury by activating mitochondrial ATP-dependent K^+ (mitoK$_{ATP}$) channels. Originally purified from inner mitochondrial membranes in beef heart, these channels are important regulators of mitochondrial matrix volume [37]. Opening of cardiac mitoK$_{ATP}$ channels leads to membrane depolarization, matrix swelling, and accelerated respiration [38]. Diazoxide has been identified as a selective mitoK$_{ATP}$ channel opener [39], and diazoxide treatment of both isolated cardiac myocytes [39] and intact myocardium [40] induces protection against ischemia-reperfusion injury. Diazoxide also reduces calcium paradox injury in isolated rat heart [41], a protective effect comparable to that observed with acute ethanol exposure [12]. 5-hydroxydecanoate (5-HD) has been identified as a selective inhibitor of mitoK$_{ATP}$ channels [39], and 5-HD pretreatment of intact rat heart abolishes ischemic preconditioning [42]. Protein kinase C appears to modulate mitoK$_{ATP}$ channel activity because treatment of isolated rabbit cardiac myocytes with the PKC activator phorbol 12-myristate 13-acetate (PMA) potentiates the effects of diazoxide [43] and because chelerythrine treatment of isolated rat heart abolishes diazoxide-induced protection [40]. Importantly, ischemic preconditioning was recently shown to redistribute ε protein kinase C to mitochondria in rabbit myocardium [44].

We recently completed a study in which we tested the hypothesis that chronic moderate alcohol consumption reduces cardiac ischemia-reperfusion injury by activation of mitoK$_{ATP}$ channels [45]. Adult male Sprague-Dawley rats received a diet of rodent chow and 18% ethanol (vol/vol) in their drinking water for 10 months, a feeding schedule previously reported to induce cardiac protection [27]. At the end of the treatment period, there were no differences in body weight, heart weight, baseline LV developed pressure, or coronary flow between ethanol-fed rats and age-matched controls. Serum ethanol levels were measured prior to each experiment and averaged 15 ± 1 mg/dL (3 mM) [45]. Hearts from control and treated rats were isolated and perfused using a modified Langendorff method. After a 20 minute equilibration period, hearts were subjected to 45 minutes of no-flow ischemia and 48 minutes of reperfusion. LV developed pressure recovered to 45% of pre-ischemic levels in hearts from ethanol-fed animals compared to only 20% in controls ($p < 0.01$). Creatine kinase release was lower from hearts of ethanol-fed animals compared with controls (14 ± 1 vs. 26 ± 1 U/min/gww, $p < 0.01$). Treatment of control hearts with 100 μM 5-HD for 10 minutes immediately prior to ischemia-reperfusion had no effect on subsequent recovery of LV developed pressure or on creatine kinase release. However, 5-HD treatment abolished resistance to ischemia-reperfusion injury in hearts from ethanol-fed rats, supporting a critical role for mitoK$_{ATP}$ channel activation in ethanol-induced protection [45]. Studies to determine how moderate alcohol exposure modulates mitoK$_{ATP}$ channel activity are currently underway.

CONCLUSIONS

Numerous epidemiological studies support a beneficial effect of light-to-moderate alcohol consumption in decreasing the risk of myocardial infarction and death due to coronary heart disease. In rodent heart models, moderate ethanol exposure directly protects cardiac myocytes through signal transduction pathways involving activation of protein kinase C. Acute exposure of hearts to low concentrations of ethanol (10 mM) rapidly induces powerful protective mechanisms against ischemia-reperfusion injury. Therefore, there may be considerable therapeutic potential for the administration of physiological concentrations of ethanol to patients prior to elective procedures that involve myocardial ischemia, such as coronary angioplasty and cardiac surgery. Chronic exposure of hearts to low concentrations of ethanol induces sustained protection against ischemia-reperfusion injury. Public health recommendations are designed to reassure current light-to-moderate drinkers but do not encourage new drinkers because of concerns regarding alcohol abuse and the exacerbation of co-existing medical conditions such as diabetes mellitus. Further examination of the cellular mediators of ethanol-induced cardiac preconditioning may lead to the development of novel therapeutic agents for the prevention and treatment of coronary heart disease.

ACKNOWLEDGMENT

Studies in the authors' laboratories were supported by National Institute on Alcohol Abuse and Alcoholism grants #AA11147 (D.M-R.) and #AA11135 (M.O.G).

REFERENCES

1 Lieber CS. Medical disorders of alcoholism. *N. Engl. J. Med.* 1995; **333**: 1058.
2 Pearson TA. AHA Medical/Scientific Statement. Alcohol and heart disease. *Circulation* 1996; **94**: 3023.
3 Friedman LA, Kimball AW. Coronary heart disease mortality and alcohol consumption in Framingham. *Am. J. Epidemiol.* 1986; **124**: 481.
4 Fuchs CS, Stampfer MJ, Colditz GA, Giovannucci EL, Manson JE, Kawachi I, Hunter DJ, Hankinson SE, Hennekens CH, Speizer FE, Willett WC. Alcohol consumption and mortality among women. *N. Engl. J. Med.* 1995; **332**: 1245.
5 Thun MJ, Peto R, Lopez AD, Monaco JH, Henley SJ, Heath CW, Doll R. Alcohol consumption and mortality among middle-aged and elderly U.S. adults. *N. Engl. J. Med.* 1997; **337**: 1705.
6 Yang T, Doherty TM, Wong ND, Detrano RC. Alcohol consumption, coronary calcium, and coronary heart disease events. *Am. J. Cardiol.* 1999; **84**: 802.
7 Gaziano JM, Gaziano TA, Glynn RJ, Sesso HD, Ajani UA, Stampfer MJ, Hennekens CH, Buring JE. Light-to-moderate alcohol consumption and mortality in the physicians' health study enrollment cohort. *J. Am. Coll. Cardiol.* 2000; **35**: 96.
8 Criqui MH, Cowan LD, Tyroler HA, Bangdiwala S, Heiss G, Wallace RB, Cohn R. Lipoproteins as mediators for the effects of alcohol consumption and cigarette smoking on cardiovascular mortality. Results from the Lipid Research Clinics Follow-up Study. *Am. J. Epidemiol.* 1987; **126**: 629.
9 Langer RD, Criqui MH, Reed DM. Lipoproteins and blood pressure as biologic pathways for the effect of moderate alcohol consumption on coronary heart disease. *Circulation* 1992; **85**: 910.
10 Renaud SC, Beswick AD, Fehily AM, Elwood PC. Alcohol and platelet aggregation: the Caerphilly Prospective Heart Disease Study. *Am. J. Clin. Nutr.* 1992; **55**: 1012.
11 Ridker PM, Vaughan DE, Stampfer MJ, Glynn RJ, Hennekens CH. Association of moderate alcohol consumption and plasma concentration of endogenous tissue-type plasminogen activator. *JAMA* 1994; **272**: 929.
12 Auffermann W, Wu S, Parmley W, Wikman-Coffelt J. Ethanol protects the heart against the calcium paradox injury. *Cell Calcium* 1990; **11**: 47.
13 Simkhovich BZ, Przyklenk K, Kloner RA. Role of protein kinase C as a cellular mediator of ischemic preconditioning: a critical review. *Cardiovasc. Res.* 1998; **40**: 9.
14 Kloner RA, Yellon D. Does ischemic preconditioning occur in patients? *J. Am. Coll. Cardiol.* 1994; **24**: 1133.
15 Billinger M, Fleisch M, Eberli FR, Garachemani A, Meier B, Seiler C. Is the development of myocardial tolerance to repeated ischemia in humans due to preconditioning or to collateral recruitment? *J. Am. Coll. Cardiol.* 1999; **33**: 1027.
16 Laskey WK. Beneficial impact of preconditioning during PTCA on creatine kinase release. *Circulation* 1999; **99**: 2085.
17 Speechly-Dick ME, Grover GJ, Yellon DM. Does ischemic preconditioning in the human involve protein kinase C and the ATP-dependent K$^+$ channel? *Circ. Res.* 1995; **77**: 1030.
18 Ping P, Zhang J, Qiu Y, Tang X-L, Manchikalapudis S, Cao X, Bolli R. Ischemic preconditioning induces selective translocation of protein kinase C isoforms ε and η in the heart of conscious rabbits without subcellular redistribution of total protein kinase C activity. *Circ. Res.* 1997; **81**: 404.

19 Gray MO, Karliner JS, Mochly-Rosen D. A selective ε-protein kinase C antagonist inhibits protection of cardiac myocytes from hypoxia-induced cell death. *J. Biol. Chem.* 1997; **49**: 30945.

20 Dorn GW, Sourojon MC, Liron T, Chen CH, Gray MO, Zhou HZ, Csukai M, Wu G, Lorenz JN, Mochly-Rosen D. Sustained cardiac protection by a rationally designed peptide that causes ε protein kinase C translocation. *Proc. Natl. Acad. Sci. USA* 1999; **96**: 12798.

21 Miyamae M, Rodriguez MM, Camacho SA, Diamond I, Mochly-Rosen D, Figueredo VM. Activation of ε protein kinase C correlates with a cardioprotective effect of regular ethanol consumption. *Proc. Natl. Acad. Sci. USA* 1998; **95**: 8262.

22 Herbert JM, Augereau JM, Gleye J, Maffrand JP. Chelerythrine is a specific inhibitor of protein kinase C. *Biochem. Biophys. Res. Comm.* 1990; **172**: 993.

23 Zhou HZ, Dulbecco FL, Gray MO. Signaling pathways of cardiac preconditioning in a mouse model of ethanol consumption. *Circulation* 2000; **102** (Suppl. S): 1318.

24 Deng XF, Rokosh DG, Simpson PC. $α_1$-adrenergic receptor subtypes activate different PKC isoforms in mouse heart. *Circulation* 1999; **100**: I-566.

25 Khasar SG, Lin YH, Martin A, Dadgar J, McMahon T, Wang D, Hundle B, Aley KD, Isenberg W, McCarter G, Green PG, Hodge CW, Levine JD, Messing RO. A novel nociceptor signaling pathway revealed in protein kinase C ε mutant mice. *Neuron* 1999; **24**: 253.

26 Wu G, Wang Y, Jantz T, Canning AM, Robbins J, Mochly-Rosen D, Dorn GW. Attenuation of cardiac growth in transgenic mice expressing the PKCε inhibitory εV1 peptide. *Circulation* 1999; **100**: I-53.

27 Miyamae M, Camacho SA, Zhou HZ, Diamond I, Figueredo VM. Alcohol consumption reduces ischemia-reperfusion injury by species-specific signaling in guinea pigs and rats. *Am. J. Physiol.* 1998; **275**: H50.

28 Gray MO, Long CS, Kalinyak JE, Li HT, Karliner JS. Angiotensin II stimulates cardiac myocyte hypertrophy via paracrine release of TGF-$β1$ and endothelin-1 from fibroblasts. *Cardiovasc. Res.* 1998; **40**: 352.

29 Souroujon MC, Mochly-Rosen D. Peptide modulators of protein–protein interactions in intracellular signaling. *Nature Biotech.* 1998; **16**: 919.

30 Ron D, Luo J, Mochly-Rosen D. C2 region-derived peptides inhibit translocation and function of β protein kinase C *in vivo. J. Biol. Chem.* 1995; **270**: 24180.

31 Liu GS, Cohen MV, Mochly-Rosen D, Downey JM. Protein kinase C-ε is responsible for the protection of preconditioning in rabbit cardiomyocytes. *J. Mol. Cell. Cardiol.* 1999; **31**: 1937.

32 Chen CH, Gray MO, Mochly-Rosen D. Cardioprotection from ischemia by a brief exposure to physiological levels of ethanol: role of epsilon protein kinase C. *Proc. Natl. Acad. Sci. USA* 1999; **96**: 12784.

33 Ping P, Zhang J, Cao X, Li RCX, Kong D, Tang XL, Qiu Y, Manchikalapudi S, Auchampach JA, Black RG, Bolli R. PKC dependent activation of p44/p42 MAPKs during myocardial ischemia-reperfusion in conscious rabbits. *Am. J. Physiol.* 1999; **276**: H1468.

34 Ping P, Zhang J, Huang S, Cao X, Tang XL, Li RCX, Zheng YT, Qiu Y, Clerk A, Sugden P, Han J, Bolli R. PKC-dependent activation of p46/p54 JNKs during ischemic preconditioning in conscious rabbits. *Am. J. Physiol.* 1999; **277**: H1771.

35 Ping P, Zhang J, Zheng YT, Li RCX, Dawn B, Takano H, Balafanova Z, Bolli R. Demonstration of selective protein kinase C-dependent activation of Src and Lck tyrosine kinases during ischemic preconditioning in conscious rabbits. *Circ. Res.* 1999; **85**: 542.

36 Csukai M, Chen CH, De Matteis MA, Mochly-Rosen D. Coatomer protein β'-COP, a selective binding protein (RACK) for epsilon protein kinase C. *J. Biol. Chem.* 1997; **272**: 29200.

37 Paucek P, Mironova G, Mahdi F, Beavis A, Woldegiorgis G, Garlid K. Reconstitution and partial purification of the glibenclamide-sensitive ATP-dependent K^+ channel from rat liver and beef heart mitochondria. *J. Biol. Chem.* 1992; **267**: 26062.

38 Holmuhamedov E, Jovanovic S, Dzeja P, Jovanovic A, Terzic A. Mitochondrial ATP-sensitive K^+ channels modulate cardiac mitochondrial function. *Am. J. Physiol.* 1998; **275**: H1567.

39 Liu Y, Sato T, O'Rourke B, Marban E. Mitochondrial ATP-dependent potassium channels: novel effectors of cardioprotection? *Circulation* 1998; **97**: 2463.

40 Wang Y, Hirai K, Ashraf M. Activation of mitochondrial ATP-sensitive K^+ channel for cardiac protection against ischemic injury is dependent on protein kinase C activity. *Circ. Res.* 1999; **85**: 731.

41 Wang Y, Ashraf M, Role of protein kinase C in mitochondrial K_{ATP} channel-mediated protection against Ca^{2+} overload injury in rat myocardium. *Circ. Res.* 1999; **84**: 1156.

42 Fryer RM, Eells JT, Hsu AK, Henry MM, Gross GJ. Ischemic preconditioning in rats: role of mitochondrial K_{ATP} channel in preservation of mitochondrial function. *Am. J. Physiol.* 2000; **278**: H305.

43 Sato T, O'Rourke B, Marban E. Modulation of mitochondrial ATP-dependent K^+ channels by protein kinase C. *Circ. Res.* 1998; **83**: 110.

44 Zhang J, Bolli R, Lalli J, Tang XL, Li RCX, Zheng Y, Pass J, Ping P. Ischemic preconditioning and phorbol ester redistribute protein kinase C ε to the nucleus, sarcolemmal membranes, and mitochondria in rabbit myocardium. *Circulation* 1999; **100**: I-325.

45 Zhou P, Zhou HZ, Gray MO. Mitochondrial K-ATP channel activation is necessary for chronic cardiac preconditioning in a rat model of moderate alcohol consumption. *Circulation* 2000; **102** (Suppl. S): 1410.

Chapter 11

Alcohol and smoking: synergism in heart disease?

Jin Zhang and Ronald Watson

INTRODUCTION

It is well known that cigarette smoking is a strong risk factor for developing cardiovascular disease (CVD) [1]. Moderate wine drinking has cardioprotective effects while alcohol abuse causes cardiomyopathy, hypertension and stroke in most cases. Epidemiologic studies suggest that current and former alcoholic adults are at greater risk for some deleterious health effects of smoking, particularly cancer and cardiovascular disease, than are members of the general smoking and nonsmoking populations. More alcoholics die from tobacco-related diseases than from alcoholism [2]. Although many studies have found individual effects of tobacco smoke or alcohol in promoting cardiovascular disease, few studies have investigated the synergisms during concomitant use of alcohol and tobacco. It is really very complicated and conditional since it depends on the dosage and types of alcohol and tobacco use, as well as other aspects of health condition. Most heavy alcohol users also smoke or have smoked superfrequently.

CIGARETTE SMOKING AND CARDIOVASCULAR DISEASE

Cigarette smoking-related cardiovascular diseases have been described widely. However, the mechanisms of their effects on cardiovascular system were not totally clear. The effects of nicotine and carbon monoxide on blood vessel walls, unfavorable lipid profiles, increased myocardial work and the decreased oxygen carrying capacity of the blood of smokers contribute to the overall effect of cigarette smoking on cardiovascular disease [3]. Of the increased cardiovascular risk caused by smoking, it is estimated that approximately one-tenth of this is due to smoking-induced changes in serum lipid [4]. The majority of studies indicate elevations in serum cholesterol, phospholipids, triglycerides, low-density lipoprotein (LDL) and increased hepatic lipase activity in smokers, with decreased serum high-density lipoprotein (HDL) cholesterol [5].

A mechanism to explain the link between smoking and some of the observed changes in serum lipid and lipoprotein concentrations includes the pharmacological effects of nicotine in stimulating sympathetic nervous activity and release of catecholamines. Catecholamines mediate lipolysis, causing an increase in plasma concentrations of free fatty acids and very low-density lipoprotein triglycerides. Free fatty acids stimulate hepatic secretion of very low-density lipoprotein and hence triglycerides and high-density lipoprotein concentrations vary inversely with low-density lipoprotein concentrations in serum [6]. On the other hand, smokers had higher levels of fibrinogen, plasminogen activator inhibitor 1 (PAI-1) activity and fasting and steady-state C-peptide levels during the clamp. They also showed insulin resistance and lipid intolerance with an impaired triglyceride clearance after a mixed test meal. Insulin resistance is an important reason for promoting the increased cardiovascular morbidity in smokers [7].

Of thousands of cigarette smoke compounds, many are capable of generating reactive oxygen species (ROS) during metabolism. ROS can initiate a serial of cellular responses, such as activation of nuclear factor kappa B (NF-κB), which plays an important role in the proinflammatory process. NF-κB can induce IL-1 beta, platelet-activating factor (PAF) and tumor necrosis factor (TNF) [8]. IL-1 beta is well known as an inducer of several other proinflammatory enzymes such as the inducible cyclooxygenase-2 (COX-2); PAF is shown to benefit platelet aggregation. These are two factors involved in atherogenesis [9]. TNF may decrease myocardial contraction through enhancing inducible nitric oxide synthase (iNOS) and nitric oxide (NO) production or by inducing myocardial apoptosis [10].

In addition, cigarette smoking is associated with unhealthy eating patterns, including increased intakes of alcohol, total fat, cholesterol, saturated fat, a lower consumption of foods with fibers such as fruits and vegetables that may lower cholesterol levels, as well as deficiencies of vitamin C, E and beta-carotene [11,12]. These factors make smokers and heavy alcohol users more predisposed to cardiovascular disease.

CARDIOPROTECTIVE EFFECT OF MODERATE WINE DRINKING

There is evidence that moderate wine consumption protects against CAD. Two studies linked the beneficial effects of moderate drinking only to wine [13,14]. Red wine contains several flavonoids and phenolic compounds with significant antioxidant properties. The protection effects against atherogenesis suggested that antioxidants in wine might play a role through modification of LDLs [15]. However, it seems unlikely that the cardioprotective effects are due solely to the antioxidant properties of these compounds, since the orally ingested phenolic antioxidants may not reach sufficiently high plasma levels to affect the oxidizability of LDL in humans [16]. Moreover, the majority of epidemiological studies have shown that all alcohol beverage types (beer, wine, and distilled spirits) confer some cardioprotective effects [17].

What is the mechanism of alcohol cardioprotection? The beneficial effects of moderate drinking have been addressed on factors involved in atherogenesis [17]. First of all, alcohol increases plasma HDL level and activity of lipoprotein lipase, which showed an inverse relationship with the risk of CAD. Secondly, in animal models, ethanol reduced atherogenic plaques by influencing the inflammatory process of endothelial lesions. Alcohol interferes with the expression of vascular adhesion molecules such as VCAM-1 and ICAM-1 by inhibiting the transcription factor NF-κB [18]. Additionally, inhibition of the enzyme HMG-CoA reductase, a key enzyme in the synthesis of cholesterol, results in the reduction of plasma cholesterol. Furthermore alcohol has antithrombotic effects which could contribute to its cardioprotective effects. Possible factors responsible for the effects of moderate alcohol consumption on clotting include an increase in the prostacyclin/thromboxane ratio, decreased platelet aggregability in response to most agonists, increased release of plasminogen activator, and lowered fibrinogen levels [19]. Certainly, some alcoholic drinks, especially wine, supply phytochemical isoflavenoids, vitamins which have powerful antioxidant effects. These effects include inhibition of low-density lipoprotein oxidation as well as reduction in coagulation and improved thrombolysis. Most importantly, the beneficial protective effects of a moderate alcohol intake are found only in non-smokers [20].

ALCOHOL ABUSE AND CARDIOVASCULAR DISEASE

Although there is considerable evidence that moderate drinking protects against mortality and morbidity from coronary heart disease [21,22], heavy consumption is shown to have deleterious cardiovascular effects. It exerts its adverse effects by increasing the risks of cardio-myopathy, hypertension, and stroke [23]. Chronic ethanol consumption has been linked to the prevalence of hypertension, which contributes to an increased incidence of stroke. Heavy drinkers have a 10 mmHg higher systolic blood pressure than non-drinkers even though the relationship may differ between men and women [24]. Stroke is a leading cause of death and morbidity. Alcohol may increase the risk of stroke through various mechanisms that include hypertension, hypercoagulable states, cardiac arrhythmias, and cerebral blood flow reductions [25]. Hypertension, including borderline hypertension, is probably the most important stroke risk factor based on degree of risk and prevalence. Furthermore, cardiac morbidity, cigarette smoking, diabetes, physical inactivity, and high levels of alcohol consumption are also strongly related to stroke risk [26]. Recently, chronic consumption of alcohol has proven detrimental to heart tissue and can lead to alcohol-induced heart muscle disease, a major cause of non-ischemic cardio-myopathy in Western society [27]. Alcohol-induced heart muscle disease yields abnormal contractile function and energy metabolism, sometimes resulting in arrhythmias, cardiomegaly, and congestive heart failure. A molecular mechanism underlying observed alcohol-induced heart failure is a nonoxidative pathway for alcohol metabolism in several target tissues including heart. Normally the mitochondria manufactures most of the cell's energy ATP via the tricarboxylic acid cycle (TCA cycle), beta-oxidation of fatty acids and oxidative phosphorylation. The very high-energy require-ments of heart muscle are mostly met by beta-oxidation of fatty acids. Fatty acids bound to albumin or from chylonmicrons and very low-density lipoproteins enter the myocyte where they are converted to acetyl CoA through beta-oxidation in the mitochondria matrix. Acetyl CoA then enters the TCA cycle. The products of TCA cycle will enter the electron transport chain of the inner mitochondrial membrane, where most of the cell's ATP is produced. In alcoholics, it turns out that nonesterified fatty acids are esterified with ethanol to produce fatty acid ethyl esters (FAEEs), which can attach to mitochondria and uncouple oxidative phosphorylation and disrupt the energy process. Furthermore, electron-microscopic and histochemical analysis have revealed shrunken, disorganized myocytes, loss of myofibrils, a dilated and disordered sarcoplasmic reticulum, excessive accumulation of lipids, and enlarged mitochondria with chaotic cristae. It has also been indicated that chronic alcohol adminis-tration decreases activity of the Na^-K^+-ATPase pump that functions in providing the necessary ionic concentrations for membrane potentials needed for cardiac muscle contrac-tion. In animal models, several weeks of chronic alcohol consumption by rats demonstrated in the myocytes a leaky sarcolemma and increases in cardiac intracellular calcium [28].

Similarly, in the alcoholic person ethanol represents on the average 50% of the total dietary energy intake [24]. Consequently, alcohol consumption displaces many normal nutri-ents of the diet, resulting in primary malnutrition and associated symptomatology, foremost that of folate, thiamine and other vitamin B deficiencies. As alcohol impairs the activation and utilization of nutrients, secondary malnutrition may result from either maldigestion or malabsorption caused by gastrointestinal complications associated with alcoholism, mainly pancreatic insufficiency. In the absence of severe liver injury, high alcohol intake results in increased levels of HDL, primarily HDL_2, but at that level of alcohol intake there is no evidence of 'protection' against CHD. While alcohol consumption is associated with severe liver disease, levels of the HDL fractions decrease. Thus, with higher alcohol intakes, adverse effects predominate.

THE CO-EFFECT OF ALCOHOL AND TOBACCO SMOKING

Alcoholics are commonly heavy smokers. There is a synergistic effect of alcohol consumption and smoking on cancer development, with long term ethanol consumption enhancing the mutagenicity of tobacco-derived product [24]. The combined ingestion of ethanol resulted in a significant formation of smoke-related DNA adducts in the esophagus and in their further, dramatic increase in the heart. Thus ethanol consumption increases the bioavailability of DNA binding of smoke components in the upper digestive tract and favors their systemic distribution. Formation of DNA adducts in the organs examined may be relevant in the pathogenesis of lung and esophageal cancers as well as in the pathogenesis of other types of chronic degenerative diseases, such as chronic obstructive pulmonary diseases and cardio-myopathies [29].

Numerous studies have indicated a correlation between ethanol intake and cigarette smoking in heavy drinkers [30]. On a pharmacological basis, an ethanol-induced potentiation of nicotinic currents may enhance the acute positive reinforcement associated with nicotine, increasing tobacco use during heavy ethanol intake. Ethanol may enhance acute nicotine-mediated receptor activation. Moreover, the opposing effect of ethanol on nicotine-induced desensitization could account for the increased tobacco use observed with excessive drinking. The dose relationship between the combined use of these two social habits and the changes in serum lipids, including high-density lipoprotein cholesterol (HDL-C), low-density lipo-protein cholesterol (LDL-C) and triglycerides, has been investigated [31]. Both social habits raised serum cholesterol levels in a dose-related manner; the more cigarettes a subject smokes and the more alcohol consumed, the higher the total serum cholesterol [31].

SUMMARY

Both cigarette smoking and alcohol drinking are involved in lipid metabolism and pro-inflammatory response. They are also related to unhealthy eating patterns. Alcohol abuse can promote the formation of smoke-related DNA adducts distributed in organs including the heart, which may be responsible for cardiomyopathies. Furthermore, ethanol intake has a correlation with nicotine addictive.

In conclusion, the abstinence of cigarette smoking should always be appropriated for prevention of heart disease. Moderate alcohol drinking may be helpful for protection of the heart. However, individuals must astain under special circumstances such as pregnancy or severe liver disorders. Cigarette smoking along with heavy alcohol drinking must be discouraged, since it is hard to prevent their adverse effects through nutritional manipulation. As there is limited research on the co-effect of alcohol and smoking on CVD, advanced studies should be done in the future with the pathway of these two factors interacting in the pathogenesis of heart disease.

ACKNOWLEDGMENT

This work was supported by NIH grant HL 63667.

REFERENCES

1 Bottcher M, Falk E. Pathology of the coronary arteries in smokers and non-smokers. *J. Cardiovas. Risk* 1999; **6**: 299–302.

2 Abrams DB, Monti PM, Niaura RS, Rohsenow DJ, Colby SM. Interventions for alcoholics who smoke. *Alcohol Health & Research World* 1996; **20**: 111–117.

3 Mitchell BE, Sobel HL, Alexander MH. The adverse health effects of tobacco and tobacco-related products, Primary Care. *Clinics in Office Practice* 1999; **26**: 463–498.

4 Craig WY, Palomaki GE, Haddow JE. Cigarette smoking and serum lipid and lipoprotein concentrations: An analysis of published data. *BMJ* 1989; **298**: 784–788.

5 Terry ML, Berkowitz HD, Kerstein MD. Tobacco: its impact on vascular disease. *Surg. Clin. N. Amer.* 1998; **78**: 409–429.

6 Muscat JE, Harris RE, Haley NJ, Wynder EL. Cigarette smoking and plasma cholesterol. *Am. Heart J.* 1991; **121**: 141–147.

7 Eliasson B, Mero N, Taskinen MR, Smith U. The insulin resistance syndrome and postprandial lipid intolerance in smokers. *Atherosclerosis* 1997; **129**: 79–88.

8 Grimble RF. Modification of inflammatory aspects of immune function by nutrients. *Nutr. Res.* 1998; **18**: 1297–1317.

9 Bkaily G, Dorleans-Juste P. Cytokine-induced free radical and their roles in myocardial dysfunctions. *Cardiovas. Res.* 1999; **42**: 576–577.

10 Ferrsri. The role of TNF in cardiovascular disease. *Pharmacol. Res.* 1999; **40**: 97–105.

11 Dallongevile J, Marecaux N, Fruchart JC. Cigarette smoking is associated with unhealthy patterns of nutrient intake: A meta-analysis. *J. Nutr.* 1998; **128**: 1450.

12 Henningfield JE, Stapleton JM, Benowitz NL. Higher levels of nicotine in arterial than in venous blood after cigarette smoking. *Drug Alcohol Depend.* 1993; **33**: 23.

13 Gronbaek M, Deis A, Sorensen TL. Mortality associated with moderate intakes of wine, beer, or spirits. *BMJ* 1995; **310**: 1165–1169.

14 St. Leger AS, Cochrane AL, Moore F. Factors associated with cardiac mortality in developed countries with particular reference to the consumption of wine. *Lancet* 1979; **1**: 1017–1020.

15 Witzum JL, Steinberge D. Role of oxidized low density lipoprotein in atherogenesis. *J. Clin. Invest.* 1991; **88**: 1785–1792.

16 DeRojke YB, Demacker PNM, Assen NA. Red wine consumption does not effect oxidizability of low-density lipoproteins in volunteers. *Am. J. Clin. Nutr.* 1996; **63**: 329–334.

17 Zakhari S, Gordis E. Moderate drinking and cardiovascular health. *Proceed. Assoc. Amer. Phys.* 1999; **111**: 148–158.

18 Zakhari S. Szabo G. NF-kappa B, a prototypical cytokine-regulated transcription factor: Implications for alcohol-mediated responses. *Alcohol Clin. Exp. Res.* 1996; **20**: 236A–242A.

19 Eagles CJ, Martin U. Non-pharmacological modification of cardiac risk factors: part 3. Smoking cessation and alcohol consumption. *J. Clin. Pharm. Therap.* 1998; **23**: 1–9.

20 Choudhury SR, Ueshima H, Kita Y, Kobayashi KM, Okayama A, Yamakawa M. Alcohol intake and serum lipids in a Japanese population. *Int. J. Epidemiol.* 1994; **23**: 940–947.

21 Coate D. Moderate drinking and coronary heart disease mortality: Evidence from NHANES I and the NHANES I follow-up. *Am. J. Publ. Health* 1993; **83**: 888–890.

22 Moore RD, Pearson TA. Moderate alcohol consumption and coronary artery disease: A review. *Medicine* 1986; **65**: 242–267.

23 Lands WEM, Zakhari S. Alcohol use as a secondary cause of hypertension. *Mil. Med.* 1988; **153**: 250–251.

24 Charles S. Lieber Hepatic and other medical disorders of alcoholism: from pathogenesis to treatment. *J. Stud. Alcohol* 1998; **59**: 9–25.

25 Sacco RL. Risk factors, outcomes, and stroke subtypes for ischemic stroke. *Neurology* 1997; **49**: PS039–PS044.

26 Sacco RL, Wolf PA, Gorelick PB. Risk factors and their management for stroke prevention: Outlook for 1999 and beyond. *Neurology* 1999; **53**: S15–S24.

27 Beckemeier ME, Bora PS. Fatty Acid Ethyl Esters: Potentially Toxic Products of Myocardial Ethanol Metabolism. *J. Mol. Cell. Cardiology* 1998; **30**(11): 2487–2494.

28 Noren GR, Stanley NA, Einzig S, Mikell FL, Asinger RW. Alcohol-induced congestive cardio-myopathy: an animal model. *Cardiovasc. Res.* 1983; **17**: 81–87.

29 Izzotti A, Balansky RM, Blagoeva PM, Mircheva ZI, Tulimiero L, Cartiglia C, De Flora S. DNA alterations in rat organs after chronic exposure to cigarette smoke and/or ethanol ingestion. *FASEB Journal* 1998; **12**(9): 753–758.

30 Marszalec W, Aistrup GL, Narahashi T. Ethanol-nicotine interactions at alpha-bungarotoxin-insensitive nicotinic acetylcholine receptors in rat cortical neurons. *Alcohol Clin. Exp. Res.* 1999; **23**: 439–445.

31 Whitehead TP, Robinson D. Allaway SL. The effects of cigarette smoking and alcohol consumption on blood lipids: a dose-related study on men. *Ann. Clin. Biochem.* 1996; **33**: 99–106.

Chapter 12

Oxidative stress, cell damage and its possible prevention by alpha-tocopherol: cardiovascular and other cells

Victor R. Preedy and Helmut Seitz

INTRODUCTION

In this review, we briefly describe the nature and origins of free radicals, and how these species cause intracellular damage, especially during ethanol metabolism. We then describe how alpha-tocopherol (ATC) has been employed in both experimental and clinical studies to reverse or ameliorate free radical-induced tissue damage in a variety of disorders. Most recent research data has focussed on the effects of ATC on the cardiovascular system, but as this review will illustrate, ATC has also been reported to have a protective role in diseases affecting a variety of tissues, including neurological disorders [1–6]. Thus, ATC can prevent cellular damage induced by exposure of rat cerebellar granule cells to cholesterol oxides *in vitro* [7]. However, the relationship between ATC intake, overall antioxidant intake and diet quality is complex, for example being related to social class [8], dietary intake of milk and fruit sugar [9], body mass index (BMI) and fat intake [10]. Life-style habits such as smoking also influence ATC status [11], although some studies (with small numbers of observations) have shown no correlation [12]. Studies on vitamin supplementation in the elderly have also shown that the physically active are more likely to take ATC (along with vitamin C and calcium) than their non-physically active counterparts [13]. Overall, the data on the potential therapeutic benefits of ATC intake suggest that even though it can increase anti-oxidant capacity and reduce lipid peroxidation *in vitro*, it may not halt disease progression or influence indices of tissue pathology in all instances. These conflicting findings probably reflect the fact that major diseases have complex etiologies in which free radical damage and/or changes in antioxidant status may represent only a single facet of the disease process. In many studies, alterations in free radical levels and/or scavenging antioxidants are measured without consideration of their functional effects. For example, dietary selenium deficiency reduces muscle glutathione peroxidase activity, but has no appreciable effects on endurance capacity in exercise, which triggers an increase in the generation of ROS [14]. We therefore conclude that the therapeutic role of this antioxidant is currently equivocal.

In the ensuing review, ATC is used synonymously with vitamin E unless specific distinction has been made between the tocopherol isomers. We propose that knowledge gained from understanding the effects and role of ATC in a variety of tissues and disease processes may be useful in devising novel therapeutic strategies, such as ameliorating the effects of excessive (i.e., greater than the moderate amounts deemed to be cardioprotective) alcohol intake on the cardiovascular system.

FREE RADICALS AND ANTIOXIDANTS

Free radicals are highly reactive transient chemical species characterized by the presence of unpaired electrons usually denoted by a point suffix ($^{\bullet}$). They are involved in a variety of metabolic and pathophysiological processes including both beneficial and detrimental reactions. They can be produced as by-products of normal metabolism, for example, in the mitochondrial electron transport system [15]. In biological systems, free radicals may be typically centered on oxygen, nitrogen, carbon or sulfur atoms. Biologically important free radicals include superoxide ($O_2^{-\bullet}$), hydroxyl ($OH^{\bullet}$), alkoxyl ($RO^{\bullet}$) and peroxyl ($RO_2^{\bullet}$) radicals and nitric oxide (Table 12.1). Hydrogen peroxide (H_2O_2) is an oxidizing species and potential source of free radicals, but is not classified as a free radical since it contains no unpaired electrons; the species $O_2^{-\bullet}$, $OH^{\bullet}$ $RO^{\bullet}$, $RO_2^{\bullet}$ and H_2O_2 are therefore conveniently classed as reactive oxygen species (ROS). In general, free radicals are continuously formed in all cells as unwanted (and potentially damaging) by-products of normal aerobic metabolism. In some instances they may perform beneficial actions e.g., $O_2^{-\bullet}$ generation during phagocytic action, and Nitric Oxide in the regulation of vascular tone. However, the beneficial effects are comparatively few compared to the damaging effects of ROS. Included in the category of ROS are singlet oxygen ($^1O_2$), ozone (O_3) [16]. Nitric oxide ($NO^{\bullet}$) is also a free radical and grouped with peroxynitrite ($ONOO^-$) and nitrogen dioxide radical ($NO_2^{\bullet}$) as reactive nitrogen species (RNS:[16]). A principal source of $O_2^{-\bullet}$ generation results from the leakage of electrons from the mitochondrial respiratory chain. It has been reported that the mitochondrial electron transport system utilizes 85% of the oxygen used by cells and 5% of oxygen consumed by mitochondria are converted to ROS [15]. In addition, $O_2^{-\bullet}$ are generated via the actions of various oxidase enzymes (e.g., xanthine oxidase, monoamine oxidase, etc.). The main source of $OH^{\bullet}$ (the most reactive of biological free radical speciess) results from the interaction of H_2O_2 and $O_2^{-\bullet}$ or H_2O_2 with metal ions, such as Fe^{2+} or Cu^{2+}, in the Fenton reaction: ($Fe^{2+}+H_2O_2 \rightarrow Fe^{3+}+OH^{\bullet}+OH^-$). Normally, Fe^{2+} or Cu^{2+} are sequestered by binding proteins *in vivo*. DNA, proteins and lipids are potential biomolecular targets for free radical attack, with lipids being particularly susceptible to peroxidative chain reactions, resulting in damage to cell membranes and subcellular organelles.

Cells are protected from free radical induced damage by a variety of free radical scavenging antioxidants. Antioxidants enzymes, which are capable of eliminating free radical species that cause tissue damage, include catalase, glutathione peroxidase and superoxide dismutase (also termed preventative antioxidants [17]). Thus, with regards the enzyme superoxide dismutase: ($2O_2^{\bullet}+2H^+\rightarrow H_2O_2+O_2$). The hydrogen peroxide generated in this or other reactions can be converted into water and oxygen ($2H_2O_2 \rightarrow 2H_2O+O_2$) via catalase, whilst glutathione peroxidase reduces peroxides ($ROOH+2GSH\rightarrow ROH+H_2O+GSSG$). These

Table 12.1 Reactive oxygen species

Superoxide radical $O_2^{-\bullet}$
Singlet oxygen $^1O_2$
Hydrogen peroxide H_2O_2
Hypochlorous acid $HOCl$
Alkoxyl radicals $RO^{\bullet}$
Peroxyl radicals $RO_2^{\bullet}$
Hydroxyl radical $OH^{\bullet}$

Source: Adapted from [228].

enzymatic reactions contrast with the non-enzyme antioxidants such as urate, biothiols such as glutathione, reduced coenzyme Q_{10}, ascorbate, carotenoids, flavonoids, lycopenes and the tocopherols which have chain-breaking or radical trapping properties and may also be capable of directly repairing anti-oxidants [17]. Some plasma proteins such as ferritin and albumin can also be considered as antioxidants as they bind metal ions such as Fe^{2+} and Cu^{2+} thereby minimizing the potential for $OH^\bullet$ generation. Histidine-containing peptides, such as the imidazole dipeptides carnosine, histidine and anserine, are also important anti-oxidants especially in muscle-containing tissues, possibly via mechanisms involving metal ion-chelation or free radical scavenging [18]. Lipids are major components in a variety of cells and organelles and for this reason adverse lipid peroxidation can be deleterious, leading to structure and functional abnormalities. Target organelle includes mitochondrion, lysosome or the sarcolemma, with implications for membrane permeability or fragility [19].

PRODUCTION OF REACTIVE OXYGEN SPECIES DURING ETHANOL METABOLISM

Most of the data available with respect to the production of ROS following ethanol administration have been obtained from studies in hepatic tissue. However, since many of the enzymes responsible for ethanol metabolism are also present in extrahepatic tissues such as the gastrointestinal mucosa, ROS can also be produced in these tissues. In the liver, alcohol consumption increases the amount of reactive oxygen species by several mechanisms:

(1) Cytochrome P450 2E1
(2) Mitochondria
(3) Xanthine oxidase and aldehyde oxidase
(4) Kupffer cells

Cytochrome P450 2E1

Alcohol consumption results in an induction of cytochrome P450 2E1 associated with enhanced activity of NADPH oxidase which leads to an extensive production of $O_2^{-\bullet}$ and H_2O_2 [20,21]. Microsomes obtained from chronically ethanol fed rats are more active in producing $O_2^{-\bullet}$, H_2O_2 and $OH^\bullet$ compared to microsomes from control animals [22]. These microsomes have an enhanced susceptibility to lipid peroxidation. This can be completely blocked by antibodies acting against cytochrome P450 2E1 [21]. NADH can replace NADPH as a cofactor in the microsomal reaction. This is important, since during ethanol oxidation NADH is produced in excess. In human hepatic microsomes, there is a significant correlation between cytochrome P450 2E1 content and NADPH oxidase activity [23].

The metabolism of ethanol via cytochrome P450 2E1 leads to the production of 1-hydroxyethyl free radical intermediates [24,25]. Increased production of cytochrome P450 2E1 enhances the production of hydroxyethyl radicals and antibodies against cytochrome P450 2E1 inhibit the production of these radicals [26]. In this context, it is of considerable importance that levels of cytochrome P450 2E1 and the capacity of microsomes to generate hydroxyethyl radicals correlate significantly when human hepatic microsomes are investigated. In addition to the cytochrome P450-dependent pathway, ethanol can be oxidized by liver microsomes to acetaldehyde through a non-enzymatic pathway involving the presence of hydroxyl radicals (OH•) originating from iron catalyzed degradation of H_2O_2 [22].

Mitochondria

Acute alcohol exposure increases superoxide production in the respiratory chain of mitochondria, which may be responsible for the damage to this subcellular organelle during alcohol consumption [27]. When hepatic mitochondria from chronically ethanol fed rats are incubated with NADH or NADPH *in vitro*, an increased production of ROS is observed [27]. It is noteworthy that ethanol stimulates the activity of rotenone-insensitive NADH cytochrome C-reductase, an enzyme of the outer mitochondrial membrane [28].

Xanthine and aldehyde oxidase

A variety of studies have shown that acute and chronic ethanol administration favors the conversion of xanthine dehydrogenase to xanthine oxidase [29,30]. This is supported by the observation that alcohol administration also leads to an increased formation of xanthine and hypoxanthine because of enhanced purine degradation via xanthine oxidase. In this context, it is important to note that allopurinol, an inhibitor of xanthine oxidase, also inhibits lipid peroxidation in the liver of ethanol-treated rats [31]. Xanthine oxidase and aldehyde oxidase metabolizes acetaldehyde with the formation of ROS. The importance of these enzymes with respect to acetaldehyde metabolism is still a matter of debate, although it has been shown that low acetaldehyde concentrations of 100 μM can induce the formation of ROS by xanthine oxidase [32]. Also, molybdenum containing aldehyde oxidase can produce superoxide anions and it is reported that its inhibition leads to decreased lipid peroxidation in the liver [33]. A novel radical has been identified during acetaldehyde oxidation by xanthine oxidase, namely methylcarbonyl species which covalently bind to proteins. This may stimulate antibody production triggered by acetaldehyde alkylation, similar to the effects of the hydroxyethyl radical [34].

In the isolated perfused canine pancreas exposed to acetaldehyde, ROS produced via the activity of xanthine oxidase might be responsible for pancreatic injury [35].

Kupffer cells

Acute ethanol administration stimulates the production of superoxide anions in the perfused rat liver [36]. Studies in rats and mice suggest that Kupffer cells may be involved in this production of free radicals [37]. It seems that the release of arachidonic acid metabolites is necessary to activate Kupffer cells by ethanol since inhibition of cyclooxygenase by ibuprofen inhibits superoxide anion production [36].

Ethanol induces the generation of a chemotactic factor for phagocytes which is formed in rat hepatocytes exposed to alcohol [38–41]. This requires free iron and depends on the oxidation of unsaturated lipids by ROS generated during acetaldehyde metabolism due to aldehyde oxidase or xanthine oxidase activities [41]. Other studies have demonstrated that protein-derived and leucotriene-derived chemotactic factors are also produced by liver cells [42,43].

It is also important to note that alcohol interferes with the expression of leukocyte adhesion molecules by endothelial cells, underlining the fact that ethanol can directly stimulate granulocyte infiltration of the tissues where it is metabolized. Activated phagocytes may produce ROS and this may not only be important in the liver, but also in the gastrointestinal tract.

TISSUES IN WHICH FREE RADICALS HAVE BEEN IMPLICATED IN PATHOLOGY

From the aforementioned section, it is clear that hepatic tissue is affected by ROS (see for example [44–46]). However, it is important to point out that virtually every mammalian tissue has the potential to be adversely affected by free radical induced damage [47]. Target tissues for ROS-induced damage include the brain and nervous tissue [48–50], eye [51–54], gastrointestinal tract [55–57], heart [58], kidney [59–61], lungs [62–65] and testes and reproductive tissue [66]. For additional reviews on the pathogenic and chemical nature of ROS and ATC, see [16,17,67–75].

ALPHA-TOCOPHEROL

Vitamin E is a fat-soluble vitamin, and compared to other fat-soluble vitamins, appears to be the least toxic in high doses. There are 8 different homologues (i.e., vitamers) of vitamin E, comprising 4 tocopherols (namely, D-alpha, D-beta, D-gamma and D-delta) and 4 tocotrienols (also D-alpha, D-beta, D-gamma and D-delta) [76]. In broad terms, vitamin E is often used synonymously with alpha-tocopherol although strictly speaking it encompasses all 8 vitamers. The tocopherols and tocotrienols differ with respect to their side chain; the former is saturated whereas the latter is unsaturated. If the biological activity of alpha-tocopherol is assigned an arbitrary value of 1.00, then the beta, gamma and delta-tocopherols have a biological activity of 0.49, 0.1 and 0.03 respectively [76]. 1 mg of pure synthetic DL-alpha-tocopherol acetate has a relative biological activity of 0.76, compared to 1.03 for both D-alpha-tocopherol acetate and D-alpha-tocopherol succinate [76]. One international unit (IU) of alpha-tocopherol is equated with 1 mg of DL-alpha-tocopherol acetate. Thus, 1 mg of D-alpha-tocopherol is equivalent to 1.49 IU. In terms of molarity, the activity of D-alpha-, D-beta-, D-gamma- and D-delta-tocopherol are 642, 313, 63 and 20 IU/mmol [76]. Absorption of dietary alpha-tocopherol occurs via the lymphatic system though its efficiency is poor, in the region of 20–40% [76,77]. ATC is transported to the parenchymal cells of the liver via chylomicrons and then secreted via very low-density lipoprotein (VLDL) [77]. ATC-binding proteins may be involved in cellular accumulation within lipid membranes [78]. Uptake is also related to the accumulation of lipoproteins within tissues accounting for its differential uptake between different tissues in ATC dosage studies [79]. At the cellular level, incorporation of ATC directly into membranes of subcellular organelles may be responsible for its potential to confer protective properties such as its ability to reduce hydrogen peroxide generation by mitochondria [15]. Both bile and pancreatic secretions are necessary for absorption; hence, patients with biliary dysfunction have limited ability to absorb ATC.

ATC is able to prevent both the initiation and propagation of lipid peroxidation via scavenging free radicals. Two electrons are donated from each tocopherol molecule during its chain-breaking activities and it is probably recycled by ascorbate [17]. Further details on the energetics of membrane damage via the oxidation of polyunsaturated lipids have been described elsewhere [17]. Metabolites of ATC, i.e., alpha-tocopheryl quinone and hydro-quinone, are able to exert potent anti-oxidant activity, albeit in the presence of ATC [80]. Due to the practical difficulties involved in directly obtaining organ biopsies, plasma levels of ATC are frequently used to indirectly reflect tissue levels. It is important to note that with regards body distribution, the most abundant reservoir source of alpha-tocopherol is skeletal muscle by virtue of the fact that this organ is a major component of the body (i.e., contributing to 40% of body weight [81]). Highest concentrations are in adipose and adrenal tissue. ATC circulates in plasma bound to beta-lipoprotein and in red cells (20% of plasma level). Levels increase in hypothyroidism, diabetes mellitus and hypercholestero-laemia, and are reduced in liver disorders and malnutrition. Dietary requirements are in the order of 15–30 IU/day.

ALPHA-TOCOPHEROL AND ETHANOL CONSUMPTION

Chronic alcohol consumption produces an increased breakdown of lipid-soluble vitamins such as hepatic alpha-tocopherol, possibly secondary to a marked increase in the formation of hepatic alpha-tocopherol quinone, a metabolite of alpha-tocopherol formed by free radical reaction [82]. Since chronic ethanol consumption has been associated with compromised antioxidant status and an increase in lipid peroxidation, the significant decrease of vitamin E compared to other lipid-soluble antioxidants may contribute, at least in part, to enhanced hepatic lipid peroxidation seen in alcoholics. Besides vitamin E, other antioxidants such as vitamin C, glutathione and selenium are also strikingly decreased following chronic ethanol ingestion [83]. It is also interesting that chronic alcohol consumption significantly alters the distribution of alpha-tocopherol and gamma-tocopherol not only in hepatic tissue but in extrahepatic tissues as well [84].

ALCOHOLIC LIVER DISEASE: ROLE OF FREE RADICALS

A substantial body of evidence exists to support the contention that ROS generated during ethanol metabolism may be involved in the pathogenesis of alcoholic liver disease (ALD). Decades ago, it was already emphasized by Lieber that the induction of cytochrome P450 is a critical event with respect to the development of ALD [85]. If free radical production and lipid peroxidation play a role in the development of ALD, depletion of dietary antioxidants such as vitamin E or an increase in oxidants such as non-heme iron in the liver, should enhance the ethanol induced liver damage. Indeed, a diet deficient in vitamin E has been shown to reduce hepatic vitamin E stores, increase lipid peroxidation and increase serum transaminase activities after alcohol feeding in rats [86]. Furthermore, iron supplementation in the diet increases ethanol-induced serum transaminase activities, lipid peroxidation and fibrosis [41]. In addition, a significant correlation between hepatic lipid peroxidation, oxid-ative stress and hepatic morphology is observed with and without iron supplementation [87,88]. Part of the mechanism may be related to the ability of ethanol-derived metabolites such as malondialdehyde and 4-hydroxynonenal to directly stimulate Ito-cells to produce collagen [87]. Further evidence for the involvement of free radicals in alcoholic liver dis-ease is supported by the fact that drugs which are metabolized by cytochrome P450 2E1 to free radicals enhance ethanol-induced liver damage. This is seen with Isoniacide [89]. On the other hand, compounds which inhibit cytochrome P4502E1 such as chlomethiazol or diallyl sulfide [90,91], also inhibit lipid peroxidation, radical production and result in an improvement of hepatic morphology.

Obviously, the degree of induction of cytochrome P4502E1 is of predominant importance with respect to ALD. It is, therefore, concluded that the ROS produced by this pathway may be especially important. This induction is diet dependent and enhanced with unsaturated fatty acids such as corn oil and low carbohydrates. In addition, iron, an important compound in the production of ROS, plays a significant role. Iron supplementation increases liver disease and administration of an iron chelator decreases ALD.

Although, the administration of vitamin E to rodents inhibits ALD to some extent, data in humans are not very encouraging. The approach of administering vitamin E together with selenium and zinc to patients with alcoholic cirrhosis did show an improvement in mortality, but the number of patients was small [92].

PANCREAS

Injury to the pancreas has important metabolic consequences, due to its central role in endocrinological and nutritional homeostasis. Susceptibility of pancreatic tissue to damage by ROS may be due to the relatively low activities of endogenous antioxidant enzymes such as glutathione peroxidase, and comparatively low cellular levels of ATC [93]. Certainly, pancreatic islet cells are profoundly sensitive to vitamin E deficiency, as reflected by reduced Mn-superoxide dismutase and increased CuZn-superoxide dismutase activities, coupled with reduced insulin secretory function [94]. Pancreatic atrophy due to dietary selenium deficiency can be reversed by high-dose vitamin E supplementation [93].

Experimental pancreatic injury in laboratory animals induced by streptozotocin is a standard model of inducing diabetes. Streptozotocin-induced diabetes alters serum lipid profiles [95], increases markers of lipid peroxidation such as hepatic thiobarbituric acid reacting substances (TBARS) and conjugated dienes [96–99], and raises serum antibodies against MDA-protein adducts [95]. In streptozotocin-induced diabetes, treatment of rats with Vitamin E reduces blood glucose levels and reduces lipid peroxidation [98,99]. At the subcellular level, ATC supplementation improves the ability of hepatic mitochondria to withstand ROS-induced damage in streptozotocin-induced diabetic rats [100].

However, in diabetes, tissue damage is not solely confined to the pancreas, and affected tissues include the eye (both cornea as well as the retina [51]), and kidney [97]. Kidney malfunction in diabetes is associated with increased diacylglycerol concentration and protein kinase C activation combined with albuminuria [97]. Injection of ATC into streptozotocin-induced diabetic animals impedes these changes, with improved rates of glomerular filtration and urinary albumin excretion rates [97]. However, ATC supplementation, whilst increasing hepatic ATC content in mitochondria, does not increase kidney mitochondrial ATC [100], emphasizing the differential uptake of ATC by individual organs.

The therapeutic administration of ATC to diabetic patients has been proposed [101]. Thus, insulin sensitivity of skeletal muscle, a key feature of Type II diabetes, may be improved by ATC supplementation, as a consequence of its ability to increase diacylglycerol kinase, and reduce the phosphatidate phosphohydrolase activity via protein kinase C [97,102]. Studies have shown that ATC supplementation for 3 months in diabetic patients reduce plasma TBARS and lipid content [103]: improvements in glucose utilization and liver response to insulin in diabetic patients treated with ATC for 4 months have also been reported [104].

GASTROINTESTINAL TRACT (INCLUDING CARCINOGENESIS)

The role of ROS in alcohol-associated gastric mucosal injury is underlined by the fact that oral administration of absolute alcohol to rats reduces glutathione and increases lipid peroxidation in the gastric mucosa [105]. Antioxidants, superoxide dismutase and hydroxyl radical scavengers prevent gastric lesions caused by alcohol, whereas inhibition of superoxide dismutase results in a deterioration [105]. It is interesting to note that the pretreatment of rats with allopurinol, a xanthine oxidase inhibitor, protects against haemorrhagic lesions due to alcohol which points to the involvement of ROS produced by xanthine oxidase in the gastric mucosa [106,107]. However, controversial results have also been published by using a stomach perfusion model with 30% alcohol [108]. In any event, cellular glutathione levels are believed to be indicators of oxidative tissue injury and it has been shown in experimental animals as well as in humans that alcohol decreases gastric mucosal glutathione concentrations.

Chronic alcohol consumption is associated with an increased risk of cancer in the upper alimentary tract and the colorectum [109]. It might be possible that the production of ROS is involved in alcohol-associated carcinogenesis since chronic alcohol consumption leads to an induction of cytochrome P450 in the oral mucosa in the esophagus and in the colon of rodents [110,111]. Such an induction can also be demonstrated in the human oral mucosa [112]. In addition, the presence of xanthine oxidase has been located in the epithelial cells of the mouse and of the esophagus [113]. In an experiment by Eskelsson and co-workers, it has been shown that the number of esophageal tumors induced by nitrosamines and stimulated by chronic alcohol administration can be significantly reduced by the concomitant application of vitamin E [114]. Furthermore, this reduction is associated with a reduction in lipid peroxidation products in the esophagus. This is indirect evidence for the involvement of ROS in alcohol associated esophageal carcinogenesis.

Mucosal hyperproliferation due to alcohol is a premalignant condition and we have recently observed that vitamin E supplementation to rats leads to a normalization of colorectal cell regeneration [115]. Thus, there is some indirect evidence that vitamin E supplementation, at least in rodents, may be helpful in alcohol-associated cancer prevention.

LIPIDS AND CARDIOVASCULAR DISEASE

There are a substantial number of large epidemiological studies examining the relationship between dietary ATC intake and cardiovascular disease mortality (reviewed in [116–118]). For example, studies carried out two decades ago showed a correlation between higher than expected mortality and very low dietary ATC intakes (as well as with very high ATC intakes [119]). The basis of its cardioprotective effects is the ability of ATC to reduce damage caused by ROS in general, and specifically to inhibit the oxidation and MDA-modification of unsaturated lipids in low-density lipoprotein (LDL) particles [116,120,121]. These oxidized products of LDL are highly damaging and initiate the formation of atherosclerotic plaques and lesions and are related to the course of myocardial infarction [116,122]. However, atherosclerotic plaque formation and the mechanisms for the ensuing increased morbidity and mortality are complex processes, which involve, for example, the production of superoxide by monocytes, and the formation of autoantibodies against oxidized LDL and MDA-LDL [123,124]. In aortic muscle or endothelial cells *in vitro*, oxidized LDL can increase collagen and fibronectin synthesis, apoptosis, intracellular calcium and TBA formation [122,125]. Moreover, concomitant pathologies such as hypertension are additional risk factors for the etiology of atherosclerosis. For example, in hypertension, ATC status as reflected by red blood cell (but not plasma), concentrations is lower than that of normotensive controls [126]. Age-related reductions in the anti-oxidant capacity of plasma, acting against peroxyl radicals, may also contribute to the atherosclerosis [127]. There is also a tentative association between dietary ATC intake and increased (deemed to be cardioprotective) serum HDL-cholesterol [128].

Apoptosis induced in smooth muscle cells *in vitro* by oxidized-LDL can be prevented with anti-oxidants [122]. ATC and Trolox (a water-soluble form of ATC), but not alpha-tocopheryl acetate or alpha-tocopheryl succinate can ameliorate these adverse changes in the levels of TBARS and intracellular calcium [125]. More recently, the novel synthetic ATC-analogue IRFI005 (i.e., a metabolite of IRFI0016) has been shown to prevent the oxidation of LDL [129].

Monocytes are involved in the formation of atherosclerotic plaque and lesions via their ability to generate ROS (for example the superoxide radical) and cytokines such as interleukin (IL)-1beta [123,124]. ATC treatment of these cells prevents IL-1-beta formation (a cytokine involved in atherosclerosis), and superoxide and hydrogen peroxide production by monocytes *in vitro* when stimulated with lipopolysaccharide [123,124]. The mechanism of this protective effect appears to be related to the ability of ATC to inhibit protein kinase C activity [123]. Studies have also shown that alpha-tocopherol, but not beta-tocopherol, is able to reduce the activation of protein-kinase C by endothelin and thrombin [130].

The potential significance of these *in vitro* data needs to be discussed in relation to the prevention of atherosclerosis by ATC *in vivo*, although consideration need to be given to the possibility that other pharmacological preparations may be equally promising in reducing the oxidation of LDL. Such candidates include analogues of tetronic acid (for example 4-(4'-chloro-1,1'-biphenyl)-2-hydroxytetronic acid), which are able to inhibit hepatic membrane lipid peroxidation and LDL oxidation *in vitro* to a greater extent than Trolox [131]. Some authors have questioned whether blood levels of lipophilic antioxidants reflect the development of atherosclerosis [132]. In a comparison between patients with coronary heart disease and controls, gamma-tocopherol levels were significantly lower in patients with coronary heart disease, although in contrast no such differences were observed for ATC [132]. In other studies, patients with coronary artery disease (for example, angina or myocardial infarction) were shown to have lower serum ATC compared to healthy controls [133,134]. It is nevertheless important to consider that the defense against ROS is represented by a number of antioxidants. Thus, alpha- and beta-carotene levels are reduced in subjects with coronary heart disease, although levels of ubiquinol-10 are not [132]. In another study of 4,802 subjects aged between 55–95 years, the risk of myocardial infarction was higher in the low intake beta-carotene group although no association of myocardial infarction with ATC (and vitamin C) intake was observed [135]. In an earlier study, antioxidant levels were examined in a cohort of patients with coronary heart disease, which were subgrouped into those with *stable* and *unstable* angina pectoris [136]. Overall, these subjects had higher levels of cholesterol, LDL-cholesterol and lipoprotein(a) and lower HDL-cholesterol [136]. However, total plasma ATC was comparable in all three groups (control, stable angina and unstable angina), except when expressed per LDL particle, whereupon it was lower in patents with unstable angina pectoris. Values in patents with stable angina pectoris were higher than the latter, but lower than controls [136]. Thus, it seems that the type of cardiovascular disorder needs to be defined and careful attention needs to be paid as to how ATC levels are expressed. Internal factors relevant to the determination of ATC status include triglycerides and apoproteins [10]. However, geographical and cultural dietary habits further compound the relationship between ATC and the etiology of heart disease. Whole grain intake and nuts correlate negatively with coronary heart disease, which is not explained by the contribution of ATC (nor fiber, folate, vitamin B6) [137,138]. Another example pertains to phenolic compounds which occur in wine and appear to be able to increase plasma ATC levels and inhibit platelet aggregation [139,140]. Resveratrol, quercetin and other phenolic compounds, which are often found in alcoholic beverages (particularly red wine) and other foodstuffs are claimed to have antioxidant properties (which may be greater than ATC). This may contribute to the French Paradox in which there is a reduced risk of cardiovascular mortality due to moderate alcohol consumption [141–145]. However, many of the studies on the role of antioxidants in red wine in reducing LDL oxidation *in vivo* have been questioned [146]. In a controlled study of 25 subjects given either red or white wine for 4 weeks, susceptibly of LDL to oxidation *in vitro* was not altered and similar negative effects were obtained for levels of plasma ATC, urate, vitamin C, glutathione and ubiquinol-10 [146].

It is clear that some epidemiological studies show beneficial correlations between ATC intake and risk of cardiovascular disease, and laboratory studies demonstrate positive effects of ATC *in vivo* and *in vitro*. These data need to be interpreted in terms of potential therapeutic benefits of ATC supplementation, and its use to reduce overall mortality has been advocated [147]. Clinical studies have shown that oxidized serum lipids in patients with hypercholesterolemia can be ameliorated with ATC [120]. In the CHAOS (Cambridge Heart Antioxidant Study), 2,002 subjects with coronary atherosclerosis (confirmed angiographically) were shown to benefit from ATC supplementation, via a reduction in the incidence of non-fatal myocardial infarction, though an increase in overall mortality (not achieving significance) was reported [148]. In a study of 11,178 subjects aged between 67 and 105, ATC supplementation reduced overall mortality (relative risk: 0.66) and mortality due to coronary disease (relative risk of 0.37) [149]. In the GISSI (Gruppo Italiano per lo Studio della Sopravvivenza nell'Infarto miocardico) trial, over 11,000 subjects were recruited and supplemented with either n-3 polyunsaturated fatty acids, ATC, both ATC and n-3 polyunsaturated fatty acids, or none [150]. n-3 polyunsaturated fatty acids were found to be of benefit, in reducing mortality and cardiovascular death [150]. However, ATC conferred no such benefit and the combined n-3 polyunsaturated fatty acid and STC therapy was similar to n-3 polyunsaturated fatty acid alone [150]. Although, some of these large studies were negative in their findings, it is important to re-emphasize that ATC intake alone is not the only nutrient or factor that correlates with reduced incidence of coronary disease. For example, increasing intake of dietary fiber, independent of fat intake, correlates with reduced incidence of cardiovascular disease as does vitamin B6 and folate [151,152].

High fat or high-cholesterol containing diets are often used in animal studies to promote atherosclerosis, as a model for examining pathogenic mechanisms in the etiology of cardiovascular disease *in vivo*. Animal studies have shown that ATC supplementation in rabbits fed high cholesterol containing diets results in reduced blood cholesterol levels [153]. A combination of dietary ATC and selenium supplementation is effective in reducing athero-sclerotic lipid deposits in myocardial vessels, as well as blood markers of oxidative stress such as MDA [139,154]. Smooth muscle cells from aorta of cholesterol-fed rabbits have increased protein kinase C levels, which are not significantly ameliorated by ATC treatment [155].

Heart tissue is also impaired in diabetes, leading to contractile dysfunction that may also result from increased cardiac lipid peroxidation and altered fatty acid profiles [98,156].

STROKE

Some clinical studies have suggested that dietary ATC does not reduce the risk of stroke [157]. In the aforementioned study in the USA, 43,738 male subjects, (without cardiovascular disease or diabetes) aged from 40–75 years were examined, and after 8 years, 210 ischaemic strokes had occurred. However, the relative risk for ischaemic stroke in the group with the top quintile with highest ATC intake (median 411 IU/d) was 1.18 compared to the group with the lowest intake of ATC (5.4 IU/d), and there was no relation between the dose or duration of ATC and the risk for total or ischaemic stroke [157].

ALCOHOL AND THE HEART

Ethanol has important effects on the cardiovascular system and particularly on anti-oxidant systems (reviewed in [75,158]). Although the relative incidence of alcohol consumption reduces the overall risk of cardiovascular disease by a number of mechanisms (for example, increasing HDL/LDL ratio, reducing platelet function and aggregation [140,159]) excessive alcohol is damaging and can lead to the development of *alcoholic cardiomyopathy* [160–163]. Paradoxically, moderate alcohol consumption has been advocated to reduce the incidence of coronary artery disease, albeit within the confines of a multifactorial approach [147]. For example, an interaction between alcohol consumption and vitamin C has been proposed to account for the reduced incidence of angina in alcohol consumers [164].

The situation regarding ATC status in alcohol studies is confusing with some reports showing higher plasma ATC in average drinkers [165] whilst others have shown reduced levels in heavy drinkers [166,167].

Apart from functional impairment, myofibrillary damage is observed in alcoholic myopathy, ranging from small, localized areas of increased osmification to loss of subcellular architecture [168]. Increased lipid peroxidation suggests free radical-mediated damage may be involved in the etiology of alcoholic cardiomyopathy [169,170]. Increased myocardial lipopigmentation and diene conjugates are observed consistent with ROS-induced damage [171]. In animal studies, cardiac lipid peroxidation increases following alcohol dosage, as does the peroxidisability index of the cardiac phospholipids (PI) and the percent content of tri-, tetra-, and hexaenoic fatty acids [172–176]. Cardiac glutathione content is also reduced [173] although cardiac ATC has been reported to be unaltered in rats chronically administered alcohol [177].

Despite, the suggestion that alcohol-induced pathologies may in part be due to the effects of ROS and/or lipid peroxidation, there is surprisingly very little information on the therapeutic effects of ATC supplementation in alcohol-exposed hearts. ATC treatment has been shown to inhibit these changes in fatty acid profile and decrease oxidized lipids and diene conjugates in cardiac tissue [173,176]. In the latter studies, ethanol feeding increased the percentage of tri-, tetra- and hexaenoic acids but were blocked by dietary ATC supplementation [176]. Glutathione content of hearts from alcohol fed rats also increases upon ATC treatment [173].

Phospholipid composition in the heart is impaired by alcohol exposure, leading to a marked increase in lysophosphatidylcholine levels when hearts are perfused with alcohol with concomitant increases in phospholipase A1 and A2 activities [178]. However, the presence of ATC in the perfusate can abolish this increase in cardiac lysophosphatidylcholine levels largely via inhibition of phospholipase A activities [178].

PROTEIN SYNTHESIS

The synthesis of tissue proteins is maintained at an optimal rate. For example, the renewal of the contractile proteins in cardiac tissue is necessary for mechanical activity, and enzymes need to be continually synthesized for a variety of metabolic functions. Protein synthesis is therefore a good parameter to assess tissue damage, as it includes many hundreds of steps, such as amino acid transport, post-receptor cascades, nucleotide availability, etc. Reduced protein synthesis occurs in virtually all mammalian tissues in response to an acute dose of ethanol. The pathogenic mechanisms are unknown but a relationship with the enhanced generation of ROS and lipid peroxidation has been proposed. For example, the shellfish toxin okadaic acid reduces protein synthesis in cultures of vero cells, by a mechanism involving increased lipid peroxidation [179]. In metabolically deranged neuronal and liver tissue *in vitro*, there are decreases in protein synthesis in response to enhanced lipid peroxidation [180,181]. In all these three tissues, reductions in protein synthesis can be prevented by ATC [179–181].

After acute ethanol administration, an increased generation of ROS has been reported [37,182–186]. It can therefore be inferred that ATC-supplementation may also have an ameliorative effect on ethanol-induced reductions in protein synthesis in cardiac muscle. For example, in the heart a single dose of ATC is able to attenuate myocardial ultrastructural damage and enzyme release into the blood, due to acute ethanol administration over 24 hours [187]. However, in our hands supplementation of rats with ATC fails to prevent the acute reduction in protein synthesis *in vivo* (Table 12.2). The failure of ATC to ameliorate acute changes in protein synthesis may reflect the complex etiology of alcohol-induced damage and more probably, the fact that ROS generation and subsequent damage is only one facet of the disease process, as discussed previously.

HAEMODIALYSIS

Lipid peroxidation is increased during haemodialysis, because of ROS generation [188–190]. Paradoxically, total antioxidant capacity increases in patients undergoing dialysis due to high serum urate levels, although this decreases after dialysis, as does serum ATC [189]. Increased ROS generation has also been reported to increase apoptosis in leukocytes [191]. Potentially, this offers the interesting possibility of using either treatment of dialysis membranes with ATC

Table 12.2 Cardiac muscle protein synthesis in vehicle-injected and α-tocopherol-supplemented rats injected with either saline or ethanol

Group	k_s (%/day)	Significance compared to corresponding saline (p)
Vehicle		
Saline	21.4 ± 0.5	
Ethanol	18.1 ± 0.8	$p < 0.05$
α-Tocopherol		
Saline	21.4 ± 0.7	
Ethanol	19.4 ± 0.6	$p < 0.05$

Rats were administered α-tocopherol in intralipid (30 mg/kg body weight/day; i.p.) for 5 days and on the 6th day, they were administered with acute (2.5 hour) doses of either ethanol (75 mmol/kg body weight, i.p.) or saline (0.15 mol/l NaCl). 150 minutes following acute i.p. bolus injections of ethanol or saline, rats were injected with a flooding dose of L-[4-3H]phenylalanine (150 mmol/l, 1 ml/100 g body weight) via a lateral tail vein. Exactly 10 minutes after injection of isotope, rats were killed by decapitation and tissues dissected out and processed for determination of tissue radioactivity. Data are means $\pm$ SEM (n = 6–8). Significance of differences between means was tested by using the pooled estimate of variance after ANOVA. From unpublished data of the authors.

or inclusion of ATC directly in the dialysate since atherosclerotic lesions are frequently found in these patients with concomitant increased oxidation of LDL and LDL-MDA formation [191]. Coating the membrane dialyser with ATC reduces oxidized products of LDL [190].

POSTNATAL DEVELOPMENT

There is some evidence that adequate dietary ATC is necessary for the optimal development of neurological and other tissues, which may be compromised in the presence of organ dysfunction such as liver disease [192–196], also reviewed in [197,198]. Thus, in children with mental impairment due to neuronal ceroid lipofuscinosis, serum ATC levels are low compared to normal controls [192]. In chronic biliary atresia, serum ATC levels are low [195,199], with the mental development of affected children correlating inversely with reduced serum ATC levels [195].

In childhood liver disease and post-natal oxygen toxicity, ATC supplementation has been advocated [200–203]. In chronic infantile cholestasis, affected patients with concomitant ATC deficiency and neurologic impairment have been treated with ATC (orally and parenterally) [194]. Such treatment leads to reductions in serum cholylglycine levels after 1.5–2.5 years without effects on other indices of hepatic function [194]. Intramuscular administration of ATC has also been assessed in cholestasis over 1.3–3.7 years with mixed results, i.e., reported as cessation of spinocerebellar degeneration without evidence of improvement [196]. Adverse effects have been observed in infants receiving intravenous ATC supplementation [204].

Studies into post-natal development and the influence of ATC deficiency and/or supplementation have been largely carried out in animal studies due to obvious limitations in obtaining adequate human tissue. The offspring of diabetic rats have raised hepatic TBARS indicative of tissue peroxidative damage by ROS [205]. However, these increases in TBARS levels are reduced with maternal vitamin E supplementation *in vivo* [205]. Vitamin E protects against lipid peroxidation during post-natal development of rat erythrocytes and liver microsomes [206] and in brain of chicks [207]. Skeletal muscle of chicks is also particularly sensitive to ATC deficiency, exhibiting characteristic lesions of myofibrillary degeneration [208].

SKELETAL MUSCLE

Skeletal muscle comprises about 40% of mammalian body weight and as such, is an important contributor to whole body physiology. Although, ATC concentration in skeletal muscle is lower than that of liver, it has a comparable (if not higher) contribution to the whole body ATC pool [81].

Various studies have shown that dietary ATC deficiency induces myopathic lesions within muscle [209,210]. Many of these studies on muscle have combined ATC deficiency with concomitant selenium deficiency [208,211]. In combined ATC-selenium deficiency, ATC supplementation alone can ameliorate myopathic lesions [212].

ATC deficiency alone causes lysis and disarray of the myofibrillary apparatus and sarcoplasmic reticulum [209,210]. Swelling of the mitochondria, and other matrix disruptions in skeletal muscle also occur [209]. These lesions are observable at both the light and electron microscopic level.

Alcoholic myopathy is arguably the most prevalent skeletal muscle disease in the Western Hemisphere, occurring in between 30–60% of all chronic alcohol misusers (see reviews in [213–215]). In a UK study, serum levels of ATC were shown lower in alcoholics with skeletal muscle myopathy compared to those alcoholics or non-alcoholic subjects without myopathy [166]. However, this has not been reproduced in Spanish alcoholics, which may reflect geographical or other differences between the patient population and/or nutritional intake [216].

Deficiencies of either alpha-tocopherol or selenium also occur naturally leading to, for example, white muscle disease which is seen in farm animals or horses where a combination of inadequate soil selenium is combined with poor dietary ATC [217–226]. Concomitant changes in this disorder include reduced plasma glutathione peroxidase activities and increased serum creatine kinase activities [221,227].

CONCLUSIONS

ROS play a complex role in the etiology of a number of disorders in which ATC supplementation seems to confer therapeutic benefits. Consideration should be given to the possibility that a failure to see beneficial effects following ATC supplementation may be a result of its synergistic action with other antioxidants, and therefore provision of one component of the endogenous repair system will be ineffectual [17].

ACKNOWLEDGMENTS

We are grateful to Dr. D Mantle (Newcastle General Hospital) for a substantial body of constructive help with this review.

ABBREVIATIONS

ATC	alpha-tocopherol
ROS	reactive oxygen species
TBARS	thiobarbituric acid reacting substances
MDA	malondialdehyde
$O_2^{-\bullet}$	superoxide radical
$OH^\bullet$	hydroxyl radical
$RO^\bullet$	alkoxyl radical
$RO_2^\bullet$	peroxyl radical
H_2O_2	hydrogen peroxide
$^1O_2$	singlet oxygen
O_3	ozone
$NO^\bullet$	nitric oxide
$ONOO^-$	peroxynitrite
$NO_2^\bullet$	nitrogen dioxide radical
RNS	reactive nitrogen species
LDL	low density lipoprotein
ALD	alcoholic liver disease

REFERENCES

1 Quintanilha AT, Packer L, Davies JM, Racanelli TL, Davies KJ. Membrane effects of vitamin E deficiency: bioenergetic and surface charge density studies of skeletal muscle and liver mitochondria. Ann. N.Y. Acad. Sci. 1982; 393: 32–47.

2 Amiel J, Maziere JC, Beucler I, Koenig M, Reutenauer L, Loux N, Bonnefont D, Feo C, Landrieu P. Familial isolated vitamin E deficiency. Extensive study of a large family with a 5-year therapeutic follow-up. J. Inherit. Metab. Dis. 1995; 18: 333–340.

3 Ouahchi K, Arita M, Kayden H, Hentati F, Ben Hamida M, Sokol R, Arai H, Inoue K, Mandel JL, Koenig M. Ataxia with isolated vitamin E deficiency is caused by mutations in the alpha-tocopherol transfer protein. Nat. Genet. 1995; 9: 141–145.

4 Hentati A, Deng HX, Hung WY, Nayer M, Ahmed MS, He X, Tim R, Stumpf DA, Siddique T, Ahmed. Human alpha-tocopherol transfer protein: gene structure and mutations in familial vitamin E deficiency. Ann. Neurol. 1996; 39: 295–300.

5 Tanyel MC, Mancano LD. Neurologic findings in vitamin E deficiency. Am. Fam. Physician. 1997; 55: 197–201.

6 Hammans SR, Kennedy CR. Ataxia with isolated vitamin E deficiency presenting as mutation negative Friedreich's ataxia. J. Neurol. Neurosurg. Psychiatry 1998; 64: 368–370.

7 Chang JY, Liu LZ. Neurotoxicity of cholesterol oxides on cultured cerebellar granule cells. Neurochem. Int. 1998; 32: 317–323.

8 Bolton Smith C, Smith WC, Woodward M, Tunstall Pedoe H. Nutrient intakes of different social-class groups: results from the Scottish Heart Health Study (SHHS). Br. J. Nutr. 1991; 65: 321–335.

9 Bolton Smith C, Woodward M. Antioxidant vitamin adequacy in relation to consumption of sugars. Eur. J. Clin. Nutr. 1995; 49: 124–133.

10 Sinha R, Patterson BH, Mangels AR, Levander OA, Gibson T, Taylor PR, Block G. Determinants of plasma vitamin E in healthy males. Cancer Epidemiol. Biomarkers Prev. 1993; 2: 473–479.

11 Dallongeville J, Marecaux N, Fruchart JC, Amouyel P. Cigarette smoking is associated with unhealthy patterns of nutrient intake: a meta-analysis. *J. Nutr.* 1998; **128**: 1450–1457.

12 Ellis NI, Lloyd B, Lloyd RS, Clayton BE. Selenium and vitamin E in relation to risk factors for coronary heart disease. *J. Clin. Pathol.* 1984; **37**: 200–206.

13 Houston DK, Johnson MA, Daniel TD, Poon LW. Health and dietary characteristics of supplement users in an elderly population. *Int. J. Vitam. Nutr. Res.* 1997; **67**: 183–191.

14 Lang JK, Gohil K, Packer L, Burk RF. Selenium deficiency, endurance exercise capacity, and antioxidant status in rats. *J. Appl. Physiol.* 1987; **63**: 2532–2535.

15 Chow CK, Ibrahim W, Wei Z, Chan AC. Vitamin E regulates mitochondrial hydrogen peroxide generation. *Free Radic. Biol. Med.* 1999; **27**: 580–587.

16 Wiseman H, Kaur H, Halliwell B. DNA damage and cancer: measurement and mechanism. *Cancer Lett.* 1995; **93**: 113–120.

17 Buettner GR. The pecking order of free radicals and antioxidants: lipid peroxidation, alpha-tocopherol, and ascorbate. *Arch. Biochem. Biophys.* 1993; **300**: 535–543.

18 Chan KM, Decker EA. Endogenous skeletal muscle antioxidants. *Crit. Rev. Food Sci. Nutr.* 1994; **34**: 403–426.

19 Warren JA, Jenkins RR, Packer L, Witt EH, Armstrong RB. Elevated muscle vitamin E does not attenuate eccentric exercise-induced muscle injury. *J. Appl. Physiol.* 1992; **72**: 2168–2175.

20 Ingelman Sundberg M, Johansson I. Mechanisms of hydroxyl radical formation and ethanol oxidation by ethanol-inducible and other forms of rabbit liver microsomal cytochromes P-450. *J. Biol. Chem.* 1984; **259**: 6447–6458.

21 Ekstrom G, Ingelman Sundberg M. Rat liver microsomal NADPH-supported oxidase activity and lipid peroxidation dependent on ethanol-inducible cytochrome P-450 (P-450 IIE1). *Biochem. Pharmacol.* 1989; **38**: 1313–1319.

22 Cederbaum AI. Oxygen radical generation by microsomes: role of iron and implications for alcohol metabolism and toxicity. *Free Radic. Biol. Med.* 1989; **7**: 559–567.

23 Ekström G, Von Bahr C, Ingelman Sundberg M. Human liver microsomal cytochrome P4502E1. Immunological evaluation of its contribution to microsomal ethanol oxidation, carbon tetrachloride reduction and NAPDH oxidase activity. *Biochem. Pharmacol.* 1989; **38**: 689.

24 Reinke LA, Lai EK, DuBose CM, McCay PB. Reactive free radical generation *in vivo* in heart and liver of ethanol-fed rats: correlation with radical formation *in vitro*. *Proc. Natl. Acad. Sci. USA* 1987; **84**: 9223–9227.

25 Albano E, Tomasi A, Goria Gatti L, Dianzani MU. Spin trapping of free radical species produced during the microsomal metabolism of ethanol. *Chem. Biol. Interact.* 1988; **65**: 223–234.

26 Albano E, Tomasi A, Persson JO, Terelius Y, Goria Gatti L, Ingelman Sundberg M, Dianzani MU. Role of ethanol-inducible cytochrome P450 (P450 IIE1) in catalysing the free radical activation of aliphatic alcohols. *Biochem. Pharmacol.* 1991; **41**: 1895–1902.

27 Kukielka E, Dicker E, Cederbaum AI. Increased production of reactive oxygen species by rat liver mitochondria after chronic ethanol treatment. *Arch. Biochem. Biophys.* 1994; **309**: 377–386.

28 Rouach H, Clément M, Orfanelli MT, Janvier B, Nordmann R. Hepatic lipid peroxidation and mitochrondrial susceptibility to peroxidative attacks during ethanol inhalation and withdrawal. *Biochim. Biophys. Acta* 1983; **753**: 439.

29 Sultatos LG. Effects of acute ethanol administration on the hepatic xanthine dehydrogenase/oxidase system in the rat. *J. Pharmacol. Exp. Ther.* 1988; **246**: 946–949.

30 Abbondanza A, Battelli MG, Soffritti M, Cessi C. Xanthine oxidase status in ethanol-intoxicated rat liver. *Alcohol Clin. Exp. Res.* 1989; **13**: 841–844.

31 Kato S, Kawase T, Alderman J, Inatomi N, Lieber CS. Role of xanthine oxidase in ethanol-induced lipid peroxidation in rats. *Gastroenterology* 1990; **98**: 203–210.

32 Puntarulo S, Cederbaum AI. Chemiluminescence from acetaldehyde oxidation by xanthine oxidase involves generation of and interactions with hydroxyl radicals. *Alcohol Clin. Exp. Res.* 1989; **13**: 84–90.

33 Rajagopalan KV, Handler P. Hepatic aldehyde oxidase. III. The substrate binding site. *J. Biol. Chem.* 1964; **239**: 2027.

34 Albano E, Clot P, Comoglio A, Dianzani MU, Tomasi A. Free radical activation of acetaldehyde and its role in protein alkylation. *FEBS Lett.* 1994; **348**: 65–69.

35 Nordback IH, MacGowan S, Potter JJ, Cameron JL. The role of acetaldehyde in the pathogenesis of acute alcoholic pancreatitis. *Ann. Surg.* 1991; **214**: 671–678.

36 Bautista AP, Spitzer JJ. Acute ethanol intoxication stimulates superoxide anion production by *in situ* perfused rat liver. *Hepatology* 1992; **15**: 892–898.

37 Bautista AP, Spitzer JJ. Postbinge effects of acute alcohol intoxication on hepatic free radical formation. *Alcohol Clin. Exp. Res.* 1996; **20**: 502–509.

38 Roll FJ, Alexander M, Perez HD. Generation of chemotactic activity for neutrophils by liver cells metabolizing ethanol. *Free Radic. Biol. Med.* 1989; **7**: 549–555.

39 Hultcrantz R, Bissell DM, Roll FJ. Iron mediates production of a neutrophil chemoattractant by rat hepatocytes metabolizing ethanol. *J. Clin. Invest.* 1991; **87**: 45–49.

40 Roll FJ, Alexander MA, Cua D, Swanson W, Perez HD. Metabolism of ethanol by rat hepatocytes results in generation of a lipid chemotactic factor: studies using a cell-free system and role of oxygen-derived free radicals. *Arch. Biochem. Biophys.* 1991; **287**: 218–224.

41 Tsukamoto H, Kamimura S, Yeager S, Chen HY, Highman TJ, Luo ZZ, Kim CM, Brittenham GM. Hepatic cirrhosis in rats fed a diet with added alcohol and iron. *Hepatology* 1992; **16**: 113A.

42 Shiratori Y, Takada H, Hai K, Kiriyama H, Nagura T, Tanaka M, Matsumoto K, Kamii K. Generation of chemotactic factor by hepatocytes isolated from chronically ethanol-fed rats. *Dig. Dis. Sci.* 1992; **37**: 650–658.

43 Shirley MA, Reidhead CT, Murphy RC. Chemotactic LTB4 metabolites produced by hepatocytes in the presence of ethanol. *Biochem. Biophys. Res. Commun.* 1992; **185**: 604–610.

44 Arteel GE, Kadiiska MB, Rusyn I, Bradford BU, Mason RP, Raleigh JA, Thurman RG. Oxidative stress occurs in perfused rat liver at low oxygen tension by mechanisms involving peroxynitrite. *Mol. Pharmacol.* 1999; **55**: 708–715.

45 Niemela O. Aldehyde-protein adducts in the liver as a result of ethanol-induced oxidative stress. *Front. Biosci.* 1999; **4**: D506–D513.

46 Rapozzi V, Comelli M, Mavelli I, Sentjurc M, Schara M, Perissin L, Giraldi T. Melatonin and oxidative damage in mice liver induced by the prooxidant antitumor drug, adriamycin. *In Vivo* 1999; **13**: 45–50.

47 Aruoma OI. Nutrition and health aspects of free radicals and antioxidants. *Food Chem. Toxicol.* 1994; **32**: 671–683.

48 van der Veen RC, Hinton DR, Incardonna F, Hofman FM. Extensive peroxynitrite activity during progressive stages of central nervous system inflammation. *J. Neuroimmunol.* 1997; **77**: 1–7.

49 Venters HD Jr, Bonilla LE, Jensen T, Garner HP, Bordayo EZ, Najarian MM, Ala TA, Mason RP, Frey WH, 2nd. Heme from Alzheimer's brain inhibits muscarinic receptor binding via thiyl radical generation. *Brain Res. Mol. Brain Res.* 1997; **764**: 93–100.

50 Tan S, Zhou F, Nielsen VG, Wang Z, Gladson CL, Parks DA. Sustained hypoxia-ischemia results in reactive nitrogen and oxygen species production and injury in the premature fetal rabbit brain. *J. Neuropathol. Exp. Neurol.* 1998; **57**: 544–553.

51 Hallberg CK, Trocme SD, Ansari NH. Acceleration of corneal wound healing in diabetic rats by the antioxidant trolox. *Res. Commun. Mol. Pathol. Pharmacol.* 1996; **93**: 3–12.

52 Longoni B, Pryor WA, Marchiafava P. Inhibition of lipid peroxidation by N-acetylserotonin and its role in retinal physiology. *Biochem. Biophys. Res. Commun.* 1997; **233**: 778–780.

53 Sohn J, Yoon YH. Iron-induced cytotoxicity in cultured rat retinal neurons. *Korean J. Ophthalmol.* 1998; **12**: 77–84.

54 Netto M, Do Carmo RJ, Martins-Ferreira H. Retinal spreading depression induced by photo-activation: involvement of free radicals and potassium. *Brain Res. Mol. Brain Res.* 1999; **827**: 221–224.

55 Chamulitrat W, Skrepnik NV, Spitzer JJ. Endotoxin-induced oxidative stress in the rat small intestine: role of nitric oxide. *Shock* 1996; **5**: 217–222.

56 Preedy VR. Alcohol and the gastrointestinal tract. *Alcohol Clin. Exp. Res.* 1996; **20**: 48A–50A.

57 Sokol RJ, Hoffenberg EJ. Antioxidants in pediatric gastrointestinal disease. *Pediatr. Clin. North Am.* 1996; **43**: 471–488.

58 Xie Z, Kometiani P, Liu J, Li J, Shapiro JI, Askari A. Intracellular reactive oxygen species mediate the linkage of Na^+/K^+-ATPase to hypertrophy and its marker genes in cardiac myocytes. *J. Biol. Chem.* 1999; **274**: 19323–19328.

59 Benito B, Wahl D, Steudel N, Cordier A, Steiner S. Effects of cyclosporine A on the rat liver and kidney protein pattern, and the influence of vitamin E and C coadministration. *Electrophoresis* 1995; **16**: 1273–1283.

60 Kavutcu M, Canbolat O, Ozturk S, Olcay E, Ulutepe S, Ekinci C, Gokhun IH, Durak I. Reduced enzymatic antioxidant defense mechanism in kidney tissues from gentamicin-treated guinea pigs: effects of vitamins E and C. *Nephron* 1996; **72**: 269–274.

61 Wallis G, Brackett D, Lerner M, Kotake Y, Bolli R, McCay PB. *In vivo* spin trapping of nitric oxide generated in the small intestine, liver, and kidney during the development of endotoxemia: a time-course study. *Shock* 1996; **6**: 274–278.

62 Schweich MD, Lison D, Lauwerys R. The role of vitamin E in the susceptibility of rat lung and liver microsomes to iron-stimulated peroxidation. *Environ. Res.* 1995; **70**: 62–69.

63 Varsila E, Pesonen E, Andersson S. Early protein oxidation in the neonatal lung is related to development of chronic lung disease. *Acta Paediatr.* 1995; **84**: 1296–1299.

64 Chung FL, Kelloff G, Steele V, Pittman B, Zang E, Jiao D, Rigotty J, Choi CI, Rivenson A. Chemopreventive efficacy of arylalkyl isothiocyanates and N-acetylcysteine for lung tumorigenesis in Fischer rats. *Cancer Res.* 1996; **56**: 772–778.

65 Lenz AG, Costabel U, Maier KL. Oxidized BAL fluid proteins in patients with interstitial lung diseases. *Eur. Respir. J.* 1996; **9**: 307–312.

66 Rosenblum ER, Gavaler JS, Van Thiel DH. Lipid peroxidation: a mechanism for alcohol-induced testicular injury. *Free Radic. Biol. Med.* 1989; **7**: 569–577.

67 Taylor DE, Piantadosi CA. Oxidative metabolism in sepsis and sepsis syndrome. *J. Crit. Care* 1995; **10**: 122–135.

68 Benzie IF. Lipid peroxidation: a review of causes, consequences, measurement and dietary influences. *Int. J. Food Sci. Nutr.* 1996; **47**: 233–261.

69 Romero FJ. Antioxidants in peripheral nerve. *Free Radic. Biol. Med.* 1996; **20**: 925–932.

70 Brooks PJ. DNA damage, DNA repair, and alcohol toxicity – a review. *Alcohol Clin. Exp. Res.* 1997; **21**: 1073–1082.

71 Diplock AT. Will the 'good fairies' please prove to us that vitamin E lessens human degenerative disease? *Free Radic. Res.* 1997; **27**: 511–532.

72 Chan AC. Vitamin E and atherosclerosis. *J. Nutr.* 1998; **128**: 1593–1596.

73 Supinski G. Free radical induced respiratory muscle dysfunction. *Mol. Cell. Biochem.* 1998; **179**: 99–110.

74 Links M, Lewis C. Chemoprotectants: a review of their clinical pharmacology and therapeutic efficacy. *Drugs* 1999 **57**: 293–308.

75 McDonough KH. The role of alcohol in the oxidant antioxidant balance in heart. *Front Biosci.* 1999; **4**: D601–D606.

76 Bender DA. Vitamin E: tocopherols and tocotrienols. In *Nutritional biochemistry of the vitamins.* Edited by DA Bender, Cambridge: Cambridge University Press, 1992; pp. 87–105.

77 Drevon CA. Absorption, transport and metabolism of vitamin E. *Free Radic. Res. Commun.* 1991; **14**: 229–246.

78 Dutta-Roy AK. Molecular mechanism of cellular uptake and intracellular translocation of alpha-tocopherol: role of tocopherol-binding proteins. *Food Chem. Toxicol.* 1999; **37**: 967–971.

79 Konneh MK, Rutherford C, Anggard E, Ferns GA. Tissue distribution of alpha-tocopherol following dietary supplementation in the rat: effects of concomitant cholesterol feeding. *Proc. Soc. Exp. Biol. Med.* 1995; **210**: 156–161.

80 Shi H, Noguchi N, Niki E. Comparative study on dynamics of antioxidative action of alpha-tocopheryl hydroquinone, ubiquinol, and alpha-tocopherol against lipid peroxidation. *Free Radic. Biol. Med.* 1999; **27**: 334–346.

81 Reilly ME, Ansell H, Marway JS, Richardson PJ, Peters TJ, Preedy VR. The effect of supplementation on alpha-tocopherol levels in liver, heart and skeletal muscle. *Biochem. Soc. Trans.* 1995; **23**: 466S.

82 Kawase T, Kato S, Lieber CS. Lipid peroxidation and antioxidant defense systems in rat liver after chronic ethanol feeding. *Hepatology* 1989; **10**: 815–821.

83 Seitz HK, Puter PM. Ethanol toxicity and nutritional status. In *Nutritional Toxicology*. Edited by FN Kotsonis, M Mackay, J Hjella. New York: Raven Press, 2000, pp. 95–116.

84 Meydani M, Seitz HK, Blumberg JB, Russell RM. Effect of chronic ethanol feeding on hepatic and extrahepatic distribution of vitamin E in rats. *Alcohol Clin. Exp. Res.* 1991; **15**: 771–774.

85 Lieber CS. Biochemical and molecular basis of alcohol-induced injury to liver and other tissues. *N. Engl. J. Med.* 1988; **319**: 1639–1650.

86 Sadrzadeh SMH, Nanji AA, Price PL, Meydani M. The effect of chronic ethanol feeding on serum and liver alpha and gamma tocopherol levels in normal and vitamin E deficient rats. *Gastroenterology* 1993; **104**: 982A.

87 Tsukamoto H, Kim CM, Horn W, Su L, Brittenham GM. Role of lipid peroxidation in in vivo and in vitro models of liver fibrogenesis. *Gastroenterology* 1993; **104**: 1012A.

88 Kamimura S, Gaal K, Britton RS, Bacon BR, Triadafilopoulos G, Tsukamoto H. Increased 4-hydroxynonenal levels in experimental alcoholic liver disease: association of lipid peroxidation with liver fibrogenesis. *Hepatology* 1992; **16**: 448–453.

89 French SW, Wong K, Jui L, Albano E, Hagbjork AL, Ingelman Sundberg M. Effect of ethanol on cytochrome P450 2E1 (CYP2E1), lipid peroxidation, and serum protein adduct formation in relation to liver pathology pathogenesis. *Exp. Mol. Pathol.* 1993; **58**: 61–75.

90 Morimoto M, Hagbjork AL, Nanji AA, Ingelman Sundberg M, Lindros KO, Fu PC, Albano E, French SW. Role of cytochrome P450 2E1 in alcoholic liver disease pathogenesis. *Alcohol* 1993; **10**: 459–464.

91 Gebhardt AC, Lucas D, Menez JF, Seitz HK. Chlormethiazole inhibition of cytochrome P450 2E1 as assessed by chlorzoxazone hydroxylation in humans. *Hepatology* 1997; **26**: 957–961.

92 Wenzel G, Kulinski B, Ruhlmann C, Ehrhardt D. Alkoholische hepatitis – eine 'freie radikale' assoziierte erkrankung. Letalitässenkung durch adjuvante antioxidantientherapie (alcoholic toxic hepatitis – a free radical associated disease. Decreased mortality by adjuvant antioxidant therapy). *Z. Gesamte Inn. Med.* 1993; 490–496.

93 Whitacre ME, Combs GF Jr, Combs SB, Parker RS. Influence of dietary vitamin E on nutritional pancreatic atrophy in selenium-deficient chicks. *J. Nutr.* 1987; **117**: 460–467.

94 Asayama K, Kooy NW, Burr IM. Effect of vitamin E deficiency and selenium deficiency on insulin secretory reserve and free radical scavenging systems in islets: decrease of islet manganosuperoxide dismutase. *J. Lab. Clin. Med.* 1986; **107**: 459–464.

95 Douillet C, Chancerelle Y, Cruz C, Maroncles C, Kergonou JF, Renaud S, Ciavatti M. High dosage vitamin E effect on oxidative status and serum lipids distribution in streptozotocin-induced diabetic rats. *Biochem. Med. Metab. Biol.* 1993; **50**: 265–276.

96 Papaccio G, Baccari GC, Frascatore S, Sellitti S, Pisanti FA. The vitamin-E derivative U-83836-E in the low-dose streptozocin-treated mouse: effects on diabetes development. *Diabetes Res. Clin. Pract.* 1995; **30**: 163–171.

97 Koya D, Lee IK, Ishii H, Kanoh H, King GL. Prevention of glomerular dysfunction in diabetic rats by treatment with d-alpha-tocopherol. *J. Am. Soc. Nephrol.* 1997; **8**: 426–435.

98 Douillet C, Bost M, Accominotti M, Borson-Chazot F, Ciavatti M. Effect of selenium and vitamin E supplements on tissue lipids, peroxides, and fatty acid distribution in experimental diabetes. *Lipids* 1998; **33**: 393–399.

99 Vannucchi H, Araujo WF, Bernardes MM, Jordao Junior AA. Effect of different vitamin E levels on lipid peroxidation in streptozotocin-diabetic rats. *Int. J. Vitam. Nutr. Res.* 1999; **69**: 250–254.

100 Sukalski KA, Pinto KA, Berntson JL. Decreased susceptibility of liver mitochondria from diabetic rats to oxidative damage and associated increase in alpha-tocopherol. *Free Radic. Biol. Med.* 1993; **14**: 57–65.

101 Rosen P, Du X, Tschope D. Role of oxygen derived radicals for vascular dysfunction in the diabetic heart: prevention by alpha-tocopherol? *Mol. Cell. Biochem.* 1998; **188**: 103–111.

102 McCarty MF. Complementary measures for promoting insulin sensitivity in skeletal muscle. *Med. Hypotheses* 1998; **51**: 451–464.

103 Jain SK, McVie R, Jaramillo JJ, Palmer M, Smith T, Meachum ZD, Little RL. The effect of modest vitamin E supplementation on lipid peroxidation products and other cardiovascular risk factors in diabetic patients. *Lipids* 1996; **31**:(Suppl.): S87–S90.

104 Caballero B. Vitamin E improves the action of insulin. *Nutr. Rev.* 1993; **51**: 339–340.

105 Mizui T, Doteuchi M. Lipid peroxidation: a possible role in gastric damage induced by ethanol in rats. *Life Sci.* 1986; **38**: 2163–2167.

106 Evangelista S, Meli A. Influence of antioxidants and radical scavengers on ethanol-induced gastric ulcers in the rat. *Gen. Pharmacol.* 1985; **16**: 285–286.

107 Mizui T, Sato H, Hirose F, Doteuchi M. Effect of antiperoxidative drugs on gastric damage induced by ethanol in rats. *Life Sci.* 1987; **41**: 755–763.

108 Albano E, Clot P. Free radicals and ethanol toxicity. In: *Alcohol and the gastrointestinal tract.* Edited by VR Preedy, RR Watson. Boca Raton, Florida: CRC Press, 1996, pp. 57–68.

109 Seitz HK, Pöschl G, Simanowski UA. Alcohol and cancer: Recent developments in alcoholism. In: *The consequences of alcoholism.* Edited by M Galanter. New York: Plenum Press, 1998, pp. 67–95.

110 Shimizu M, Lasker JM, Tsutsumi M, Lieber CS. Immunohistochemical localization of ethanol-inducible P450 IIE1 in the rat alimentary tract. *Gastroenterology* 1990; **99**: 1044–1053.

111 Hakkak R, Korourian S, Ronis MJ, Ingelman Sundberg M, Badger TM. Effects of diet and ethanol on the expression and localization of cytochromes P450 2E1 and P450 2C7 in the colon of male rats. *Biochem. Pharmacol.* 1996; **51**: 61–69.

112 Baumgarten G, Waldherr RB, Stickel F et al. Enhanced expression of cytochrome P450 2E1 in the oropharyngeal mucosa in alcoholics with cancer. Annual Meeting International Society of Biomedical Research on Alcoholism, Washington DC, June 22–27, (abstract), 1996.

113 Gossrau R, Frederiks WM, van Noorden CJ. Histochemistry of reactive oxygen-species (ROS)-generating oxidases in cutaneous and mucous epithelia of laboratory rodents with special reference to xanthine oxidase. *Histochemistry* 1990; **94**: 539–544.

114 Eskelson CD, Odeleye OE, Watson RR, Earnest DL, Mufti SI. Modulation of cancer growth by vitamin E and alcohol. *Alcohol Alcohol.* 1993; **28**: 117–125.

115 Vincon P, Wunderer J, Simanowski UA, Preedy VR, Peters TJ, Waldherr R, Seitz HK. Inhibition of alcohol-associated hyperregeneration in the rat colon by alpha-tocopherol. *Alcohol Clin. Exp. Res.* 2000; **24**(Suppl.): 213A.

116 Holvoet P, Collen D. Oxidation of low density lipoproteins in the pathogenesis of atherosclerosis. *Atherosclerosis* 1998; **137**(Suppl.): S33–S38.

117 Suzukawa M, Ayaori M, Shige H, Hisada T, Ishikawa T, Nakamura H. Effect of supplementation with vitamin E on LDL oxidizability and prevention of atherosclerosis. *Biofactors* 1998; **7**: 51–54.

118 Stocker R. The ambivalence of vitamin E in atherogenesis. *Trends Biochem. Sci.* 1999; **24**: 219–223.

119 Enstrom JE, Pauling L. Mortality among health-conscious elderly Californians. *Proc. Natl. Acad. Sci. USA* 1982; **79**: 6023–6027.

120 Ihara Y, Nobukuni K, Namba R, Kamisaka K, Kibata M, Kajinami K, Fujita H, Mabuchi H, Shirabe T, Ohshima K et al. A family of familial hypercholesterolemia with cerebral infarction and without coronary heart disease. An unusual case with corneal opacity, polyneuropathy and carpal tunnel syndrome in the family: therapy with probucol and tocopherol nicotinate. J. Neurol. Sci. 1991; 106: 10–18.

121 Bowry VW, Ingold KU, Stocker R. Vitamin E in human low-density lipoprotein. When and how this antioxidant becomes a pro-oxidant. Biochem. J. 1992; 288: 341–344.

122 Bachem MG, Wendelin D, Schneiderhan W, Haug C, Zorn U, Gross HJ, Schmid-Kotsas A, Grunert A. Depending on their concentration oxidized low density lipoproteins stimulate extracellular matrix synthesis or induce apoptosis in human coronary artery smooth muscle cells. Clin. Chem. Lab. Med. 1999; 37: 319–326.

123 Devaraj S, Li D, Jialal I. The effects of alpha tocopherol supplementation on monocyte function. Decreased lipid oxidation, interleukin 1 beta secretion, and monocyte adhesion to endothelium. J. Clin. Invest. 1996; 98: 756–763.

124 Cachia O, Leger CL, Descomps B. Monocyte superoxide production is inversely related to normal content of alpha-tocopherol in low-density lipoprotein. Atherosclerosis 1998; 138: 263–269.

125 Mabile L, Fitoussi G, Periquet B, Schmitt A, Salvayre R, Negre-Salvayre A. Alpha-tocopherol and trolox block the early intracellular events (TBARS and calcium rises) elicited by oxidized low density lipoproteins in cultured endothelial cells. Free Radic. Biol. Med. 1995; 19: 177–187.

126 Wen Y, Killalea S, McGettigan P, Feely J. Lipid peroxidation and antioxidant vitamins C and E in hypertensive patients. Ir. J. Med. Sci. 1996; 165: 210–212.

127 Aejmelaeus RT, Holm P, Kaukinen U, Metsa-Ketela TJ, Laippala P, Hervonen AL, Alho HE. Age-related changes in the peroxyl radical scavenging capacity of human plasma. Free Radic. Biol. Med. 1997; 23: 69–75.

128 Slattery ML, Jacobs DR Jr, Dyer A, Benson J, Hilner JE, Caan BJ. Dietary antioxidants and plasma lipids: the Cardia Study. J. Am. Coll. Nutr. 1995; 14: 635–642.

129 Iuliano L, Pedersen JZ, Camastra C, Bello V, Ceccarelli S, Violi F. Protection of low density lipoprotein oxidation by the antioxidant agent IRFI005, a new synthetic hydrophilic vitamin E analogue. Free Radic. Biol. Med. 1999; 26: 858–868.

130 Martin-Nizard F, Boullier A, Fruchart JC, Duriez P. Alpha-tocopherol but not beta-tocopherol inhibits thrombin-induced PKC activation and endothelin secretion in endothelial cells. J. Cardiovasc. Risk 1998; 5: 339–345.

131 Mak IT, Murphy A, Hopper A, Witiak D, Ziemniak J, Weglicki WB. Potent inhibitory activities of hydrophobic aci-reductones (2-hydroxytetronic acid analogs) against membrane and human low-density lipoprotein oxidation. Biochem. Pharmacol. 1998; 55: 1921–1926.

132 Kontush A, Spranger T, Reich A, Baum K, Beisiegel U. Lipophilic antioxidants in blood plasma as markers of atherosclerosis: the role of alpha-carotene and gamma-tocopherol. Atherosclerosis 1999; 144: 117–122.

133 Torun M, Avci N, Yardim S. Serum levels of vitamin E in relation to cardiovascular diseases. J. Clin. Pharm. Ther. 1995; 20: 335–340.

134 Kim SY, Lee-Kim YC, Kim MK, Suh JY, Chung EJ, Cho SY, Cho BK, Suh I. Serum levels of antioxidant vitamins in relation to coronary artery disease: a case control study of Koreans. Biomed. Environ. Sci. 1996; 9: 229–235.

135 Klipstein-Grobusch K, Geleijnse JM, den Breeijen JH, Boeing H, Hofman A, Grobbee DE, Witteman JC. Dietary antioxidants and risk of myocardial infarction in the elderly: the Rotterdam Study. Am. J. Clin. Nutr. 1999; 69: 261–266.

136 Kostner K, Hornykewycz S, Yang P, Neunteufl T, Glogar D, Weidinger F, Maurer G, Huber K. Is oxidative stress causally linked to unstable angina pectoris? A study in 100 CAD patients and matched controls. Cardiovasc. Res. 1997; 36: 330–336.

137 Hu FB, Stampfer MJ, Manson JE, Rimm EB, Colditz GA, Rosner BA, Speizer FE, Hennekens CH, Willett WC. Frequent nut consumption and risk of coronary heart disease in women: prospective cohort study. *BMJ* 1998; **317**: 1341–1345.

138 Liu S, Stampfer MJ, Hu FB, Giovannucci E, Rimm E, Manson JE, Hennekens CH, Willett WC. Whole-grain consumption and risk of coronary heart disease: results from the Nurses' Health Study. *Am. J. Clin. Nutr.* 1999; **70**: 412–419.

139 Rozewicka L, Barcew-Wiszniewska B, Wojcicki J, Samochowiec L, Krasowska B. Protective effect of selenium and vitamin E against changes induced in heart vessels of rabbits fed chronically on a high-fat diet. *Kitasato. Arch. Exp. Med.* 1991; **64**: 183–192.

140 Ruf JC. Wine and polyphenols related to platelet aggregation and atherothrombosis. *Drugs Exp. Clin. Res.* 1999; **25**: 125–131.

141 Abu Amsha R, Croft KD, Puddey IB, Proudfoot JM, Beilin LJ. Phenolic content of various beverages determines the extent of inhibition of human serum and low-density lipoprotein oxidation *in vitro*: identification and mechanism of action of some cinnamic acid derivatives from red wine. *Clin. Sci. Colch.* 1996; **91**: 449–458.

142 Soleas GJ, Diamandis EP, Goldberg DM. Wine as a biological fluid: history, production, and role in disease prevention. *J. Clin. Lab. Anal.* 1997; **11**: 287–313.

143 Constant J. Alcohol, ischemic heart disease, and the French paradox. *Coron. Artery. Dis.* 1997; **8**: 645–649.

144 Serafini M, Maiani G, Ferro-Luzzi A. Alcohol-free red wine enhances plasma antioxidant capacity in humans. *J. Nutr.* 1998; **128**: 1003–1007.

145 Paganga G, Miller N, Rice-Evans CA. The polyphenolic content of fruit and vegetables and their antioxidant activities. What does a serving constitute? *Free Radic. Res.* 1999; **30**: 153–162.

146 de Rijke YB, Demacker PN, Assen NA, Sloots LM, Katan MB, Stalenhoef AF. Red wine consumption does not affect oxidizability of low-density lipoproteins in volunteers. *Am. J. Clin. Nutr.* 1996; **63**: 329–334.

147 Borghi C, Ambrosioni E. Primary and secondary prevention of myocardial infarction. *Clin. Exp. Hypertens.* 1996; **18**: 547–558.

148 Stephens NG, Parsons A, Schofield PM, Kelly F, Cheeseman K, Mitchinson MJ. Randomised controlled trial of vitamin E in patients with coronary disease: Cambridge Heart Antioxidant Study (CHAOS). *Lancet* 1996; **347**: 781–786.

149 Losonczy KG, Harris TB, Havlik RJ. Vitamin E and vitamin C supplement use and risk of all-cause and coronary heart disease mortality in older persons: the Established Populations for Epidemiologic Studies of the Elderly. *Am. J. Clin. Nutr.* 1996; **64**: 190–196.

150 Anonymous. Dietary supplementation with n-3 polyunsaturated fatty acids and vitamin E after myocardial infarction: the results of the GISSI-Prevention Trial. Gruppo Italiano per lo Studio della Sopravvivenza nell'Infarto miocardico. *Lancet* 1999; **354**: 447–455.

151 Rimm EB, Ascherio A, Giovannucci E, Spiegelman D, Stampfer MJ, Willett WC. Vegetable, fruit, and cereal fiber intake and risk of coronary heart disease among men. *JAMA* 1996; **275**: 447–451.

152 Rimm EB, Willett WC, Hu FB, Sampson L, Colditz GA, Manson JE, Hennekens C, Stampfer MJ. Folate and vitamin B6 from diet and supplements in relation to risk of coronary heart disease among women. *JAMA* 1998; **279**: 359–364.

153 Phonpanichrasamee C, Komaratat P, Wilairat P. Hypocholesterolemic effect of vitamin E on cholesterol-fed rabbit. *Int. J. Vitam. Nutr. Res.* 1990; **60**: 240–244.

154 Wojcicki J, Rozewicka L, Barcew Wiszniewska B, Samochowiec L, Juzwiak S, Kadlubowska D, Tustanowski S, Juzyszyn Z. Effect of selenium and vitamin E on the development of experimental atherosclerosis in rabbits. *Atherosclerosis* 1991; **87**: 9–16.

155 Sirikci O, Ozer NK, Azzi A. Dietary cholesterol-induced changes of protein kinase C and the effect of vitamin E in rabbit aortic smooth muscle cells. *Atherosclerosis* 1996; **126**: 253–263.

156 Jain SK, Levine SN. Elevated lipid peroxidation and vitamin E-quinone levels in heart ventricles of streptozotocin-treated diabetic rats. *Free Radic. Biol. Med.* 1995; **18**: 337–341.

157 Ascherio A, Rimm EB, Hernan MA, Giovannucci E, Kawachi I, Stampfer MJ, Willett WC. Relation of consumption of vitamin E, vitamin C, and carotenoids to risk for stroke among men in the United States. *Ann. Intern. Med.* 1999; **130**: 963–970.

158 Friedman HS. Cardiovascular effects of alcohol. *Recent Dev. Alcohol* 1998; **14**: 135–166.

159 Freedman JE, Farhat JH, Loscalzo J, Keaney JF Jr. Alpha-tocopherol inhibits aggregation of human platelets by a protein kinase C-dependent mechanism. *Circulation* 1996; **94**: 2434–2440.

160 Richardson P, McKenna W, Bristow M, Maisch B, Mautner B, O'Connell J, Olsen E, Thiene G, Goodwin J, Gyarfas I, Martin I, Nordet P. Report of the 1995 World Health Organization/International Society and Federation of Cardiology Task Force on the Definition and Classification of cardiomyopathies. *Circulation* 1996; **93**: 841–842.

161 Preedy VR, Richardson PJ. Alcoholic cardiomyopathy: clinical and experimental pathological changes. *Herz.* 1996; **21**: 241–247.

162 Preedy VR, Richardson PJ. Alcohol and the heart. In: *Current issues in cardiovascular therapy.* Edited by HL Elliott. London: Martin Dunitz, 1997, pp. 83–95.

163 Richardson PJ, Patel VB, Preedy VR. Alcohol and the myocardium. *Novartis Found Symp.* 1998; **216**: 35–45.

164 Simon JA, Hudes ES. Serum ascorbic acid and cardiovascular disease prevalence in U.S. adults: the Third National Health and Nutrition Examination Survey (NHANES III). *Ann. Epidemiol.* 1999; **9**: 358–365.

165 Simonetti P, Brusamolino A, Pellegrini N, Viani P, Clemente G, Roggi C, Cestaro B. Evaluation of the effect of alcohol consumption on erythrocyte lipids and vitamins in a healthy population. *Alcohol Clin. Exp. Res.* 1995; **19**: 517–522.

166 Ward RJ, Peters TJ. The antioxidant status of patients with either alcohol-induced liver damage or myopathy. *Alcohol Alcohol.* 1992; **27**: 359–365.

167 Simonetti P, Cestaro B, Porrini M, Viani P, Roggi C, Testolin G. Effect of alcohol intake on lipids and fat-soluble vitamins in blood. *Minerva Med.* 1993; **84**: 447–452.

168 Hibbs RG, Ferrans VJ, Black WC, Weilbaecher DG, Walsh JJ, Burch GE. Alcoholic cardiomyopathy. An electron microscopy study. *Am. Heart J.* 1965; **69**: 766–769.

169 Garcia Bunuel L. Lipid peroxidation in alcoholic myopathy and cardiomyopathy. *Med. Hypotheses* 1984; **13**: 217–231.

170 Tsiplenkova VG, Vikhert AM, Cherpachenko NM. Ultrastructural and histochemical observations in human and experimental alcoholic cardiomyopathy. *J. Am. Coll. Cardiol.* 1986; **8**: 22A–32A.

171 Jaatinen P, Saukko P, Hervonen A. Chronic ethanol exposure increases lipopigment accumulation in human heart. *Alcohol Alcohol.* 1993; **28**: 559–569.

172 Antonenkov VD, Pirozhkov SV, Popova SV, Panchenko LF. Effect of chronic ethanol, catalase inhibitor 3-amino-1,2,4-triazole and clofibrate treatment on lipid peroxidation in rat myocardium. *Int. J. Biochem.* 1989; **21**: 1313–1318.

173 Edes I, Toszegi A, Csanady M, Bozoky B. Myocardial lipid peroxidation in rats after chronic alcohol ingestion and the effects of different antioxidants. *Cardiovasc. Res.* 1986; **20**: 542–548.

174 Nordmann R, Ribiere C, Rouach H. Involvement of oxygen free radicals in the metabolism and toxicity of ethanol. *Prog. Clin. Biol. Res.* 1987; **241**: 201–213.

175 Coudray C, Boucher F, Richard MJ, Arnaud J, De Leiris J, Favier A. Zinc deficiency, ethanol, and myocardial ischemia affect lipoperoxidation in rats. *Biol. Trace Elem. Res.* 1991; **30**: 103–118.

176 Pirozhkov SV, Eskelson CD, Watson RR, Hunter GC, Piotrowski JJ, Bernhard V. Effect of chronic consumption of ethanol and vitamin E on fatty acid composition and lipid peroxidation in rat heart tissue. *Alcohol* 1992; **9**: 329–334.

177 Ribiere C, Hininger I, Rouach H, Nordmann R. Effects of chronic ethanol administration on free radical defence in rat myocardium. *Biochem. Pharmacol.* 1992; **44**: 1495–1500.

178 Choy PC, O K, Man RY, Chan AC. Phosphatidylcholine metabolism in isolated rat heart: modulation by ethanol and vitamin E. *Biochim. Biophys. Acta* 1989; **1005**: 225–232.

179 Matias WG, Traore A, Bonini M, Sanni A, Creppy EE. Oxygen reactive radicals production in cell culture by okadaic acid and their implication in protein synthesis inhibition. *Hum. Exp. Toxicol.* 1999; **18**: 634–639.

180 Uto A, Dux E, Kusumoto M, Hossmann KA. Delayed neuronal death after brief histotoxic hypoxia *in vitro. J. Neurochem.* 1995; **64**: 2185–2192.

181 Fraga CG, Zamora R, Tappel AL. Damage to protein synthesis concurrent with lipid peroxidation in rat liver slices: effect of halogenated compounds, peroxides, and vitamin E1. *Arch. Biochem. Biophys.* 1989; **270**: 84–91.

182 Zloch Z. Temporal changes of the lipid peroxidation in rats after acute intoxication by ethanol. *Z. Naturforsch. C.* 1994; **49**: 359–362.

183 Lecomte E, Herbeth B, Pirollet P, Chancerelle Y, Arnaud J, Musse N, Paille F, Siest G, Artur Y. Effect of alcohol consumption on blood antioxidant nutrients and oxidative stress indicators. *Am. J. Clin. Nutr.* 1994; **60**: 255–261.

184 Kurose I, Higuchi H, Miura S, Saito H, Watanabe N, Hokari R, Hirokawa M, Takaishi M, Zeki S, Nakamura T, Ebinuma H, Kato S, Ishii H. Oxidative stress-mediated apoptosis of hepatocytes exposed to acute ethanol intoxication. *Hepatology* 1997; **25**: 368–378.

185 Reinke LA, Moore DR, McCay PB. Free radical formation in livers of rats treated acutely and chronically with alcohol. *Alcohol Clin. Exp. Res.* 1997; **21**: 642–646.

186 Reinke LA, McCay PB. Spin trapping studies of alcohol-initiated radicals in rat liver: influence of dietary fat. *J. Nutr.* 1997; **127**: 899S–902S.

187 Redetzki JE, Griswold KE, Nopajaroonsri C, Redetzki HM. Amelioration of cardiotoxic effects of alcohol by vitamin E. *J. Toxicol. Clin. Toxicol.* 1983; **20**: 319–331.

188 Peuchant E, Carbonneau MA, Dubourg L, Thomas MJ, Perromat A, Vallot C, Clerc M. Lipoperoxidation in plasma and red blood cells of patients undergoing haemodialysis: vitamins A, E, and iron status. *Free Radic. Biol. Med.* 1994; **16**: 339–346.

189 Jackson P, Loughrey CM, Lightbody JH, McNamee PT, Young IS. Effect of hemodialysis on total antioxidant capacity and serum antioxidants in patients with chronic renal failure. *Clin. Chem.* 1995; **41**: 1135–1138.

190 Mune M, Yukawa S, Kishino M, Otani H, Kimura K, Nishikawa O, Takahashi T, Kodama N, Saika Y, Yamada Y. Effect of vitamin E on lipid metabolism and atherosclerosis in ESRD patients. *Kidney Int. Suppl.* 1999; **71**: S126–S129.

191 Galli F, Canestrari F, Buoncristiani U. Biological effects of oxidant stress in haemodialysis: the possible roles of vitamin E. *Blood Purif.* 1999; **17**: 79–94.

192 Westermarck T. Selenium content of tissues in Finnish infants and adults with various diseases, and studies on the effects of selenium supplementation in neuronal ceroid lipofuscinosis patients. *Acta Pharmacol. Toxicol. Copenh.* 1977; **41**: 121–128.

193 Werlin SL, Harb JM, Swick H, Blank E. Neuromuscular dysfunction and ultrastructural pathology in children with chronic cholestasis and vitamin E deficiency. *Ann. Neurol.* 1983; **13**: 291–296.

194 Sokol RJ, Heubi JE, McGraw C, Balistreri WF. Correction of vitamin E deficiency in children with chronic cholestasis. II. Effect on gastrointestinal and hepatic function. *Hepatology* 1986; **6**: 1263–1269.

195 Stewart SM, Uauy R, Waller DA, Kennard BD, Andrews WS. Mental and motor development correlates in patients with end-stage biliary atresia awaiting liver transplantation. *Pediatrics* 1987; **79**: 882–888.

196 Perlmutter DH, Gross P, Jones HR, Fulton A, Grand RJ. Intramuscular vitamin E repletion in children with chronic cholestasis. *Am. J. Dis. Child.* 1987; **141**: 170–174.

197 Sokol RJ. Vitamin E deficiency and neurologic disease. *Annu. Rev. Nutr.* 1988; **8**: 351–373.

198   Kaufman SS, Murray ND, Wood RP, Shaw BW Jr, Vanderhoof JA. Nutritional support for the infant with extrahepatic biliary atresia. *J. Pediatr.* 1987; **110**: 679–686.

199   Tazawa Y, Nakagawa M, Yamada M, Konno T, Tada K, Ohi R, Kasai M. Serum vitamin E levels in children with corrected biliary atresia. *Am. J. Clin. Nutr.* 1984; **40**: 246–250.

200   Neu J, Valentine C, Meetze W. Scientifically-based strategies for nutrition of the high-risk low birth weight infant. *Eur. J. Pediatr.* 1990; **150**: 2–13.

201   Cywes C, Millar AJ. Assessment of the nutritional status of infants and children with biliary atresia. *S. Afr. Med. J.* 1990; **77**: 131–135.

202   Boudreaux JP, Hayes DH, Mizrahi S, Maggiore P, Blazek J, Dick D. Use of water-soluble liquid vitamin E to enhance cyclosporine absorption in children after liver transplant. *Transplant Proc.* 1993; **25**: 1875.

203   Sokol RJ, Butler Simon N, Conner C, Heubi JE, Sinatra FR, Suchy FJ, Heyman MB, Perrault J, Rothbaum RJ, Levy J *et al*. Multicenter trial of d-alpha-tocopheryl polyethylene glycol 1000 succinate for treatment of vitamin E deficiency in children with chronic cholestasis. *Gastroenterology* 1993; **104**: 1727–1735.

204   Lorch V, Murphy D, Hoersten LR, Harris E, Fitzgerald J, Sinha SN. Unusual syndrome among premature infants: association with a new intravenous vitamin E product. *Pediatrics* 1985; **75**: 598–602.

205   Siman CM, Eriksson UJ. Vitamin E decreases the occurrence of malformations in the offspring of diabetic rats. *Diabetes* 1997; **46**: 1054–1061.

206   Suarez A, Ramirez-Tortosa M, Gil A, Faus MJ. Addition of vitamin E to long-chain polyunsaturated fatty acid-enriched diets protects neonatal tissue lipids against peroxidation in rats. *Eur. J. Nutr.* 1999; **38**: 169–176.

207   Surai PF, Noble RC, Speake BK. Relationship between vitamin E content and susceptibility to lipid peroxidation in tissues of the newly hatched chick. *Br. Poult. Sci.* 1999; **40**: 406–410.

208   Van Vleet JF, Ferrans VJ. Ultrastructural changes in skeletal muscle of selenium-vitamin E-deficient chicks. *Am. J. Vet. Res.* 1976; **37**: 1081–1089.

209   Van Vleet J, Ferrans VJ. Ultrastructural alterations in skeletal muscle of ducklings fed selenium-vitamin E-deficient diet. *Am. J. Vet. Res.* 1977; **38**: 1399–1405.

210   Dahlin KJ, Chan AC, Benson ES, Hegarty PV. Rehabilitating effect of vitamin E therapy on the ultrastructural changes in skeletal muscles of vitamin E-deficient rabbits. *Am. J. Clin. Nutr.* 1978; **31**: 94–99.

211   Van Vleet JF, Ruth G, Ferrans VJ. Ultrastructural alterations in skeletal muscle of pigs with selenium-vitamin E deficiency. *Am. J. Vet. Res.* 1976; **37**: 911–922.

212   Niyo Y, Glock RD, Ramsey FK, Ewan RC. Effects of intramuscular injections of selenium and vitamin E on selenium-vitamin E deficiency in young pigs. *Am. J. Vet. Res.* 1977; **38**: 1479–1484.

213   Preedy VR, Reilly M, Mantle D, Peters TJ. Free radicals and antioxidants in the pathogenesis of alcoholic myopathy. In: *Free radicals and skeletal muscle*. Edited by AE Reznick, DL Packer, CK Sen, JO Holloszy, MJ Jackson. Basel: Birkhauser Verlag, 1998, pp. 283–293.

214   Preedy VR, Reilly ME, Peters TJ. A current and retrospective analysis of whether the animal model of alcoholic myopathy is suitable for studying its clinical counterpart. *Addict. Biol.* 1999; **4**: 241–242.

215   Preedy VR, Reilly ME, Patel VB, Richardson PJ, Peters TJ. Protein metabolism in alcoholism: effects on specific tissues and the whole body. *Nutrition* 1999; **15**: 604–608.

216   Fernandez Sola J, Villegas E, Nicolas JM, Deulofeu R, Antunez E, Sacanella E, Estruch R, Urbano Marquez A. Serum and muscle levels of alpha-tocopherol, ascorbic acid, and retinol are normal in chronic alcoholic myopathy. *Alcohol Clin. Exp. Res.* 1998; **22**: 422–427.

217   Wilson TM, Morrison HA, Palmer NC, Finley GG, van Dreumel AA. Myodegeneration and suspected selenium/vitamin E deficiency in horses. *J. Am. Vet. Med. Assoc.* 1976; **169**: 213–217.

218   Whanger PD, Weswig PH, Schmitz JA, Oldfield JE. Effects of selenium and vitamin E on blood selenium levels, tissue glutathione peroxidase activities and white muscle disease in sheep fed purified or hay diets. *J. Nutr.* 1977; **107**: 1298–1307.

219 Turner RJ, Wheatley LE, Beck NF. Impaired mitogen responses in lambs with white muscle disease. *Res. Vet. Sci.* 1984; **37**: 357–358.

220 Higuchi T, Ichijo S, Osame S, Ohishi H. Studies on serum selenium and tocopherol in white muscle disease of foal. *Nippon Juigaku Zasshi* 1989; **51**: 52–59.

221 Hoshino Y, Ichijo S, Osame S, Takahashi E. Studies on serum tocopherol, selenium levels and blood glutathione peroxidase activities in calves with white muscle disease. *Nippon Juigaku Zasshi* 1989; **51**: 741–748.

222 Osame S, Ohtani T, Ichijo S. Studies on serum tocopherol and selenium levels and blood glutathione peroxidase activities in lambs with white muscle disease. *Nippon Juigaku Zasshi* 1990; **52**: 705–710.

223 de Gritz BG, Rahko T, Korpela H. Diet-induced lipofuscin and ceroid formation in growing pigs. *J. Comp. Pathol.* 1994; **110**: 11–24.

224 de Gritz BG. Copper-zinc superoxide dismutase (CuZnSOD) in antioxidant deficient pigs. *Zentralbl Veterinarmed* A 1995; **42**: 561–573.

225 Dickerson B, McKnight A, Middleton J, Tyler JW, Bagley R, Valdez R. Electromyographic evaluation of a calf with white muscle disease. *Vet. Rec.* 1997; **140**: 431–432.

226 Lofstedt J. White muscle disease of foals. *Vet. Clin. North Am. Equine Pract.* 1997; **13**: 169–185.

227 Walsh DM, Kennedy DG, Goodall EA, Kennedy S. Antioxidant enzyme activity in the muscles of calves depleted of vitamin E or selenium or both. *Br. J. Nutr.* 1993; **70**: 621–630.

228 Halliwell B, Aeschbach R, Loliger J, Aruoma OI. The characterization of antioxidants. *Food Chem. Toxicol.* 1995; **33**: 601–617.

Chapter 13

Alcohol and platelet function

Adam K. Myers, Kabita Das and Qing-Hui Zhang

INTRODUCTION

Coronary heart disease (CHD) and its manifestations account for approximately half a million deaths annually in the United States, 25% of the nation's total mortality [1]. Much progress has been made in defining the mechanisms involved in the pathogenesis and progression of CHD, devising new therapeutic approaches for the treatment and prevention of CHD, and identifying factors that promote susceptibility to this disease. Important lifestyle factors affecting CHD risk include exercise, smoking, diet and alcohol consumption [2]. Moderate drinking reduces risk of CHD mortality, and although it is generally accepted that about half of the risk reduction might be due to a beneficial effect of moderate consumption of alcohol or alcoholic beverages on plasma lipids [3–5], the effects of alcohol on other parameters undoubtedly contribute. Although there are many definitions of 'moderate alcohol consumption' the United States Departments of Agriculture and Health and Human Services define moderate drinking as 'no more than one drink per day for women and no more than two drinks per day for men' (a standard drink contains approximately 12 grams of ethanol, which is the amount present in a 12 oz bottle of beer, a 5 oz serving of table wine, or 1.5 ounces of 80 proof distilled spirits) [6]. The effects of alcohol on platelet aggregation and subsequent thrombus formation have been studied by several laboratories including our own [7–14], and is the topic of the present review. Platelets are of substantial interest because of their role in CHD-related mortality. Myocardial infarction (MI) most often results from thrombotic occlusion of stenosed coronary vessels. In this scenario, the blockage is due to the rupture of an atherosclerotic plaque, which exposes a thrombogenic surface to platelets. Adherence of platelets and subsequent thrombus formation eventually blocks flow through the affected coronary artery, causing ischemia, acute MI and potentially death [15]. An inhibitory effect of alcohol on platelet aggregation is therefore a potential factor in the reduced risk of CHD-related death with moderate drinking. In addition, studies have suggested that alcohol consumption might have a role in inhibiting the progression of atherosclerosis, a process that involves both plasma lipids and platelets [16]. While this chapter focuses mainly on the possibly beneficial aspects of moderate alcohol consumption on the hemostatic system, it is recognized that there are complex issues associated with drinking, which can vary from individual to individual. Some of these are discussed elsewhere in this volume.

MECHANISMS OF HEMOSTASIS

In order to consider the effects of alcohol on platelet aggregation and their mechanisms, it is first necessary to provide a brief background on the coagulation and fibrinolytic systems responsible for normal hemostasis.

Vascular injury leads to activation of platelets and adhesion to the vessel wall. Platelet receptors for subendothelial components such as collagen, fibronectin, or laminin promote adhesion to the injured vessel wall; under high shear conditions, these interactions are not adequate and von Willebrand factor and its platelet receptor are required for adhesion [17]. During primary hemostasis, this adhesion of platelets to the vascular wall produces activation, which is characterized by platelet morphological and biochemical changes, aggregation of platelets to each other, and the secretion of platelet granule contents (the platelet release reaction). The end result is the primary hemostatic plug. The subsequent formation of fibrin around the primary platelet plug constitutes secondary hemostasis, and is the end result of a series of biochemical reactions involving the coagulation factors of plasma and the platelet surface.

Stimulation of platelets involves multiple pathways of activation. One major biochemical pathway, which can be activated by receptor binding of several agonists including collagen, thrombin, platelet activating factor, and thromboxane A2, is the phospholipase C-mediated second messenger system. Phosphatidylinositol (4,5) bis-phosphate is broken down to inositol triphosphate (IP3) and diacylglycerol by phospholipase C when such agonists bind to their receptors. IP3 causes an increase in cytosolic-free calcium, a central event in platelet activation and aggregation, initially resulting in platelet shape change from a discoid-shaped formed element to a spherical body with pseudopods. Diacylgylcerol activates protein kinase C directly, which in concert with the elevated calcium is responsible for platelet aggregation and secretion of granule contents. These granule contents are numerous and serve a variety of functions, important among them support of hemostasis and vascular repair. Notably, amine storage granules release ADP, which is a platelet agonist and therefore recruits further platelets for aggregation [17].

A second major stimulatory pathway is mediated by phospholipase A2, an enzyme that is activated when intraplatelet Ca^{2+} is elevated and to some extent by agonist-receptor interactions. This enzyme releases the fatty acid from the sn-2 position of membrane phospholipids; when the fatty acid is arachidonic acid, it is metabolized rapidly in platelets to thromboxane A2 (TXA2), a potent platelet agonist. Thus, TXA2 amplifies platelet responses. Arachidonic acid can also be released subsequent to the activation of phospholipase C, as a result of the breakdown of diacylglycerol by diglyceride lipase, but this pathway probably contributes a minor amount of arachidonic acid compared to the phospholipase A2 pathway [18].

Platelet activation can be inhibited by both the cAMP and cGMP signal transduction pathways. A major physiological agonist for adenylyl cyclase activation and cAMP production in platelets is prostacyclin. Although platelets do not synthesize prostacyclin, its production by vascular endothelium inhibits platelet activation. Nitric oxide produced by vascular tissues activates guanylyl cyclase in platelets and stimulates cGMP production; platelets can also directly produce nitric oxide as a negative feedback mechanism during activation [19]. Interestingly, alcohol stimulates vascular prostacyclin synthesis under some experimental conditions [20], although the relevance of this to the *in vivo* hemostatic system has not been adequately demonstrated.

Regardless of the mechanism or stimulus for platelet activation, the final common pathway involves expression of glycoprotein (Gp) IIb-IIIa on the platelet surface, which results in binding and cross-linking of platelets with fibrinogen [17]. Activation also produces the expression on the platelet surface of binding sites for coagulation factors and enzymes, accelerating the rate of thrombin formation. Thrombin converts fibrinogen to fibrin, which adheres to damaged surfaces of blood vessels enmeshing platelets, blood cells, and plasma to form the secondary hemostatic plug. During the process of platelet activation, the initial stage of aggregation (primary platelet aggregation) is reversible, but once platelets have undergone secondary aggregation and release of granule contents, the aggregation is irreversible.

The platelet-fibrin plug can eventually be broken down and removed through the process of fibrinolysis, which involves the plasmin/plasminogen system. Plasminogen is converted to plasmin by activators generated by endothelial and smooth muscle cells: tissue type plasminogen activator (t-PA) and urokinase type plasminogen activator (u-PA). Plasmin is a proteolytic enzyme resembling trypsin, which digests fibrin fibers as well as fibrinogen and clotting factors [21]. By secreting plasminogen activator inhibitor (PAI-1), platelets serve to protect the clot from degradation and inhibit fibrinolysis.

Thus, many sites exist at which alcohol might interact with the hemostatic system, and possibly affect parameters related to risk of CHD. The following is an overview of work done to date by our laboratory, as well as a review of the field in general. In many of these studies, the primary methodology used was optical density platelet aggregometry, in which platelet rich plasma or platelets resuspended in buffer are stimulated by agonists and changes in optical density of the platelet preparation are measured as platelets become activated and form aggregates. In our own studies, we have also incorporated whole blood platelet aggregometry. In this technique, whole blood is stimulated with a platelet agonist, and increased electrical impedance is measured as platelets aggregate on a pair of metal electrodes. Specifically, our interest has been in the effects of ethanol itself on platelets, as opposed to effects of other biologically active compounds contained in various alcoholic beverages (the latter are considered elsewhere in this volume).

ACTIONS OF *IN VITRO* ALCOHOL ON PLATELETS

The immediate functional effect of ethanol usually observed under experimental conditions is inhibition of platelet aggregation in response to most agonists such as thrombin, ADP, epinephrine and collagen [7–9]. This effect has been generally consistent across both animal and human studies in *in vitro*, *in vivo* and *ex vivo* preparations with various methods of ethanol administration. Despite such broad evidence, questions have remained regarding the relevance of the effect to moderate alcohol consumption in humans, due to the doses of alcohol used in those studies, the method of administration, and various other factors. For this reason, our own laboratory has sought to systematically evaluate the effects of ethanol in animal and human studies, with both *in vitro* addition of alcohol and alcohol consumption, using multiple platelet agonists and multiple concentrations of alcohol. Here, we review our own findings, in the context of the broader literature.

In vitro platelet studies in several species including man have generally [13,22,23] but not always [12,24,25] demonstrated an inhibitory effect of alcohol on aggregation or other measures of activation. In the first study in our laboratory, we actually observed that alcohol could promote platelet aggregation under some experimental conditions [12]. We made the serendipitous observation that when alcohol was added directly to whole blood but not platelet rich plasma (PRP), it directly induced aggregation of platelets at final concentrations as low as 34 mM, as measured by impedance aggregometry. This concentration is equivalent to blood alcohol of 156 mg%; lower concentrations were not tested. Further experiments demonstrated that the pro-aggregatory action of alcohol in whole blood was dependent upon the direct injection of ethanol into whole blood, achieving a locally high concentration of alcohol that produces lysis of red blood cells. Consequently, the ADP released during hemolysis activates platelets. Thus, that early study had limited relevance to health effects of moderate alcohol consumption, but may be related to the hematological abnormalities occurring as a result of binge drinking and acute alcohol toxicity [23]. Observations that alcohol might activate platelets *in vitro* under some circumstances have been usually made when platelets were exposed to the ethanol in high final concentrations (inconsistent with blood alcohol levels attained during consumption) or, as discussed above, high local concentrations during alcohol delivery [12,24,25]. When working with a multifunctional and potentially toxic agent such as ethanol, careful interpretations of results, taking into account the physiological and pharmacological relevance of alcohol concentrations and delivery modality, is obviously important.

Our subsequent study [13] is an example of the more commonly observed, inhibitory effect of *in vitro* alcohol on platelets. We systematically examined a more 'physiologically relevant' range of alcohol concentrations (1–85 mM, equivalent to 5–391 mg%), added as a dilute solution (7.8% w/v) to human and rat PRP and whole blood. Aggregation responses to collagen, ADP and arachidonic acid were studied. Collagen-induced platelet aggregation was inhibited by the short term exposure to alcohol, at concentrations as low as 4.25 mM (20 mg%) in rat whole blood (higher concentrations were required for significant effects in human samples, perhaps owing to the small sample size of 6 in this study).

It is generally accepted that the major mechanism for the inhibitory effect of ethanol (though not necessarily for other components of alcoholic beverages) on platelet aggregation involves inhibition of phospholipase A2 and, as a result, inhibition of thromboxane A2 synthesis [18,26]. For this reason, most studies, including ours [13], have observed a greater effect when secondary aggregation (which involves thromboxane A2 synthesis) is induced, by agonists such as collagen or in human platelets, higher concentrations of ADP. Alcohol does not influence platelet shape change or primary aggregatory responses to ADP because these activities are not closely associated with phospholipase A2 activity but rather with phospholipase C (in fact, concentrations of ethanol well beyond physiological levels can actually induce shape change in human platelets) [25]. When arachidonic acid is used as the platelet agonist, the phospholipase A2 step is bypassed and alcohol is a less efficacious inhibitor [13]. An interesting possibility has been noted regarding the inhibition of phospholipase A2 activity by alcohol, in that increased membrane fluidity could be a factor in this inhibition because this enzyme is membrane bound. If increased platelet membrane fluidity is associated with drinking [26], this may be especially beneficial in subjects who consume a diet high in saturated fats, contributing to the well-known effects of the French paradox of low incidence of CHD despite a diet rich in saturated fats [7].

Another platelet signal transduction system that is modulated *in vitro* by ethanol is the nitric oxide (NO)-cGMP system. We originally performed studies based on the hypothesis that alcohol might inhibit platelet aggregation and release reaction in part by enhancing cGMP production, but instead observed that platelet guanylyl cyclase activity and cGMP production in response to the nitric oxide donor sodium nitroprusside is actually inhibited by alcohol [10]. Such an action would theoretically potentiate platelet activation (contrary to the inhibition by alcohol actually observed), suggesting that other actions of ethanol in platelets (for example, inhibition of phospholipase A2) are functionally more important, because the actual effect of alcohol *in vitro* is to inhibit platelet activation.

IN VIVO ALCOHOL EXPOSURE IN ANIMALS AND PLATELET FUNCTION

In the next phase of our systematic evaluation of ethanol and platelet function, our laboratory investigated the effects of acute, *in vivo* exposure of rats to ethanol through inhalation [11]. We focused on effects on whole blood platelet aggregation, based on the apparent sensitivity of this technique in the earlier *in vitro* experiments [13]. By varying alcohol delivery rate and time of exposure, blood alcohol concentrations (BAC) can be controlled. *Ex vivo* platelet aggregation tests were performed after animals had been exposed to a specific atmospheric ethanol environment for either 3, 6, or 9 hours which produced to BAC of 127 ± 15, 259 ± 21 mg%, and 453 ± 16 respectively. At the highest BAC (453 ± 16 mg%), responses to three doses of collagen (1, 3 or 5μg/ml) were significantly inhibited, with the effects of the two lower concentrations being inhibited by more than 50%. At 259 ± 21 mg/%, responses to the two lower collagen concentrations were inhibited, while at BAC of 127 ± 15 mg/%, the response to the low collagen concentration was significantly attenuated. Results with ADP and arachidonic acid were less consistent and less marked. Thus, these results illustrated that acute *in vivo* alcohol exposure had effects very similar to those observed with *in vitro* addition of alcohol to whole blood or PRP, although the BACs tested in our study are substantially higher than those associated with moderate alcohol consumption in humans.

Littleton *et al.* had previously studied the chronic effects on ethanol vapor inhalation in rats [27]. When ethanol was given to the rats over a period of 5–7 days to attain plasma level of 50 mM (230 mg%) *ex vivo* aggregation responses to collagen were reduced in PRP. More profound platelet inhibition and thrombocytopenia were observed after 30 days of inhalation; plasma ethanol concentrations in those rats ranged from 80–120 mM (368–552 mg%). Although these early experiments of Littleton *et al.* involved long-term intoxication associated with high plasma alcohol levels, the general result (inhibition of platelet aggregation after *in vivo* alcohol exposure by various routes, particularly in response to collagen) has been confirmed in several studies including ours described above.

Ex vivo platelet aggregation measurements can be a simple and convenient surrogate for analysis of thrombotic tendency *in vivo*, but, importantly, studies on the effects of alcohol consumption on aggregation have been supported by results of *in vivo* thrombosis models, for example, in a rabbit experimentally induced arterial thrombosis model [28]. Rabbits were given alcohol by gastric intubation, resulting in blood levels of 48 or 100 mM (221 or 460 mg%), and a catheter was used to produce arterial wall injury to stimulate platelet activation and thrombosis. The dry weights of thrombi were reduced in alcohol-treated rabbits compared to controls. In addition to testing the effects of ethanol, Rand *et al.* in a previous study demonstrated that it is the aggregation and not adhesion to the vessel wall that is inhibited by ethanol [22].

ALCOHOLIC BEVERAGE CONSUMPTION AND HUMAN PLATELET FUNCTION

As discussed elsewhere in this volume, quite a few epidemiological studies have examined the association between morbidity and mortality from CHD and moderate alcoholic beverage consumption, and an inverse association has been established in studies involving nearly a million subjects [29]. One example of such reports is a study of American Cancer Society volunteers, which showed that the rate of death from all cardiovascular diseases was 30–40% lower among men and women who consumed at least one alcoholic drink daily than among nondrinkers. While it should be emphasized that alcohol consumption is associated with higher death rates from injuries, violence, suicide, cirrhosis, certain cancers and hemorrhagic stroke [30], the incidence of death from heart disease is much greater compared to these other causes, making any role of platelets potentially important.

Cross-cultural studies have shed light onto the French paradox involving the Mediterranean diet. A Mediterranean diet typically consists of high fruit, vegetable, and grain intake, while also including one to two drinks per day. The daily intake of fats and meat is also higher among those who consume this type of diet, but yet, the rate of coronary heart disease is low [31]. This has led to studies such as the Caerphilly Prospective Heart Disease Study [32] of 1600 men aged 49–66 years. This study is particularly noteworthy in the present context, because along with other parameters related to CHD risk, platelet responses in PRP were measured using thrombin, collagen and ADP. There was a decreased CHD risk associated with increased alcohol consumption, and secondary aggregation to ADP was the aggregation test most closely associated with the occurrence of MI. In contrast, there was no inhibitory effect of alcohol against thrombin induced aggregation; in fact, for each level of alcohol intake, the response of platelets to thrombin was higher than in nondrinkers [32]. The effects of alcohol or drinking on thrombin-induced platelet aggregation are complex; withdrawal from alcohol in alcoholics as well as binge drinking has been associated with a platelet-rebound effect [33,34], with hypersensitivity of platelets to physiological agonists, particularly thrombin.

The rebound effect may explain the rate of sudden death and ischemic stroke in this subset of the population. In a related animal study performed by Ruf et al. [35], rats drank diluted alcohol, and aggregation to thrombin was reduced substantially. However, after deprivation of alcohol for 18 hours, platelet activation by thrombin was more than doubled compared to the original response. This was also observed among men in the Caerphilly study, with the rebound effect also seen in ADP-induced aggregation one to two hours after consumption of alcohol.

The issue of how drinking affects platelet function is complicated even more by the fact that the non-alcoholic components of alcoholic beverages may also have effects on platelets (this aspect is discussed more fully elsewhere). Among wine drinking farmers lower platelet response to thrombin was observed compared to non-drinkers, even after alcohol deprivation for 10 hours [37]. Similarly, in rats, the rebound to thrombin-induced aggregation does not occur when animals are fed red wine as opposed to ethanol before deprivation [38]. This may be related to a reduction in lipid peroxidation by grape tannins.

Pikaar and colleagues investigated the effect of moderate red wine consumption on twelve male volunteers [5]. Four standardized amounts of wine were consumed during 5-week intervals in randomized order. The doses consisted of 0, 2, and 4 glasses of red wine a day (corresponding to 0, 23, and 46 grams of alcohol a day). The effects of 'binge drinking' were also tested (14 glasses consumed over three days). Little difference was seen between binge and daily drinking, but collagen-induced aggregation was reduced with wine consumption compared to abstention. Some studies have specifically examined the potential role of red wine flavanoids such as quercetin and resveratrol in platelet inhibition and potential reduction of CHD risk by wine consumption, based in part on the observation that the compounds may prevent lipid oxidation [37]. Bertellini *et al.* demonstrated a dose-dependent inhibition of collagen induced aggregation by *in vitro* exposure of platelets to resveratrol [38]. The mechanisms involved have been postulated to involve suppression of TXA2 production by trans-resveratrol and an inhibition of phospholipase C by quercetin. The *in vivo* relevance of various red wine components to platelet functional parameters is only now being sorted out, and is discussed in more depth elsewhere in this volume.

SPECIFIC EFFECTS OF ETHANOL CONSUMPTION ON PLATELETS

From the foregoing, although it is clear that consumption of alcoholic beverages inhibits platelet function in humans, several questions remain regarding the nature of the effect. Duration of the effect and dose–response relationships, for example, are not established, and even the fundamental question of whether ethanol itself has a direct role in the effects of alcoholic beverages on platelet function has not been sufficiently investigated. Thus, we recently performed a study in human volunteers, who consumed ethanol in the form of grain alcohol, at doses equivalent to one or two alcoholic beverages (0.25 or 0.5 ml ethanol/kg, respectively) [14]. Aggregation of platelets was measured in both PRP and whole blood, collected before and one hour after consumption, in response to ADP, arachidonic acid and collagen, with sample size of at least 16 for each statistical comparison. This study demonstrated that alcohol itself, at levels relevant to moderate consumption, dose-dependently inhibited platelet aggregation. The response was most pronounced when collagen was the agonist and aggregation was measured in whole blood, at the higher alcohol dose (blood alcohol concentration one hour after consumption was only 38 mg%). Interestingly, we observed that the effects were more evident in women than in men.

While these observations suggest that an anti-platelet effect of ethanol could contribute to the reduced risk of CHD-related mortality in drinkers, it must be emphasized that any contribution of a platelet action of ethanol must be viewed in the context of other actions of ethanol and alcoholic beverage components. Furthermore, the duration of the antiplatelet effect is not known, nor are the effects of chronic vs. acute alcohol consumption or pattern of consumption (regular consumption vs. binge drinking). Nonetheless, this is the first clear demonstration of dose-dependent, inhibitory effects of acute, moderate alcohol consumption on platelet function.

EFFECTS OF ACETALDEHYDE ON PLATELETS

An obvious question when considering effects of drinking on platelet function is whether the degradation products of alcohol, particularly acetaldehyde, have a role in the observed effects. Insufficient work has been published to support firm conclusions, but some studies in rat and human suggest that acetaldehyde, like ethanol, might reduce platelet responses to agonists [39,40]. We have been recently performing studies on acetaldehyde, and find little if any effect of acetaldehyde, added *in vitro*, on human platelet aggregation at concentrations consistent with levels in humans after ethanol consumption (unpublished data from our laboratory). More work is needed in this area.

ETHANOL AND OTHER ASPECTS OF HEMOSTASIS

Because a variety of hemostatic factors beyond those associated with platelets also contribute to the complications associated with coronary heart disease, it is important to consider the above information on platelets in the context of some of these other observations. One of the strongest risk factors for myocardial infarction is elevated plasma fibrinogen level [41]. The association of fibrinogen and alcohol consumption was evaluated by Mennen and colleagues [42]. Alcohol consumption was associated with plasma fibrinogen levels in a U-shaped fashion for men only, with fibrinogen being the lowest in those subjects who drank 20–59 grams of alcohol per day. Fibrinogen levels were greater for nondrinkers and those who consumed over 60 grams of alcohol per day. The type of alcohol consumed also apparently played a role, with a lower level of fibrinogen in those who drank wine and spirits as opposed to those who drank beer and cider (in which no association was found).

Endothelial cells provide a stage for both coagulation and fibrinolysis by synthesizing proteins involved in both processes. With regard to other factors involved in hemostasis, an association has been observed between alcohol exposure and the transcription of t-PA, u-PA and PAI-1 [43]. It was demonstrated that a relatively low concentration of ethanol (0.01– 0.10%, v/v) increased surface-localized fibrinolytic activity, as well as t-PA and u-PA antigen and mRNA levels, while decreasing PAI-1 antigen and mRNA levels. Pre-incubation of cultured endothelial cells produced time- and concentration-dependent effects; notably, increased fibrinolytic activity could be sustained for a full 24 hours after a brief exposure of endothelial cells to less than 0.1% ethanol. If this mechanism is operant *in vivo*, frequent consumption of a moderate amount of alcohol could result in a reduced risk of vascular disorders by effects on the fibrinolytic system.

CONCLUSIONS

In conclusion, a broad array of circumstantial evidence now suggests that platelet inhibitory effects of alcohol might contribute to the reduced risk of CHD mortality among moderate drinkers. This evidence includes epidemiological data, *in vitro* data on effects of alcohol on platelets, and studies on *ex vivo* platelet function after alcohol consumption in animal models and human volunteers. While the effects of multiple components of alcoholic beverages might contribute, it is likely that ethanol itself is partially responsible for the inhibition of platelet function after consumption. The primary mechanism of this inhibition likely involves effects of ethanol on platelet mediators and signaling, due to inhibition of phospholipase A2, and consequently reduced thromboxane synthesis.

Despite the circumstantial evidence, however, there is a need for definitive studies of several aspects of this issue. Specifically, studies must be performed to more fully define the time-action and dose-dependence of ethanol's effects on the hemostatic system. Furthermore, the relative balance between platelet inhibition and possible rebound effects after alcohol consumption should be fully examined, and the role of pattern of drinking behavior must be elucidated. Ultimately, there is a need for prospective human studies on the relationship between alcoholic beverage consumption and CHD mortality and morbidity.

Finally, caution must be exercised in interpreting findings of potential benefits of drinking. Risks associated with alcohol consumption are substantial, and vary considerably between individuals and populations. Although CHD-related risk is reduced in moderate drinkers, and although it is important to define the mechanisms involved, development of any specific recommendations regarding appropriate levels of individual alcohol consumption will be a difficult task.

REFERENCES

1 American Heart Association. *Heart and Stroke Facts: 1995 Statistical Supplement.* American Heart Association, Dallas, TX, 1994.

2 Hennekens CH. Alcohol and risk of coronary events. In '*Alcohol and the Cardiovascular System*', Research Monograph-31, Zakhari S, Wassef M. (Eds.) National Institute of Health, Washington DC 1996, pp. 15–24.

3 Fraser GE, Anderson JT, Foster N, Goldberg R, Jacobs D, Blackburn H. The effect of alcohol on serum high density lipoprotein (HDL): A controlled experiment. *Atherosclerosis* 1983; **46**: 275–286.

4 Willet W, Hennekens CH, Siegel AJ, Adner MM, Castelli WP. Alcohol consumption and high-density lipoprotein cholesterol in marathon runners. *New Eng. J. Med.* 1980; **303**: 1159–1162.

5 Pikkar NA, Wedel M, van der Beek EJ, van Dokkum W, Kempen HJM, Kluft C, Ockhuizen T, Hermus RJJ. Effect of moderate alcohol consumption on platelet aggregation, fibrinolysis, and blood lipids. *Metabolism* 1987; **36**: 538–543.

6 Zakhari S, Gordis E. Moderate drinking and cardiovascular health. *Proc. Assoc of Amer. Physicians* 1999; **111**: 148–158.

7 Renaud SC, Ruf JC. Effects of alcohol on platelet functions. *Clin. Chim. Acta* 1996; **246**: 77–89.

8 Rubin R. Effect of ethanol on platelet function. *Alcohol Clin. Exp. Res.* 1999; **23**: 1114–1118.

9 Rubin R, Rand ML. Alcohol and platelet function. *Alcoholism: Clin. Exp. Res.* 1994; **18**: 105–110.

10 Dong QS, Wroblewska B, Myers AK. Inhibitory effect of alcohol on cyclic GMP accumulation in human platelets. *Thromb. Res.* 1995; **80**: 143–151.

11 Dong QS, Karanian JW, Wesely L, Myers AK. Inhibition of platelet aggregation in whole blood after exposure of rats to alcohol inhalation. *Alcohol* 1997; **14**: 49–54.

12 Abi-Younes SA, Ayers ML, Myers AK. Mechanism of ethanol-induced aggregation in whole blood. *Thromb. Res.* 1991; **63**: 481–489.

13 Torres-Duarte AP, Dong QS, Young J, Abi-Younes S, Myers AK. Inhibition of platelet aggregation in whole blood by alcohol. *Thromb. Res.* 1995; **78**: 107–115.

14 Zhang QH, Das K, Siddiqui S, Myers AK. Effects of acute, moderate ethanol consumption on human platelet aggregation in platelet-rich plasma and whole blood. *Alcoholism: Clin. Exp. Res.* 2000; **24**: 528–534.

15 Fuster V. Mechanisms leading to myocardial infarction: insights from studies of vascular biology. *Circulation* 1994; **90**: 2126–2140.

16 Ducimetiere P, Guize L, Marciniak A, Milon H, Richard J, Rufat P. Arteriographically documented CAD and alcohol consumption in French men. The Corali Study. *Eur. Heart J.* 1993; **14**: 727–733.

17 Bennett JS. Mechanisms of platelet adhesion and aggregation: an update. *Hospital Practice* 1992: 70–86.

18 Stubbs CD, Rubin R. Effect of ethanol on platelet phospholipase A_2. *Lipids* 1992; **27**: 255–260.

19 Riddel DR, Owens JS. Nitric oxide and platelet aggregation. *Vitamins Hormones* 1999; **57**: 25–48.

20 Landolfi R, Steiner M. Ethanol raises prostacyclin *in vivo* and *in vitro*. *Blood* 1984; **64**: 679–682.

21 Kwaan HC. The biological role of components of the plasminogen–plasmin system. *Prog. in Cardiovasc. Dis.* 1992; **34**: 309–316.

22 Rand ML, Groves HM, Kinlough-Rathbone RL, Packham MA, Mustard JF. Effects of ethanol on rabbit platelet responses to collagen *in vitro* and *ex vivo* and on platelet adhesion to de-endothelialized aortae *in vivo*. *Thromb. Res.* 1987; **48**: 379–388.

23 Haut MJ, Cowan DH. The effect of ethanol on hemostatic properties of human blood platelets. *Amer. J. Med.* 1974; **56**: 22–33.

24 Rubin R, Hoek JB. Alcohol-induced stimulation of phospholipase C in human platelets requires G-protein activation. *Biochem. J.* 1988; **254**: 147–153.

25 Rubin R, Ponnappa BC, Thomas AP, Hoek JB. Ethanol stimulates shape change in human platelets by activation of phosphoinositide-specific phospholipase C_1. *Arch. Biochem. Biophy.* 1988; **260**: 480–492.

26 Rubin R. Ethanol interferes with collagen-induced platelet activation by inhibition of arachidonic acid mobilization. *Arch. Biochem. Biophys.* 1989; **270**: 99–113.

27 Littleton JM, Fenn CG, Ummney ND, Yazdanbakhsh M. Effects of ethanol administration on platelet function in the rat. *Alcoholism: Clin. Exp. Res.* 1982; **6**: 512–519.

28 Rand ML, Groves HM, Packham MA, Mustard JF, Kinlough-Rathbone RL. Acute administration of ethanol to rabbits inhibits thrombus formation induced by indwelling aortic catheters. *Lab. Invest.* 1990; **63**: 742–745.

29 Renaud S, Criqui MH, Farchi G, Veenstra J. Alcohol drinking and coronary heart disease. In 'Health Issues Related to Alcohol Consumption', Verschuren PM (Ed.), ILSI Press, Washington DC 1993, pp. 81–123.

30 Thun MJ, Peto R, Lopez AD, Monaco JH, Henley SJ, Heath CW, Doll R. Alcohol consumption and mortality among middle-aged and elderly U.S. adults. *New Eng. J. Med.* 1997; **337**: 1705–1714.

31 Rimm EB, Ellison RC. Alcohol in the Mediterranean diet. *Amer. J. Clin. Nutr.* 1995; **61**: 1378S–1382S.

32 Renaud SC, Beswick AD, Fehily AM, Sharp DS, Elwood PC. Alcohol and platelet aggregation: the Caerphilly prospective heart disease study. *Amer. J. Clin. Nutr.* 1992; **55**: 1012–1017.

33 Hillbom M, Kangasaho M, Kaste M, Numminen H, Vapaatalo H. Acute ethanol ingestion increases platelet reactivity: is there a relationship to stroke? *Stroke* 1985; **16**: 19–23.

34 Hillbom M, Kangasaho M, Hjelm-Jager M. Platelet aggregation and thromboxane B2 formation after ethanol abuse: is there a realtionship to stroke? *Acta Neurol. Scand.* 1984; **70**: 432–437.

35 Ruf JC, Berger J, Renaud S. Platelet rebound effect of alcohol withdrawal and wine drinking in rats. *Arterioscler. Thromb. Vasc. Biol.* 1995; **15**: 140–144.

36 Renaud S, Dumont E, Godsey F, Supplisson A, Thevenon C. Platelet functions in relation to dietary fats in farmers from two regions of France. *Thromb. and Haemostas.* 1979; **40**: 518–531.

37 Ruf JC. Wine and polyphenols related to platelet aggregation and atherothrombosis. *Drugs Exper. Clin. Res.* 1999; **25**: 125–131.

38 Bertelli AAE, Giovannini L, De Caterina R, Bernin W, Migliori M, Fregoni M, Bavaresco L, Bertelli A. Antiplatelet activity of *cis*-resveratrol. *Drugs Exper. Clin. Res.* 1996; **22**: 61–63.

39 Zoucas E, Bengmark S. Effects of acetaldehyde on rat platelet aggregation *in vivo* and *in vitro*. *Res. Exp. Med.* 1987; **187**: 43–48.

40 Spertini O, Hauert J, Bachmann F. Reaction of acetaldehyde with human platelets. *Thromb. Haemostas.* 1992; **67**: 126–130.

41 Ma J, Hennekens CH, Ridker PM, Stampfer MJ. A prospective study of fibrinogen and risk of myocardial infarction in the Physicians Health Study. *Journal of the Amer. Coll. Cardiol.* 1999; **33**: 1347–1352.

42 Mennen LI, Balkau B, Vol S, Caces E, Eschwege E. Fibrinogen a possible link between alcohol consumption and cardiovascular disease? *Arteriosclerosis Thromb. Vascular Biol.* 1999; **19**: 887–892.

43 Booyse FM, Aikens ML, Grenett HE. Endothelial cell fibrinolysis: transcriptional regulation of fibrinolytic protein gene expression (t-PA, u-PA, and PAI-1) by low alcohol. *Alcoholism: Clin. Exp. Res.* 1999; **23**: 1119–1124.

Chapter 14

Fatty acid ethyl esters: role in alcohol cardiotoxicity

Leo Hsu, Mary E. Beckemeier and Puran S. Bora

INTRODUCTION

Alcohol is the most frequently used mind-altering drug except for caffeine. Half of Americans, aged 12 years and older, use alcohol on a regular basis and approximately 10% of these Americans are regarded to be alcoholics [1]. More pertinent to the heart, chronic alcohol abuse has been found to be the chief source of secondary cardiomyopathy (termed alcoholic cardiomyopathy or alcohol-induced heart muscle disease) in the Western world [2,3]. Furthermore, patients with alcohol-induced heart muscle disease who continue in chronic alcohol abuse have 50% mortality rates [4]. Despite, the severity and prevalence of alcohol's role in cardiotoxicity, research was previously hindered due to a lack of knowledge of any existing biochemical mechanisms. The most commonly known catabolic pathway for alcohol is catalyzed by the enzyme alcohol dehydrogenase (ADH) to the toxic metabolite acetyl-aldehyde. Although this mechanism may partially explain liver damage associated with alcohol intake, it does not account for the presence of extrahepatic damage. Only the liver possesses this oxidative metabolic pathway to a sufficient degree [5].

A connection between extrahepatic organ damage and chronic abuse of alcohol has been made with the discovery of a nonoxidative pathway for alcohol metabolism. This pathway has been identified in the heart, pancreas, brain, and tissues such as blood [6–16]. Further-more, the pathway creates a toxic metabolite named fatty acid ethyl ester (FAEE). FAEEs are neutral molecules that are thought to accumulate in the mitochondria and have been shown to produce mitochondrial dysfunction *in vitro* in rabbit hearts, and *in vitro* and *in vivo* in rat hearts. The uncoupling of the mitochondria's energy transduction process can result in an inefficient energy production as well as cell damage, providing a link between ethanol ingestion and the subsequent development of alcohol-induced end-organ damage. In addition, the FAEEs are able to induce myocardial cell damage in rat and rabbit hearts. [11,12,16,17]

The enzyme responsible for the production of the potentially toxic ethyl esters, named fatty acid ethyl ester synthase (FAEES), exhibits its highest activity in heart, brain, and pancreas, those extrahepatic organs most commonly damaged by alcohol abuse [18,19]. Four FAEESs, labeled synthase-I, synthase-II, synthase-III and synthase/carboxylesterase have been purified to homogeneity and have also been characterized [6–10,12–14,20,21]. This chapter will discuss the potential toxicity of FAEEs, and examine the role of synthase/carboxylesterase on cardiotoxicity and its genetics. Further information on the other FAEESs can be found in a recent review article [22].

FATTY ACID ETHYL ESTERS

The majority of ingested alcohol is rapidly absorbed from the small intestine into the blood-stream, and is distributed to tissues that possess high water content and blood flow, e.g., myocardium [5]. Once ethanol has reached myocardium, it has been shown to affect both the sarcolemma (muscle cell membrane) and the sarcoplasmic reticulum (SR). In rat myocytes, chronic alcohol intake creates sarcolemma leaking along with an intracellular calcium increase [23,24]. Several studies also exhibited decreased Ca^{2+} binding and uptake by the SR [25–29]. Normal function of these components is essential for proper contraction of the heart. Indeed, several investigators have reported depressed cardiac function with acute and chronic exposure to ethanol [26,30–34].

A decreased capacity to produce metabolic energy was observed in many investigations [30–35]. It was noted that ethanol increases basal metabolic rates and oxygen consumption [35]. Changes in phosphate/O_2 and respiratory control ratios was also demonstrated with ethanol intake [30,36–38]. In addition, mitochondrial cristae disruption, swelling, and existence of dense inclusion bodies was detected in laboratory animals receiving chronic ethanol intake [26,39–41]. The toxic metabolite acetylaldehyde does not appear to cause these results for reasons discussed above. However, recent research on FAEEs may help elucidate the mechanism for ethanol's effect on the sarcolemma, SR, and cellular respiration.

It was previously thought that the heart was unable to metabolize ethanol. More recently, however, isolated perfused hearts have exhibited a non-oxidative metabolism of ethanol [16]. As shown in Figure 14.1, ethanol (ETOH) is esterified with fatty acids to produce the neutral molecule, FAEE. FAEE synthesis and accumulation of ethyl esters was observed in organs commonly damaged by chronic ethanol abuse [18]. This putative toxic metabolite is produced in the myocardium, brain, pancreas and blood [6–16]. Furthermore, uncoupling of oxidative phosphorylation was shown to linearly decrease with concentrations of ethyl oleate (a FAEE) below 40–50 μM [17].

Although fatty acids are known uncouplers of oxidative phosphorylation, they are usually bound to fatty acid binding proteins as seen in Figure 14.1. Therefore, they are unable to produce the uncoupling effect under physiological conditions. However, it was hypothesized that FAEEs act as a shuttle for the toxic fatty acids to reach mitochondria [17]. FAEEs are less likely to bind fatty acid binding proteins compared to fatty acids due to their lack of negative charge. Once the FAEEs are produced, they are believed to bind mitochondria. This is supported by the finding that 72% of the FAEEs produced intracellularly were bound to mitochondria [17]. Furthermore, 60 minute incubation of rabbit myocardium in ethyl [^{3}H] oleate resulted in a linear increase in mitochondrial binding of the FAEE [11].

After the FAEEs bind to mitochondria, they are thought to be hydrolyzed into fatty acids. These fatty acids have been shown to uncouple oxidative phosphorylation in concentrations $\geq 5\,\mu$M [17,42,43]. Bora *et al.* have indeed demonstrated that when ethyl [^{3}H] oleate was injected into rat myocardium, the ratio of ethyl [^{3}H] oleate:[^{3}H] oleate (FAEE:FA) was 1:8. In addition, miniscule amounts of [^{3}H] oleate were formed in the absence of mitochondria [11]. These results were confirmed by Szczepiokowski *et al.*, who revealed that 90% of FAEEs were hydrolyzed to fatty acids in HepG2 cells [44]. Therefore, it was concluded that the majority of the uncoupling effect was due to the fatty acids, and that mitochondria possess an esterase that substantially hydrolyzes FAEEs into toxic fatty acids. Carboxylesterase was also noted to be partly responsible for this hydrolysis [20].

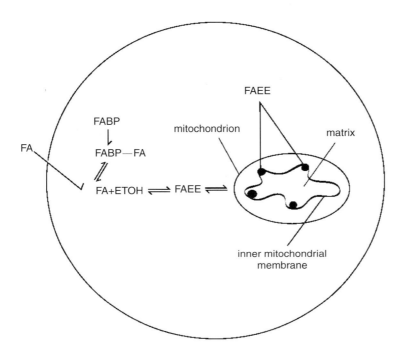

Figure 14.1 Fatty acids (FA) are found linked to fatty acid binding proteins (FABP) and are therefore prevented from entering the mitochondria. However, FA can react with ethanol (ETOH) to produce fatty acid ethyl esters (FAEE) via fatty acid ethyl ester synthase. Once inside the mitochondria, FAEE can cause direct damage, but also their hydrolysis to fatty acids can lead to uncoupling of oxidative phosphorylation.

To determine the accumulation of FAEEs in the body, Lange *et al.* have measured the amount of the ethyl esters in autopsy samples [18]. They have reported FAEE concentrations ranging from 9–115 μM in human left ventricles. The autopsy samples were taken from patients exposed to acute or chronic alcohol. In addition, ventricles from patients that had abstained from alcohol contained no ethyl esters [45]. Presence of FAEE persisted in the autopsy samples despite undetectable alcohol levels in the blood. Furthermore, the biological half life ($t_{1/2}$) has been estimated to be between 20–24 hours [17]. Therefore, FAEEs are thought to collect in tissues, such as the heart, with chronic ethanol intake and may play a pathologic role. This has been further corroborated by Yamazaki *et al.*'s finding that heart FAEE concentrations in autopsy samples were higher in alcoholics despite low blood ethanol concentrations [46].

Besides its uncoupling effect, evidence of FAEE's toxicity has been reported by several other studies. One such study revealed that FAEEs can be a direct cause of membrane fluidity aberrations [47]. In addition, pancreatic lysosomes incubated with FAEEs have shown increased instability [48]. Decreases in protein synthesis and cell formation were also observed in HepG2 cells which had taken in ethanol [44]. Histologic changes were also observed by light microscopy just 4 days after 30–50 μL injections of 50 μM oleic acid ethyl ester solution. 30 days after the injection, myocytes had further increased in size and deformity [11] (Figure 14.2).

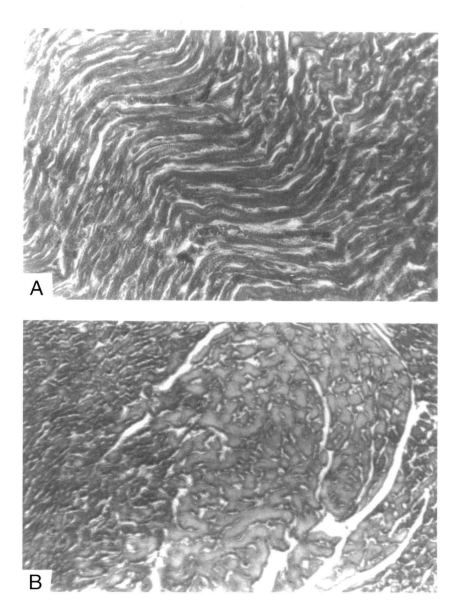

Figure 14.2 (A) Histopathological analyses of control rat myocardium with 30 μl phosphate-buffered saline (PBS) + 0.01% dimethylsulfoxide. Sections stained with Mason trichrome. No cell damage is observed (original magnification × 300). (B) Histopathological analyses of rat myocardium injected with 30 μL of 50 μM FAEE. Sections stained with Mason trichrome. The significant cell damage was observed after 30 days. The cells were enlarged and irregular in shape (original magnification × 300).

Szczepiorkowski *et al.* reported a histologic distinction between human hepatoblastoma cells with and without FAEEs [44]. *In vivo* damage to pancreatic tissue was also noted. FAEEs in reconstituted LDLs were infused intra-arterially to rats. Pancreatic injury from the infused ethyl esters was indicated by pancreatic trypsinogen-activation peptide increases, creation of pancreatic edema, and acinar cell ultrastructural changes [49]. It is important to point out, however, that no histological alterations or edema were observed in the myocardium. These results may be confounded due to the nonuse of ethanol in the study. If ethanol was given to the rats, it is reasonable to believe that FAEE concentrations would be significantly higher due to endogenous synthesis of FAEEs.

Although, the oxidative metabolite, acetylaldehyde, exists in low concentrations in blood [50], notable concentrations of FAEEs have been located in human blood serum following ethanol intake [51]. In fact, FAEEs in the circulation have been commonly proposed as a marker for ethanol exposure. Furthermore, a recent study suggests that plasma FAEEs are produced by lipoprotein lipase [52], rather than in tissue or cells as Doyle [51] and Gorski [15] hypothesize. Lipoprotein lipase (LPL) was previously reported to have fatty acid ethyl ester synthase (FAEES) capability [53]. After perfusion of isolated rat hearts with chylomicrons (a LPL substrate), Chang *et al.* observed that the majority of the ethyl esters were found in the perfusate rather than in the myocardium itself. Apo CII (co-factor for LPL) levels were significantly increased, supporting the hypothesis that plasma FAEEs are synthesized by LPL [52].

Serum FAEE appear to favor lipoprotein vs. albumin binding during increased concentrations of the ethyl esters. FAEEs also display a lack of competition with free fatty acids for albumin binding [54]. Gorski *et al.* have shown that FAEES ability also exists within leukocytes. The highest synthase levels were measured in the natural killer (NK) cells. CD4$^+$ T cells had 50% of the FAEES levels as CD8$^+$ T cells [15]. Interestingly, alcoholics were measured to have approximately half the leukocyte FAEES levels as non-alcoholics. This may suggest that alcoholics possess a genetic predisposition to chronic alcohol abuse due to a reduced ability to produce toxic metabolites. An alternate conclusion, however, is that alcoholics possess a smaller FAEES capability due to an adaptive response [15].

FATTY ACID ETHYL ESTER SYNTHASE

As shown in Figure 14.1, FAEEs are produced by an enzyme named fatty acid ethyl ester synthase (FAEES). This enzyme has four forms, named synthase-I, synthase-II, synthase-III, and synthase/carboxylesterase. Each of these enzymes has been purified and characterized from human myocardium [6–10,12–14,20,21]. FAEES has also been reported in rat pancreas [55], murine brain [47], and rabbit myocardium [56,57]. These enzymes have been extensively reviewed [6–14]. For further details, please read the review [22].

CHARACTERIZATION OF SYNTHASE/ CARBOXYLESTERASE

Dual activity of synthase/carboxylesterase

A FAEES enzyme purified from human heart exhibited FAEE synthesis as well as carboxylesterase hydrolytic activity [20]. Homology between carboxylesterase and FAEES was found by Tsujita and Okuda [58], who demonstrated that the FAEES obtained from adipose tissue, lung, and testis possessed both hydrolytic and FAEE synthetic activities. Furthermore, a 62 Kda FAEES, isolated from human heart by Bora *et al.* was revealed to have 88% homology to the first 17 N-terminal residues in rat liver and adipose tissue carboxylesterase [20]. The purified synthase/carboxylesterase demonstrated a PNPB-hydrolyzing activity of 620 µmol/mg/h and a FAEES activity of 3700 nmol/mg/h, providing evidence that this human heart FAEES exhibits dual carboxylesterase and FAEE synthesis functions [20]. In addition, a 62 KDa synthase/carboxylesterase band was detected, via Western blot with antibody against pure human synthase/carboxylesterase, in human heart cytosolic, microsomal and mitochondrial fractions,which suggests that synthase/carboxylesterase may be present in the human heart mitochondria. Furthermore, the FAEEs produced are thought to be hydrolyzed to fatty acids. As mentioned above, *in vitro* experiments show that fatty acids are known uncouplers of mitochondrial oxidative phosphorylation [11,42,17]. Hence, a mechanism for the onset of alcohol-induced cardiomyopathy via FAEE formation by synthase/carboxylesterase, has been provided. The purified enzyme was designated FAEES/carboxylesterase, establishing a link between synthase/carboxylesterase and alcohol-induced end-organ damage.

Structure of synthase/carboxylesterase

There are many structural features of the amino-acid sequence that are highly conserved among most carboxylesterase isoenzymes, such as the serine esterase active site discussed previously, an endoplasmic reticulum-retention signal, and one Asn-Xxx-Thr site for N-linked carbohydrate addition. The primary structure of the carboxylesterase family indicates that these proteins should be localized to the endoplasmic reticulum, with most of the hydrolytic activity occurring in the microsomal fraction of the liver [59]. Many of the carboxylesterases retained in the lumen of the endoplasmic reticulum contain a hydrophobic signal peptide sequence which will initiate a secretory pathway [60]. Yet, the retention of some of these proteins in the endoplasmic reticulum, as suggested by Munro and Pelham, may be due to the C-terminal amino acid residues [61,62]. The C-terminal dipeptide Glu–Leu was discovered in various carboxylesterases to be part of a directant for intracellular retention [60–64]. A recent investigation by Potter *et al.* (1998) shows this same Glu–Leu dipeptide directant in two homologous carboxylesterase cDNAs [65]. The group truncated the C-terminal and N-terminal ends, separately and together, of rabbit liver and human alveolar macrophage carboxylesterases. Through PCR-mediated mutagenesis of the cDNAs and expression in Cos7 cells with subsequent immunohistochemical localization, C-terminal residues, which include the characteristic Glu–Leu dipeptide, were determined to prevent secretion of the proteins from the cell.

The group also concluded that the hydrophobic 18-amino acid NH_2-terminal end of the carboxylesterase cDNAs is responsible for the localization of these proteins to the endoplasmic reticulum. Enzymatic activity was lost when the N-terminal was truncated, yet activity could be detected in the culture media of the C-terminally truncated cells. When the investigators treated Cos7 cells expressing C-terminal truncated carboxylesterase with brefeldin A, a fungal derived antibiotic that causes reversible loss of the endoplasmic reticulum in mammalian cells, a prevention of the secretion of the carboxylesterases was observed. This confirmed that these carboxylesterase enzymes were processed and released from cells via exocytosis mediated by the endoplasmic reticulum. As the investigators pointed out, the data suggest that modification by the endoplasmic reticulum may be required to generate active carboxylesterases, regardless of whether the enzyme is retained in the cell or secreted.

The important roles that have been established for the carboxylesterase enzyme family have prompted a look into its gene structure. Identification of the respective genes of the carboxylesterase enzyme family will offer insight into the structural and functional tenets of its many enzymes as well as making it feasible to establish a genetic link between alcohol abuse and alcohol-induced heart muscle disease.

Since, a large portion of the carboxylesterase activity in the body occurs in the liver, numerous liver and liver microsomal carboxylesterases have been purified and characterized by several investigators [68–78]. Furthermore, various carboxylesterase cDNAs have been purified from other tissues including human heart [20], human intestine [79], rat adipose tissue [58], and rat kidney [80] to name a few. Since key serine, histidine, and glutamine residues have been conserved in the active sites of the various carboxylesterases, mutagenesis studies of these particular residues have shown decreased enzyme activities [68–71].

Genetics of synthase/carboxylesterase

The determination of the genetics underlying carboxylesterase enzyme family function has proven critical as the complex and diverse substrate specificity of the enzyme family unravels. Studies have been completed on various carboxylesterase substrates and inhibitors in order to create a library for characterizing the numerous carboxylesterase enzymes present in mammalian tissues [81]. Carboxylesterase is a multigene family belonging to the serine esterase superfamily of enzymes. To date, there have been numerous proteins identified with amino acid sequences homologous with carboxylesterase. The serine esterase superfamily is characterized by multigene families, such as carboxylesterase, or single-copy genes that have similar sequences, but divergent functions [82]. Shibata et al. (1993) in their isolation and characterization of a human carboxylesterase gene encoding a human liver carboxylesterase, put together a phylogenetic tree of 12 mammalian members of the esterase super family. Analysis of the sequence alignments of these proteins, including human carboxylesterase, revealed a separation of these proteins as a possible result of gene duplications into at least 4 groups: thyroglobin, cholinesterase, lipase, and carboxylesterase [82].

Shibata et al. furthermore examined the amino acid alignment of eight different mammalian carboxylesterases, including human carboxylesterase, rabbit liver 60 kD carboxylesterase 1 [83], pig carboxylesterase, rat pI 6.1 esterase [84], mouse carboxylesterase Es-N [85], rat carboxylesterase E1, mouse esterase-22 (egasyn) [86], and rabbit liver 60 kD carboxylesterase 2 [87]. Analysis of this alignment allowed the investigators to put these carboxylesterases into three groups. The characteristic C-terminal contained the amino acids HXEL in groups I and III and TEHX in group II. A motif of tetrapeptides, more notably the E-L dipeptide, has been recognized for endoplasmic reticulum retention. Since, group II does not exhibit this motif it has been characterized as secretory [88]. The researchers proposed that the data from the phylogenetic tree and the data from the carboxylesterase amino acid alignment suggests that there are at least 2 types of microsomal carboxylesterases (group 1 and III) and one type of serum carboxylesterase (group II) in various species of mammals. The determination of the variant physiological roles of serum and microsomal carboxylesterases is currently underway.

Identification of the respective carboxylesterase genes will provide insight into the regulation and biosynthesis of this enzyme family. Investigators have isolated a carboxylesterase gene, 31 kb in size with 14 exons and 13 introns [66,82]. Langmann and investigators examined the 5′ flanking sequence of the carboxylesterase gene in order to identify sequences relevant for promoter activity. A promoter region was identified in the 945-bp long DNA-sequence preceding the transcription start point. No classical TATA box was located and the proximal region of the carboxylesterase was revealed to be rich in guanine and cytosine [66]. In the DNA sequence preceding the transcription start point, several potential binding sites for various transcription factors were found. As the investigators point out, the nature of the promoter region is, therefore, consistent with the broad distribution of carboxyl-esterase expression in various tissues.

CONCLUSIONS

Previous research on ethanol's effect on cardiotoxicity was hindered by a lack of a known metabolic pathway in the heart. Recent research, however, has revealed that ethanol can be metabolized with fatty acids to produce FAEEs. It has been observed that FAEEs may act as a toxic shuttle for fatty acids to reach the mitochondria within myocytes. These FAEEs may then be hydrolyzed into fatty acids causing cellular and tissue damage due to the uncoupling of oxidative phosphorylation. The enzyme which catalyzes this reaction (FAEES), has been purified and characterized in each of its four forms: synthase-I, II, III, and synthase/carboxylesterase. The discovery of FAEEs in human myocardium, and the putative toxicity of these molecules has provided a model for ethanol's damaging effect on the heart. Continued investigation on this non-oxidative metabolic pathway of ethanol will provide further understanding to the ethyl ester's role in cardiotoxicity.

It has been suggested that alcohol metabolism may be under genetic control and related to the presence of different amounts or types of ethanol-metabolizing enzymes [89,90]. FAEES could be a likely candidate for the underlying genetic vulnerability to the effects of alcohol since no other significant alcohol metabolizing pathway is known to exist in the heart. This FAEES gene opens up new possibilities for mapping a gene for alcoholism or alcohol-induced myocardial damage. Further sequence analysis of this gene may provide insight into the domain and functional structure of FAEES, offering promise for establishing a genetic link between alcohol abuse and end-organ damage such as that observed in the heart.

ACKNOWLEDGMENT

The study was supported by V.A. Merit grant to PSB. We thank Gloria Skelton for the help in preparing this book chapter for publication, Nicole Lee for the critical review and Samantha Son for the graphical design.

REFERENCES

1 Substance Abuse and Mental Health Services Administration, Office of Applied Studies, In: *Preliminary estimates from the 1993 National Household Survey on Drug Abuse. Advance report no. 7.* Department of Health and Human Services, Maryland, 1994.

2 Andersson B, Waagstein F. Spectrum and outcome of congestive heart failure in a hospitalized population. *Am. Heart J.* 1993; **126**: 632–640.

3 Roberts WC, Siegel RJ, McManus BM. Idiopathic dilated cardiomyopathy: analysis of 152 necropsy patients. *Am. J. Cardiol.* 1987; **60**: 1340–1355.

4 Demakis JG, Proskey A, Rahimtola SH *et al.* The natural course of alcoholic cardiomyopathy. *Ann. Intern. Med.* 1974; **80**: 293–297.

5 Goldstein D. Effects of alcohol on neuronal membranes. In: *The Pharmacology of Alcohol.* Eds. Henri Begleiter and Benjamin Kissin. Oxford University Press, New York, 1974.

6 Bora PS, Spilburg C, Lange LG. Identification of a satellite fatty acid ethyl ester synthase from human myocardium as a glutathione S-transferase. *J. Clin. Invest.* 1989a; **84**: 1942–1946.

7 Bora PS, Spilburg C, Lange LG. Purification of homogeneity and characterization of major fatty acid ethyl ester synthase from human myocardium. *FEBS Lett.* 1989b; **258**: 236–239.

8 Bora PS, Spilburg C, Lange LG. Metabolism of ethanol and carcinogens by glutathione transferases. *Proc. Natl. Acad. Sci. USA* 1989c; **86**: 4470–4473.

9 Bora PS, Bora NS, WU X, Lange LG. Molecular cloning, sequencing and expression of human myocardial fatty acid ethyl ester synthase-III cDNA. *J. Biol. Chem.* 1991; **266**: 12670–12673.

10 Bora PS, Wu X, Spilburg C, Lange LG. Purification and characterization of fatty acid ethyl ester synthase-II from human myocardium. *J. Biol. Chemistry* 1992a; **267**: 13217–13221.

11 Bora PS, Farrar MA, Miller DD, Chaitman BR, Guruge BL. Myocardial cell damage by fatty acid ethyl esters. *J. Cardiovascular Pharmacol.* 1996a; **27**: 1–6.

12 Bora PS, Lange LG. Fatty acid ethyl esters and heart disease. *Alcohol Health Res. World* 1990; **14**: 285–288.

13 Bora PS, Lange LG. Fatty acid ethyl ester, alcohol and liver changes. *Alcohol and Drug Abuse Reviews* 1991a; **II**: 150–165.

14 Bora PS, Lange LG. Homogenous synthase-I from human myocardium is a glutathione S-transferase. *Ann. New York Acad. Sci.* 1991b; **625**: 827–829.

15 Gorski NP, Nouraldin H, Dube DM, Preffer FI, Dombkowski DM, Villa EM, Lewandrowsk KB, Weiss RD, Hufford C, Laposata M. Reduced fatty acid ethyl ester synthase activity in the white blood cells of alcoholics. *Alcohol Clin. Exp. Res.* 1996; **20**: 268–274.

16 Lange LG, Bergman SR, Sobel BE. Identification of fatty acid ethyl esters as products of rabbit myocardial ethanol metabolism. *J. Biol. Chem.* 1981; **256**: 12968–12973.

17 Lange LG, Sobel BE. Mitochondrial dysfunction induced by fatty acid ethyl esters, myocardial metabolites of ethanol. *J. Clin. Invest.* 1983a; **72**: 724–731.

18 Laposata EA, Lange LG. Presence of non-oxidative ethanol metabolism in human organs commonly damaged by ethanol abuse. *Science* 1986; **231**: 487–499.

19 Laposata EA, Scherre DE, Mazow C, Lange LG. Metabolism of ethanol by human brain to fatty acid ethyl esters. *J. Biol. Chem.* 1987; **262**: 4653–4657.

20 Bora PS, Guruge BL, Miller DD, Chaitman B, Ruyle M. Purification and characterization of human heart fatty acid ethyl ester synthase/carboxylesterase. *J. Mol. Cell Cardiol.* 1996b; **28**: 2027–2032.

21 Bora PS, Wu X, Lange LG. Site-specific mutagenesis of two histidine residues in fatty ethyl ester synthase-III. *Biochem. Biophys. Res. Commun.* 1992b; **184**: 706–711.

22 Beckemeier ME, Bora PS. Fatty acid ethyl esters: potentially toxic products of myocardial ethanol metabolism. *J. Mol. Cell Cardiol.* 1998; **30**: 2487–2494.

23 Polimeni PI, Otten MD, Hoeschen LE. *In vivo* effects of ethanol on the rat myocardium: evidence for a reversible, non-specific increase of sarcolemmal permeability. *J. Mol. Cell Cardiol.* 1983; **15**: 113–122.

24 Noren GR, Staley NA, Einzig S, Mikell FL, Asinger RW. Alcohol-induced congestive cardiomyopathy: an animal model. *Cardiovasc. Res.* 1983; **17**: 81–87.

25 Bing RJ, Tillmanns H, Fauvel JM, Seeler K, Mao JC. Effect of prolonged alcohol administration on calcium transport in heart muscle of the dog. *Circ. Res.* 1974; **35**: 33–38.

26 Sarma JSM, Ikeda S, Fischer R, Maruyama Y, Weishaar R, Bing RJ. Biochemical and contractile properties of heart muscle after prolonged alcohol administration. J. Mol. Cell Cardiol. 1976; **8**: 951–972.

27 Segel LD, Rendig SV, Choquet Y, Chacko K, Amsterdam EA, Mason DT. Effects of chronic graded ethanol consumption on the metabolism ultrastructure and mechanical function of the rat heart. Cardiovasc. Res. 1975; **9**: 649–663.

28 Olsen C, Piano MR, Schwertz DW, Solaro JR, Ferguson J. Ethanol's subcellular effect on the heart: the beginning of alcoholic cardiomyopathy [abstract]. Alcohol Clin. Exp. Res. 1991; **15**: 348.

29 Segel LD, Rendig SV, Mason DT. Alcohol-induced hemodynamic and Ca^{++} flux dysfunctions are reversible. J. Mol. Cell Cardiol. 1981; **13**: 443–455.

30 Pachinger OM, Tillmanns H, Mao JC, Fauvel JM, Bing RJ. The effect of prolonged administration of ethanol on cardiac metabolism and performance in the dog. J. Clin. Invest. 1973; **52**: 2690–2696.

31 Ettinger PO, Lyons M, Oldewurtel HA, Regan TJ. Cardiac conduction abnormalities produced by chronic alcoholism. Am. Heart J. 1976; **91**: 66–78.

32 Hastillo AH, Poland J, Hess ML. Mechanical and subcellular function of rat myocardium during chronic ethanol consumption. Proc. Soc. Exp. Biol. Ed. 1980; **164**: 415–420.

33 Regan TJ, Levinson GE, Oldewurtel HA, Frank MJ, Weisse AB, Moschos CB. Ventricular function in noncardiacs with alcoholic fatty liver: role of ethanol in the production of cardiomyopathy. J. Clin. Invest. 1969; **48**: 397–407.

34 Gimeno AL, Gimeno MF, Webb JL. Effects of ethanol on cellular membrane potentials and contractility of isolated rat atrium. Am. J. Physiol. 1962; **203**: 194–196.

35 Higgins H. Effect of alcohol on the respiration and the gaseous metabolism in man. J. Pharmacol. Exp. Ther. 1971; **9**: 441–472.

36 Rossi M. Alcohol and malnutrition in the pathogenesis of experimental alcoholic cardiomyopathy. J. Pathol. 1980; **130**: 105–116.

37 Weishaan R, Sarma JSM, Maruyama Y, Fisher R, Bertuglia S, Bing RJ. Reversibility of mitochondrial and contractile changes in the myocardium after cessation of prolonged ethanol intake. Am. J. Cardiol. 1977; **40**: 556–562.

38 Bottenus RE, Spach PI, Filns S, Cunningham CC. Effect of chronic ethanol consumption on energy-linked processes associated with oxidative phosphorylation. Biochem. Biophys. Res. Commun. 1982; **105**: 1368–1373.

39 Ferrans VJ, Hibbs RG, Weilbaecher DG, Black WC, Walsh JJ, Burch GE. Alcoholic cardiomyopathy: a histochemical study. Am. Heart J. 1965; **69**: 766–779.

40 Alexander CS. Electron microscopic observations in alcoholic heart disease. Br. Heart J. 1967; **29**: 200–206.

41 Segel L, Rendig S, Mason D. Left ventricular dysfunction of isolated working rat hearts after chronic alcohol consumption. Cardiovasc. Res. 1979; **13**: 136–146.

42 Borst R, Loos JA, Christ EF, Slater EC. Uncoupling activity of long chain fatty acids. Biochim. Biophys. Acta 1962; **62**: 509–517.

43 Jezek P, Freisleben HJ. Fatty acid binding site of the mitochondrial uncoupling protein. Demonstration of its existence by EPR spectroscopy of 5-DOXYL-stearic acid. FEBS Lett. 1994; **343**: 22–26.

44 Szczepiorkowski ZM, Dickersin RG, Laposata M. Fatty acid ethyl ester decreases human hepatoblastoma cell proliferation and protein synthesis. Gastroenterology 1995; **108**: 515–522.

45 Lange LG, Sobel BE. Myocardial metabolites of ethanol. Circulation Research 1983b; **52**: 479–482.

46 Yamazaki K, Gilg T, Kauert G, von Meyer L, Eisenmenger W. Nonoxidative ethanol and methanol changes in the heart and brain tissue of alcohol abusers. Nippon Hoigaku Zasshi – Japanese Journal of Legal Medicine 1997; **51**: 380–387.

47 Hungund BL, Goldstein DB, Villegas F, Cooper CP. Formation of fatty acid ethyl esters during chronic ethanol treatment in mice. Biochem. Pharmacol. 1988; **37**: 3001–3004.

48 Haber PS, Wilson JS, Apte MV, Pirola RC. Fatty acid ethyl esters increase rat pancreatic lysosomal fragility. *J. Lab. Clin. Ed.* 1993; **121**: 759–764.

49 Werner J, Laposata M, Castillo CF, Saghir M, Iozzo RV, Lewandrowski KB, Warshaw AL. Pancreatic injury in rats induced by fatty acid ethyl ester, a nonoxidative metabolite of alcohol. *Gastroenterology* 1997; **113**: 286–294.

50 Eriksson CJ, Sippel HW. The distribution and metabolism of acetaldehyde in rats during ethanol oxidation. *Biochem. Pharmacol.* 1977; **26**: 241–247.

51 Doyle KM, Bird DA, Al-Salihi S, Hallaq Y, Cluette-Brown JE, Goss KA, Laposata M. Fatty acid ethyl esters are present in human serum after ethanol ingestion. *J. Lipid Res.* 1994; **35**: 428–437.

52 Chang W, Waltenbaugh C, Borensztajn J. Fatty acid ethyl ester synthesis by the isolated perfused rat heart. *Metabolism* 1997; **46**: 926–929.

53 Tsujita T, Okuda H. Fatty acid ethyl ester-synthesizing activity of lipoprotein lipase from rat postheparin plasma. *J. Biol. Chem.* 1994; **269**: 5884–5889.

54 Bird DA, Kabakibi A, Laposata M. The distribution of fatty acid ethyl esters among lipoproteins and albumin in human serum. *Alcoholism: Clinical and Experimental Research* 1997; **21**: 602–605.

55 Hamamoto T, Yamada S, Murawaki Y, Kawasaki H. Effect of ethanol feeding on fatty acid ethyl ester synthase in the liver and pancreas of rats fed a nutritionally adequate diet or a low protein diet. *Biochem. Pharmacol.* 1991; **42**: 1148–1150.

56 Mogelson S, Lange LG. Nonoxidative ethanol metabolism in rabbit myocardium: Purification to homogeneity of fatty acid ethyl ester synthase. *Biochemistry* 1984; **23**: 4075–4081.

57 Mogelson S, Pieper SJ, Lange LG. Thermodynamic bases for fatty acid ethyl ester synthase catalyzed esterification of free fatty acid ethyl esters. *Biochemistry* 1984; **23**: 4082–4087.

58 Tsujita T, Okuda H. Fatty acid ethyl ester synthase in rat adipose tissue and its relationship to carboxylesterase. *J. Biol. Chem.* 1992; **267**: 23489–23494.

59 Mentlein R, Heymann E. Hydrolysis of retinyl esters by non-specific carboxylesterases from rat liver endoplasmic reticulum. *Biochem. J.* 1987; **245**: 863–867.

60 Kroetz D, McBride O, Gonzalez F. Glycosylation-dependant activity of baculovirus-expressed human liver carboxylesterases: cDNA cloning and characterization of two highly similar enzyme forms. *Biochemistry* 1993; **32**: 11606–11617.

61 Munro S, Pelham HRB. A C-terminal signal prevents secretion of luminal ER proteins. *Cell* 1987; **48**: 899–907.

62 Munro S, Pelham HRB. An Hsp70-like protein in the ER: identity with the 78 kd glucose-regulated protein and immunoglobulin heavy chain binding protein. *Cell* 1986; **46**: 291–300.

63 Andres DA, Dickerson IM, Dixon JE. Variants of the carboxy-terminal KDEL sequence direct intracellular retention. *J. Biol. Chem.* 1990; **265**: 5952–5955.

64 Robbi M, Beaufay H. The COOH terminus of several liver carboxylesterase targets these enzymes to the lumen of the endoplasmic reticulum. *J. Biol. Chem.* 1991; **266**: 20498–20503.

65 Potter PM, Wolverton JS, Morton CL, Wierdl M, Danks MK, Potter PM. Cellular localization domains of a rabbit and a human carboxylesterase: influence of irinotecan (CPT-11) metabolism by the rabbit enzyme. *Cancer Research* 1998; **58**: 3627–3632.

66 Langmann T, Becker A, Aslanidis C, Notka F, Ulrich H, Schwer H, Schmitz G. Stuctural organization and characterization of the promoter region of a human carboxylesterase gene. *Biochimica et Biophysica Acta* 1997; **1350**: 65–74.

67 Shibata F, Takagi Y, Kitajima A, Kuroda T, Omura T. Molecular cloning and characterization of a human carboxylesterase gene. *Genomics* 1993; **17**: 79–82.

68 Alexon SE, Mentlein R, Werstedt C, Hellman U. Isolation and characterization of microsomal acyl-CoA thioesterase. A member of the rat liver microsomal carboxylesterase multi-gene family. *Eur. J. Biochem.* 1993; **214**: 719–727.

69 Hosokawa M. Differences in the functional roles of hepatic microsomal carboxylesterase isozymes in various mammals and humans. *Xenobiotic Metab. Dispos.* 1990; **5**: 185–195.

70 Hosokawa M, Maki T, Satoh T. Characterization of molecular species of liver microsomal carboxylesterases of several animal species and humans. *Arch. Biochem. Biophys.* 1990; **277**: 219–227.

71 Hosokawa M, Maki T, Satoh T. Multiplicity and regulation of hepatic microsomal carboxylesterases in rats. *Mol. Pharmacol.* 1987; **31**: 579–584.

72 Ketterman AJ, Bowles MR, Pond SM. Purification and characterization of two human liver carboxylesterases. *Int. J. Biochem.* 1989; **21**: 1303–1312.

73 Mentlein R, Heiland S, Heymann E. Simultaneous purification and comparative characterization of six serine hydolases from rat liver microsomes. *Arch. Biochem. Biophys.* 1980; **200**: 547–559.

74 Hsiang Y-H, Lihou MG, Liu LF. Arrest of replication forks by drug-stabilized topoisomerase I-DNA cleavable complexes as a mechanism of cell killing by camptothecin. *Cancer Res.* 1989; **49**: 5077–5082.

75 Robbi M, Beaufay H. Purification and characterization of various esterases from rat liver. *Eur. J. Biochem.* 1983; **137**: 293–301.

76 Sone T, Zukowski K, Land SJ, King CM, Marin BM *et al.* Characteristics of a purified dog hepatic microsomal N,O-acyltransferase. *Carcinogenesis* 1994; **15**: 595–599.

77 Takagi Y, Morohashi K, Kawabata S, Go M, Omure T. Molecular cloning and nuleotide sequence of cDNA of microsomal carboxylesterase E1 of rat liver. *J. Biochem.* 1988; **104**: 801–806.

78 Van Lith HA, Den Bieman M, Van Zutphen BF. Purification and molecular properties of rabbit liver esterase Es-1A. *Eur. J. Biochem.* 1989; **184**: 545–551.

79 Schwer H, Langmann T, Diag R, Becker A, Aslandis C, Schmitz G. Molecular cloning and characterization of a novel putative carboxylesterase, present in human intestine and liver. *Biochem. Biophys. Res. Comm.* 1997; **233**: 117–120.

80 Tsujita T, Miyada T, Okuda H. Purification of rat kidney carboxylesterase and its camparison with other tissue esterases. *J. Biochem.* 1988; **103**: 327–331.

81 Huang TL, ShioTsuki T, Uematsu T, Borhan B, Li QX, Hammock BD. Structure-activity relationships for substrates and inhibitors of mammalian liver microsomal carboxylesterases. *Pharm. Res.* 1996; **13**: 1495–1500.

82 Stryer L. *Biochemistry.* W.H. Freeman and Co., New York, 1988.

83 Korza G, Ozols J. Complete covalent structure of 60-kDa esterase isolated from 2,3,7,8-tetrachlorodibenzo-p-dioxin-induced rabbit liver microsomes. *J. Biol. Chem.* 1988; **263**: 3486–3495.

84 Robbi M, Beaufay H, Octave J-N. Nucleotide sequence of a cDNA coding for a rat liver pI 6.1 esterase (ES-10), a carboxylesterase located in the lumen of the endoplasmic reticulum. *Biochem. J.* 1990; **269**: 451–458.

85 Ovnic M, Tepperman K, Medda S, Elliot RW, Stephenson DA, Grant SG, Ganschow RE. Characterization of a murine cDNA encoding a member of the carboxylesterase multigene family. *Genomics* 1991b; **9**: 344–354.

86 Ovnic M, Swank RT, Fletcher C, Zhen L, Novak EK, Baumann H, Heintz N, Ganschow RE. Characterization and functional expression of a cDNA encoding egasyn (esterase-22): The endoplasmic reticulum-targeting protein of B-glucuronidase. *Genomics* 1991a; **11**: 956–967.

87 Ozols J. Isolation, properties, and the complete amino acid sequence of a second form of 60 kDa glycoprotein esterase. *J. Biol. Chem.* 1989; **264**: 12533–12545.

88 Murakami K, Takagi Y, Mihara K, Omura T. An isozyme of microsomal carboxylesterases, carboxylesterase Sec, is secreted form rat liver into the blood. *J. Biochem.* 1993; **113**: 61–66.

89 Cloninger C, Bohman M, Sigvardsson D. Inheritance of alcohol abuse. Cross-fostering analysis of adopted men. *Arch. Gen. Psychiatry* 1981; **38**: 861–868.

90 Goodwin D. Genetic factors in the development of alcoholism. *Adv. Intern. Med.* 1987; **31**: 383–398.

Chapter 15

Alcohol and apolipoproteins

Mark Deeg

INTRODUCTION

Moderate alcohol intake is associated with a reduction in cardiovascular events (see Part III of this book). Alcohol consumption has numerous effects on various risk factors for cardiovascular disease including lipoprotein metabolism. Generally, alcohol consumption is associated with increased serum levels of very low density lipoproteins (VLDL) and high density lipoproteins (HDL) [1,2]. The increase in HDL cholesterol has been estimated to account for half of the beneficial effects of alcohol consumption on cardiovascular events [3]. Lipoproteins consist of lipids (cholesterol, triglycerides, and phospholipids) and proteins. The proteins on the surface can serve as ligands or co-ligands for receptors, activators or inhibitors of enzymes involved in lipid metabolism. Other chapters address the effect of alcohol intake on serum lipids and lipoproteins. This chapter will review some of the epidemiological studies on alcohol consumption and apolipoproteins as well as the effect of alcohol intake on the production and catabolism of various apolipoproteins in humans and various animal models.

APOLIPOPROTEIN A-I

Human and non-human primate studies

Apolipoprotein A-I is the most abundant protein in HDL and plays an important role in maintaining the structure of HDL and activating lecithin cholesterol acyltransferase (LCAT), an enzyme involved in converting cholesterol to cholesterol ester. HDL appears to be primarily cardioprotective by transporting cholesterol from the periphery to the liver for export as bile acids. This process is termed reverse cholesterol transport. From epidemiological studies, higher levels of HDL cholesterol are associated with a decrease in cardiovascular disease risk. Similar studies have shown that apolipoprotein A-I levels show a similar inverse relationship with risk for cardiovascular disease [4].

Consumption of moderate amounts of alcohol is associated with an increase in HDL cholesterol and apolipoprotein A-I. The increases occur in a dose-dependent fashion. As little as 15 g of alcohol/day can increase apolipoprotein A-I levels in humans [5]. Hojnacki *et al.* [6] examined the dose response of alcohol on lipids and apolipoproteins in male squirrel monkeys. Comparing diets containing 0, 6, 12, 18, 24, 30, and 36% of calories derived from alcohol, there was a dose dependent increase in apolipoprotein A-I levels (and HDL cholesterol) with a significant increase detectable at 24%.

Acute administration of alcohol has no or little effect on apolipoprotein A-I levels. Valimaki *et al.* examined the time course of 60 g/day of alcohol (16% of total calories were derived from alcohol) for 3 weeks in men on total apolipoprotein A-I levels [7]. Apolipoprotein A-I levels did not increase until after 1 week of alcohol consumption.

In contrast, in a study using young, healthy men consuming 160 g/day of alcohol in three divided doses over three days did not change total apolipoprotein A-I levels or total HDL cholesterol. However, there were pronounced changes in the HDL subfractions. The apolipoprotein A-I content of HDL_2 increased which was mitigated by the decrease in apolipoprotein A-I content of HDL_3 [8]. The lipid composition of both subfractions was characterized by a relative increase in phospholipids but decrease in cholesterol. These changes in HDL composition likely have important effects on HDL function, since the conformation of apolipoprotein A-I on the surface of HDL is dependent upon the lipid composition of the particle [9,10]. Alcoholics (male and female) also have increases in the apolipoprotein A-I and A-II of HDL compared to controls [11].

Other environmental factors can influence the effect of alcohol on apolipoprotein levels including level of physical activity [12] and diet. Rumpler *et al.* [13] examined the effect of adding alcohol to the diet of women consuming either a high fat (38% fat calories) or low fat (18% fat calories). Alcohol (5% of calories) only increased HDL cholesterol while on the high fat diet. This effect was confined to the HDL_2 subfraction. Diet influences the metabolism of most apolipoproteins and is the major confounding factor in interpreting the effects of alcohol on apolipoproteins in human and animals.

The steady state concentration of apolipoprotein A-I is a balance between synthesis and catabolism. Alcohol appears to affect both processes. In a study with healthy men consuming 60–70 g/alcohol/day for two weeks, alcohol increased apolipoprotein A-I synthesis by nearly 50% [14]. Apolipoprotein A-I is synthesized and secreted primarily in the intestine and liver. No studies have examined the effect of alcohol on apolipoprotein A-I secretion in intestinal cells. *In vitro*, alcohol has been shown to stimulate apolipoprotein A-I secretion from two human hepatoma cell lines, HepG2 and Hep3B [15]. As little as 10 mM alcohol (equivalent to 46 mg/dl) stimulated apolipoprotein A-I synthesis and secretion in HepG2 cells [16]. This effect on synthesis appears to be a post-translational effect, since alcohol has little effect on apolipoprotein A-I mRNA steady state levels. The alcohol effect was not blocked by 4-methylphyrazole, an aldehyde dehydrogenase inhibitor, or aminotriazole, a catalase inhibitor, but was inhibited by metyrapone, a microsomal alcohol oxidizing system [15]. These results suggest that acetylaldehyde is responsible to this effect and that metabolism via cytochrome P450 2E1 is required. However, the mechanism for this alcohol effect on apolipoprotein A-I synthesis and secretion has not been elucidated. One possibility is that alcohol may increase the fraction of translatable apolipoprotein A-I mRNA. This mechanism appears to account for the effect of high fat diets to increase apolipoprotein A-I synthesis [17].

In addition, alcohol also increases the catabolism of apolipoprotein A-I. Consuming 60–70 g/day in healthy mean increased the fractional catabolic rate of apolipoprotein A-I by 30% [14]. Hence, there was an increase in the turnover of apolipoprotein A-I.

In contrast to humans, feeding male squirrel monkeys with a diet consisting of 24% alcohol-derived calories for 18 months had no effect on apolipoprotein A-I synthesis but *decreased* the FCR by nearly 50% [18]. It is unclear whether this represents a difference in time of treatment and/or a species differences in response to alcohol feeding.

No published work has been done to determine the mechanism for alcohol increasing catabolism of apolipoprotein A-I. It is possible that the changes in lipid composition of

HDL induced by alcohol could increase the catabolism of apolipoprotein A-I. In addition, no studies have examined the effect of alcohol on various HDL receptors including SR-B1 and cubulin.

In summary, the HDL raising effects of alcohol consumption in humans appears to derive from an increase in apolipoprotein A-I secretion from hepatocytes and decreased catabolism from serum.

Animal models

The effect of alcohol consumption in various animal models can vary significantly from the effect in humans. In rats, like humans, alcohol consumption increases apolipoprotein A-I levels in serum. Lakshman *et al.* fed male Wistar rats a high fat (40% of calories) with or without high doses of alcohol (36% of total calories) [19]. Over a 6 week feeding period, alcohol nearly doubled the total apolipoprotein A-I in serum. However, when apolipoprotein A-I synthesis was examined in perfused liver, the alcohol-fed rats had a 50% decrease in apolipoprotein A-I synthesis. This suggests that apolipoprotein A-I catabolism must have also decreased to account for the increase in serum apolipoprotein. In a study using rats, inclusion of 35% ethanol-derived calories on a high fat diet (40%) increases apolipoprotein A-I levels. However, when the fat calories were replaced with fish oil (enriched in Ω-3 fatty acids), the alcohol effect was blunted [20].

Mice appear to have an entirely different response to alcohol than rats. Some, but not all studies in C57BL/6 mice have shown that including alcohol in liquid diets does not increase and may even decrease serum total apolipoprotein A-I levels. The differences likely represent differences in the dietary components. C57BL/6 mice have become the standard strain for studying atherosclerosis, since this strain develops atherosclerosis when fed a high fat diet containing cholate. The cholate in the diet results in a decrease in HDL cholesterol and apolipoprotein A-I levels. This appears to occur by increasing the expression of ARP-1, a repressor protein that inhibits apolipoprotein A-I promoter activity [21]. C57BL/6 mice fed a high fat (34% fat calories) containing cholate have a decrease in HDL cholesterol compared to mice fed a low fat (12% fat). In one study utilizing a liquid diet based upon the classic Lieber-DeCarli diet which included moderate (18% of total calories) or high (36% of calories) doses of alcohol over 22 weeks, there was no effect on apolipoprotein levels except at the highest dose of alcohol in the high fat group, where apolipoprotein A-I levels decreased [22].

A second study with the same strain of mice, but utilizing a modified AIN '76 liquid diet with 36% alcohol-derived calories, showed that alcohol had no effect on apolipoprotein A-I levels [23]. This AIN '76 diet differed from the Lieber-DeCarli diet in that it lacks essential fatty acids and has approximately 2% of the vitamin A content. Since retinoic acid regulates apolipoprotein A-I expression [24], it is conceivable that the vitamin A content may modify the ethanol response, however this has not been examined.

Genetics may also play a role in the ethanol effect. LDL receptor knockout mice fed the modified AIN '76 diet for 6 weeks did demonstrate an approximate 50% decrease in apolipoprotein A-I levels [23]. However, inclusion of alcohol (36% of calories) raised apolipoprotein A-I levels to control levels. This effect does not appear to be secondary to an increase in hepatic apolipoprotein A-I synthesis (unpublished observation). However, alcohol does not increase apolipoprotein A-I levels in these mice if a diet containing essential fatty acids and vitamin A levels used in the classic Lieber-DeCarli diet (Yuan *et al.*, manuscript submitted). These studies emphasize that the alcohol effect on apolipoprotein levels can vary depending upon dietary and genetic factors.

One possible site of action that has not been examined is the effect of alcohol on apolipoprotein A-I synthesis from the intestine. Intestinal-derived apolipoprotein A-I may be important in the atherogenic protective effect of HDL; this is based upon the observation that staggerer mice (sg/sg), which lack the retinoic acid receptor-related orphan receptor α (RORα), have an increased atherogenic response to a high fat diet in association with decreased levels of apolipoprotein A-I [25]. RORα regulates apolipoprotein A-I expression within the intestine but not the liver [26]. LDL receptor knockout mice fed the modified AIN '76 diet show no change in steady state levels of apolipoprotein A-I mRNA (unpublished observation). However, this does not eliminate an alcohol effect on synthesis as described above.

It is very interesting to note that although alcohol did not increase HDL cholesterol or apolipoprotein A-I levels in the C57BL/6 mice fed a modified Lieber-DeCarli diet, atherosclerotic plaque size decreased [22]. Similarily, the LDL receptor knockout mice fed either the modified AIN '76 or Lieber-DeCarli diet with or without alcohol for 6 weeks showed that alcohol intake was associated with a decrease in atherosclerotic plaque size after 6 weeks. However, if the feeding on the modified AIN '76 diet was continued for an additional 6 weeks (12 weeks total), the plaque size was comparable in the control and alcohol fed animals despite normal apolipoprotein A-I levels [23]. These data suggest that alcohol may inhibit plaque development by factors other than raising HDL.

APOLIPOPROTEIN B

Apolipoprotein B is the major structural protein for triglyceride-rich particles including chylomicrons and very low density lipoprotein (VLDL) as well as intermediate density lipoproteins (IDL) and low density lipoproteins (LDL). VLDL is sequentially metabolized to IDL and LDL by hydrolysis of the triglycerides. There are two forms of apolipoprotein B, apolipoprotein B100 and apolipoprotein B48. Apolipoprotein B48 derives from mRNA editing of apolipoprotein B100 mRNA. In the intestine, where chylomicrons are formed, apolipoprotein B48 is synthesized. In the liver, apolipoprotein B is produced and secreted as VLDL. In humans, only apolipoprotein B100 is produced in the liver. The apolipoprotein B on these various lipoproteins serves as the ligand for various receptors including the LDL receptor.

VLDL secretion from liver is regulated by a number of factors including the availability of lipid for packaging and the production of apolipoprotein B. If excess apolipoprotein B is produced, it is degraded. Microsomal triglyceride transfer protein (MTP) assembles VLDL within the endoplasmic reticulum. MTP appears to regulate the number of apolipoprotein B-containing lipoproteins secreted and not the lipid composition.

Epidemiological studies in humans have shown that the effect of alcohol consumption on total serum apolipoprotein B is varied. This discordance may reflect the fact that total serum apolipoprotein B does not differentiate between apolipoprotein B-containing lipoproteins, i.e., VLDL-apolipoprotein B may increase while LDL-apolipoprotein B decreases. In addition, dietary and genetic factors may influence the response to alcohol. Like apolipoprotein A-I, the alcohol effect on total serum apolipoprotein B may be dose dependent. In squirrel monkeys, total serum apolipoprotein B levels increase in a dose-dependent fashion with significant elevations seen when alcohol constituted 18% of the calories consumed for 3 months.

VLDL apolipoprotein B

Human studies

Alcoholics have a higher VLDL protein mass than nonalcoholics [27]. However, this does not differentiate between the various apolipoproteins associated with VLDL, which include apolipoproteins B, E, and C's. During a four day abstinence, there was a downward trend of VLDL mass toward nonalcoholic levels. Whether these changes reflect a change in synthesis and/or catabolism is unknown. Alcohol enhances the production and catabolism of VLDL triglycerides in chronic alcoholics [28]. However, the metabolism of VLDL triglycerides and apolipoprotein B may be regulated differently [29]. Hence, alcohol effects on VLDL-triglyceride may not apply to the protein portion of this lipoprotein. Alcohol effects on VLDL apolipoprotein B secretion have been examined in animal models but not humans.

In vitro studies have shown that alcohol increases apolipoprotein B secretion in a concentration-dependent fashion. At low concentrations of alcohol (0.01% v/v), alcohol inhibits apolipoprotein B secretion from HepG2 cells [30]. The effect of alcohol appears to be related to a decrease in expression of MTP via a negative response element in the MTP promoter. Treating rats with 1 or 3 g/kg of ethanol lowered hepatic expression of MTP. Other studies with higher concentrations of alcohol have shown that incubating HepG2 and Hep3B with increasing concentrations of alcohol stimulates apolipoprotein B secretion with as little as 25 mM [31]. This increase in secretion is associated with increases in intracellular accumulation of apolipoprotein B as well suggesting increased synthesis. Apolipoprotein B mRNA levels did increase [32].

Animal models

There are a number of significant differences in apolipoprotein B metabolism in animals compared to humans. The most pronounced differences occur in rodents. In rats, both apolipoprotein B100 and B48 are secreted from liver. VLDL apoB100 is converted to LDL but VLDL apolipoprotein B48 cannot be converted to LDL [33]. Hence, considerable differences in alcohol effects can be observed between animal models and humans.

In a rat model examining VLDL protein metabolism, consumption of moderate amounts of alcohol (3.6% of total calories) with a high fat diet for 6 weeks had no effect on VLDL protein synthesis [19]. However, increasing the alcohol content of the diet to 36% of total calories was associated with a 55% decrease in synthesis. In addition, alcohol feeding is associated with a decrease in the catabolism of VLDL and chylomicrons proteins of 28% and 47%, respectively [34]. In contrast, in the cholesterol-fed rabbit model, including 30% of calories in a liquid diet had no effect on VLDL apolipoprotein production or catabolism [35].

In rodents, a significant amount of apolipoprotein B100 mRNA undergoes editing leading to secretion of VLDL with apolipoprotein B48. Rats fed a nonalcoholic diet have about 50% apolipoprotein B100 mRNA and about 50% of the secreted apolipoprotein B is in the form of apolipoprotein B100. On feeding rats an alcohol-containing liquid diet, the proportion of apolipoprotein B48 mRNA increased to greater than 99% with concomitant synthesis of only apoB48 from liver [36]. The mechanism for this alcohol effect has not been elucidated. Apolipoprotein B mRNA editing is catalyzed the cytidine deaminase, APOBEC-1. *In vitro* studies with primary rat hepatocytes and the rat hepatoma cell line, McArdle RH7777 cells, but not the human HepG2 hepatoma cell line also demonstrated an alcohol dose-dependent increase apolipoprotein B editing [37]. The effect occurred without changes in the levels of apobec-1 mRNA. This alcohol effect could derive from altered mRNA synthesis or degradation and or changes in the proteins within the editsome.

Hence, alcohol may regulate most of the steps involved in VLDL assembly: lipid synthesis, MTP expression and apolipoprotein B expression and editing.

Another potential alcohol effect to alter lipoprotein metabolism is chemical modification of the apolipoproteins. Acetaldehyde-modified lipoproteins have been identified in alcoholics [38]. Acetaldehyde modification of VLDL proteins has a biphasic effect [39]. The metabolism of VLDL modified with a range of acetaldehyde (2–8 mM) was examined in rabbits. With 2 mM acetaldehyde, a reduced conversion of VLDL to LDL was observed; in contrast, with high levels of modification, increased conversion was seen. Therefore, at low levels seen in alcoholics, this might be one mechanism to explain the lower levels of LDL seen in the context of higher VLDL levels.

LDL apolipoprotein B

Human and nonhuman primates

Alcohol consumption is generally associated with decreases in LDL levels [2]. The etiology of this effect is unknown. In a study of alcoholic patients, there was no difference in the catabolism of LDL apolipoprotein B isolated during drinking or after 7 days of abstinence [27]. This raises the possibility that in this group of patients, modifications of LDL with drinking do not account for the LDL effect. However, alcohol effects on the removal mechanism cannot be eliminated. In another study of LDL binding activity, LDL from heavy drinkers had reduced binding affinity for LDL receptors [40].

A study examining the kinetics of LDL apolipoprotein B in healthy males consuming 60–70 g/day of alcohol for two weeks resulted in a small increase in total serum apolipoprotein B levels. Alcohol consumption was associated with both an increase in LDL-apolipoprotein B synthesis (which suggests increased conversion of VLDL-apolipoprotein B to LDL) and increased catabolism [14]. The mechanism for altered catabolism of LDL apolipoprotein B is unknown. One possibility is an effect on the LDL receptor. Feeding rats a diet containing 36% of calories as alcohol increases expression of the LDL apolipoprotein B/E receptor [41]. Alternatively, modification of the apolipoprotein B in LDL may affect its metabolism.

Modification of apolipoprotein B in LDL with acetaldehyde resulted in a concentration-dependent increase in LDL catabolism in humans. The degree of LDL catabolism was positively correlated with the percentage of modified amino groups in LDL [42]. Alcohol itself will incorporate into lipoproteins. Incubating LDL with 300 mM alcohol induces a conformation in apolipoprotein B [38]. Whether with apolipoprotein B structure or conformation occurs *in vivo* and whether the catabolism via the LDL B/E receptor and/or scavenger receptors is unknown.

When the kinetics of LDL-apolipoprotein B were examined in the squirrel monkey model, consumption of alcohol with 24% of calories for 18 months was associated with an increase in LDL levels with no change in LDL-apolipoprotein B synthesis and a decrease in LDL-apolipoprotein B catabolism [18].

Animal models

In rabbits fed a liquid diet containing 30% of calories as alcohol, a 55% increase in LDL apolipoprotein B production occurred [35]. This increase occurred in the presence of no increase in VLDL apolipoprotein production suggesting either reduced removal of VLDL or increased secretion of LDL directly from the liver.

APOLIPOPROTEIN E

Apolipoprotein E is synthesized primarily in liver and brain but is expressed in most cell types. In the liver, apolipoprotein E is secreted with VLDL and plays a major role in catabolism of VLDL by serving as a ligand for various receptors that bind VLDL. As the triglycerides in the VLDL are hydrolyzed, the apolipoprotein E and phospholipids redistributes to HDL. In addition, apolipoprotein E plays a role in reverse cholesterol transport.

Human studies

Little information is available about the effects of alcohol consumption on apolipoprotein E metabolism in humans. In one study, comparing apolipoprotein E levels among low (<20 g alcohol/day), moderate (20–50 g/day), heavy (>50 g/day) and alcoholic (>100 g/day) drinkers showed no difference in serum apolipoprotein E levels between groups [43]. Conversely, other studies have shown that alcohol intake is associated with increases or decreases in apolipoprotein E [11,44]. Interestingly, there may be a gender difference in the alcohol effect on apolipoprotein E in that male alcoholics have a higher level of apolipoprotein E levels compared to controls whereas this difference does not exist between female alcoholics and controls [11]. In examining the distribution of apolipoprotein E between VLDL and HDL, Lin et al. found that alcoholics have a lower level of VLDL apolipoprotein E and higher level of HDL apolipoprotein E than controls [11].

Animal models

In rats and mice, adding alcohol to a liquid diet does not change the total serum apolipoprotein E levels [20,23]. Alcohol also reduces the secretion of apolipoprotein E from hepatocytes both in vivo [19] and in vitro [45], suggesting that catabolism in serum also decreases to maintain steady state levels. Alcohol feeding has no effect on steady state levels of apolipoprotein E mRNA. However, alcohol feeding does reduce the glycosylation of apolipoprotein E resulting in increased degradation of the synthesized protein [45]. The apolipoprotein E that is secreted also has a decrease in sialylation content.

Alcohol decreases the expression of sialyltransferase in the liver and affects all sialylated proteins secreted from liver including apolipoprotein J [45]. This same effect occurs in macrophages [45]. The decrease in sialylation of apolipoprotein E has two effects on the function of apolipoprotein E. First, a decrease in the sialylation of apolipoprotein E decreases the affinity of apolipoprotein E for HDL [46]. This may explain the observation that although alcohol has no effect on total serum apolipoprotein E, the apolipoprotein E content of VLDL increases and HDL decreases in rats. The apolipoprotein E content of HDL can be restored by adding small amount of Ω-3 fatty acids (2.8% of calories) to the diet [47]. Second, it decreases the ability of HDL to bind to the liver [48] and remove cholesterol from macrophages [45]. This is an important observation as this may be one mechanism by which alcohol increases HDL cholesterol levels. It also raises the possibility that this HDL may be 'dysfunctional' in that it cannot complete the first step in reverse cholesterol transport. Dysfunctional HDL is associated with an increased risk of atherosclerosis in both humans and animal models of atherosclerosis [49]. Clearly, this needs further evaluation.

OTHER APOLIPOPROTEINS

Apolipoprotein A-II

Apolipoprotein A-II is the second major protein present in HDL. Alcohol intake is associated with increases in apolipoprotein A-II levels in a dose-dependent fashion [7,11]. This may be secondary to a decrease in the catabolism of apolipoprotein A-II [50].

Apolipoproteins C-II and C-III

Apolipoproteins C-II and C-III both play a major role in VLDL metabolism. Apolipoprotein C-II and C-III stimulate and inhibit, respectively, lipoprotein lipase, the enzyme responsible for hydrolyzing the triglycerides in VLDL. In one study comparing apolipoprotein E levels among low (<20 g alcohol/day), moderate (20–50 g/day), heavy (>50 g/day) and alcoholic (>100 g/day) drinkers showed a significant increase in serum apolipoprotein C-III levels with increasing alcohol consumption [43]. Incubating human hepatoma cells with alcohol with concentrations up to 50 mM had no effect on apolipoprotein C-II or apolipoprotein C-III secretion [43].

SUMMARY

Alcohol consumption affects the metabolism of most apolipoproteins resulting in changes in serum levels. Most of the effects appear to be post-transcriptional with effects on synthesis or secretion. Mechanisms involving catabolism of apolipoprotein degradation have not been elucidated. The response to alcohol can be influenced by diet, lifestyle differences, and genetics.

ACKNOWLEDGEMENT

Studies conducted in the author's laboratory have been supported by NIH grant AA06991.

REFERENCES

1 Frohlich JJ. Effects of alcohol on plasma lipoprotein metabolism. *Clin. Chim. Acta* 1996; **246**: 39–49.

2 Savolainen MJ, Kesaniemi YA. Effects of alcohol on lipoproteins in relation to coronary heart disease. *Curr. Opin. Lipidol.* 1995; **6**: 243–250.

3 Criqui MH, Cowan LD, Tyroler HA, Bangdiwala S, Heiss G, Wallace RB, Cohn R. Lipoproteins as mediators for the effects of alcohol consumption and cigarette smoking on cardiovascular mortality: results form the Lipid Research Clinics Follow-up Study. *Am. J. Epidemiol.* 1987; **126**: 629–637.

4 Rader DJ, Hoeg JM, Brewer HB Jr. Quantitation of plasma apolipoproteins in the primary and secondary prevention of coronary artery disease [see comments]. *Ann. Intern. Med.* 1994; **120**: 1012–1025.

5 Rimm EB, Williams P, Fosher K, Criqui M, Stampfer MJ. Moderate alcohol intake and lower risk of coronary heart disease: meta-analysis of effects on lipids and haemostatic factors. *BMJ* 1999; **319**: 1523–1528.

6 Hojnacki JL, Cluette-Brown JE, Deschenes RN, Mulligan JJ, Osmolski TV, Rencricca NJ, Barboriak JJ. Alcohol produces dose-dependent antiatherogenic and atherogenic plasma lipoprotein responses. *Proc. Soc. Exp. Biol. Med.* 1992; **200**: 67–77.

7 Valimaki M, Taskinen MR, Ylikahri R, Roine R, Kuusi T, Nikkila EA. Comparison of the effects of two different doses of alcohol on serum lipoproteins, HDL-subfractions and apolipoproteins A-I and A-II: a controlled study. *Eur. J. Clin. Invest.* 1988; **18**: 472–480.

8 Taskinen MR, Valimaki M, Nikkila EA, Kuusi T, Ylikahri R. Sequence of alcohol-induced initial changes in plasma lipoproteins (VLDL and HDL) and lipolytic enzymes in humans. *Metab.* 1985; **34**: 112–119.

9 Sparks DL, Phillips MC, Lund-Katz S. The conformation of apolipoprotein A-I in discoidal and spherical recombinant high density lipoprotein particles. 13C NMR studies of lysine ionization behavior. *J. Biol. Chem.* 1992; **267**: 25830–25838.

10 Sparks DL, Lund-Katz S, Phillips MC. The charge and structural stability of apolipoprotein A-I in discoidal and spherical recombinant high density lipoprotein particles. *J. Biol. Chem.* 1992; **267**: 25839–25847.

11 Lin RC, Miller BA, Kelly TJ. Concentrations of apolipoprotein AI, AII, and E in plasma and lipoprotein fractions of alcoholic patients: gender differences in the effects of alcohol. *Hepatology* 1995; **21**: 942–949.

12 Hartung GH, Foreyt JP, Reeves RS, Krock LP, Patsch W, Patsch JR, Gotto AM Jr. Effect of alcohol dose on plasma lipoprotein subfractions and lipolytic enzyme activity in active and inactive men. *Metab.* 1990; **39**: 81–86.

13 Rumpler WV, Clevidence BA, Muesing RA, Rhodes DG. Changes in women's plasma lipid and lipoprotein concentrations due to moderate consumption of alcohol are affected by dietary fat level. *J. Nutr.* 1999; **129**: 1713–1717.

14 Malmendier CL, Delcroix C. Effect of alcohol intake on high and low density lipoprotein metabolism in healthy volunteers. *Clin. Chim. Acta* 1985; **152**: 281–288.

15 Tam SP. Effect of ethanol on lipoprotein secretion in two human hepatoma cell lines, HepG2 and Hep3B. *Alcohol Clin. Exp. Res.* 1992; **16**: 1021–1028.

16 Amarasuriya RN, Gupta AK, Civen M, Horng YC, Maeda T, Kashyap ML. Ethanol stimulates apolipoprotein A-I secretion by human hepatocytes: implications for a mechanism for atherosclerosis protection. *Metab.* 1992; **41**: 827–832.

17 Azrolan N, Odaka H, Breslow JL, Fisher EA. Dietary fat elevates hepatic apoA-I production by increasing the fraction of apolipoprotein A-I mRNA in the translating pool. *J. Biol. Chem.* 1995; **270**: 19833–19838.

18 Hojnacki JL, Cluette-Brown JE, Dawson M, Deschenes RN, Mulligan JJ. Alcohol delays clearance of lipoproteins from the circulation. *Metab.* 1992; **41**: 1151–1153.

19 Lakshman MR, Chirtel SJ, Chambers LC, Campbell BS. Hepatic synthesis of apoproteins of very low density and high density lipoproteins in perfused rat liver: influence of chronic heavy and moderate doses of ethanol. *Alcohol Clin. Exp. Res.* 1989; **13**: 554–559.

20 Lakshman MR, Chirtel SJ, Chambers LL. Roles of omega 3 fatty acids and chronic ethanol in the regulation of plasma and liver lipids and plasma apoproteins A1 and E in rats. *J. Nutr.* 1988; **118**: 1299–1303.

21 Srivastava RA, Srivastava N, Averna M. Dietary cholic acid lowers plasma levels of mouse and human apolipoprotein A-I primarily via a transcriptional mechanism. *Eur. J. Biochem.* 2000; **267**: 4272–4280.

22 Emeson EE, Manaves V, Singer T, Tabesh M. Chronic alcohol feeding inhibits atherogenesis in C57BL/6 hyperlipidemic mice. *Am. J. Pathol.* 1995; **147**: 1749–1758.

23 Dai J, Miller BA, Lin RC. Alcohol feeding impedes early atherosclerosis in low-density lipoprotein receptor knockout mice: factors in addition to high-density lipoprotein-apolipoprotein A1 are involved. *Alcohol Clin. Exp. Res.* 1997; **21**: 11–18.

24 Hargrove GM, Junco A, Wong NC. Hormonal regulation of apolipoprotein AI. *J. Mol. Endocrinol.* 1999; **22**: 103–111.

25 Mamontova A, Seguret-Mace S, Esposito B, Chaniale C, Bouly M, Delhaye-Bouchaud N, Luc G, Staels B, Duverger N, Mariani J, Tedgui A. Severe atherosclerosis and hypoalphalipoproteinemia in the staggerer mouse, a mutant of the nuclear receptor RORalpha. *Circ.* 1998; **98**: 2738–2748.

26 Vu-Dac N, Gervois P, Grotzinger T, De Vos P, Schoonjans K, Fruchart JC, Auwerx J, Mariani J, Tedgui A, Staels B. Transcriptional regulation of apolipoprotein A-I gene expression by the nuclear receptor RORalpha. *J. Biol. Chem.* 1997; **272**: 22401–22404.

27 Kervinen K, Savolainen MJ, Kesaniemi YA. Multiple changes in apoprotein B containing lipo-proteins after ethanol withdrawal in alcoholic men. *Ann. Med.* 1991; **23**: 407–413.

28 Sane T, Nikkila EA, Taskinen MR, Valimaki M, Ylikahri R. Accelerated turnover of very low density lipoprotein triglycerides in chronic alcohol users. A possible mechanism for the up-regulation of high density lipoprotein by ethanol. *Athero.* 1984; **53**: 185–193.

29 Melish J, Le NA, Ginsberg H, Steinberg D, Brown WV. Dissociation of apoprotein B and triglyceride production in very-low-density lipoproteins. *Am. J. Physiol.* 1980; **239**: E354–E362.

30 Lin MC, Li JJ, Wang EJ, Princler GL, Kauffman FC, Kung HF. Ethanol down-regulates the transcription of microsomal triglyceride transfer protein gene. *FASEB J.* 1997; **11**: 1145–1152.

31 Dashti N, Franklin FA, Abrahamson DR. Effect of ethanol on the synthesis and secretion of apoA-I- and apoB-containing lipoproteins in HepG2 cells. *J. Lipid Res.* 1996; **37**: 810–824.

32 Wang TW, Byrne CD, Hales CN. Effect of ethanol on hepatic apolipoprotein B synthesis and secretion *in vitro*. *Biochim. Biophys. Acta* 1994; **1211**: 234–238.

33 Van't Hooft FM, Hardman DA, Kane JP, Havel RJ. Apolipoprotein B (B-48) of rat chylomicrons is not a precursor of the apolipoprotein of low density lipoproteins. *Proc. Natl. Acad. Sci. USA* 1982; **79**: 179–182.

34 Lakshmanan MR, Ezekiel M. Effect of chronic ethanol feeding upon the catabolism of protein and lipid moieties of chylomicrons and very low density lipoproteins *in vivo* and in the perfused heart system. *Alcohol Clin. Exp. Res.* 1985; **9**: 327–330.

35 Latour MA, Patterson BW, Kitchens RT, Ostlund RE Jr, Hopkins D, Schonfeld G. Effects of alcohol and cholesterol feeding on lipoprotein metabolism and cholesterol absorption in rabbits. *Arterioscler. Thromb. Vasc. Biol.* 1999; **19**: 598–604.

36 Lau PP, Cahill DJ, Zhu HJ, Chan L. Ethanol modulates apolipoprotein B mRNA editing in the rat. *J. Lipid Res.* 1995; **36**: 2069–2078.

37 Van Mater D, Sowden MP, Cianci J, Sparks JD, Sparks CE, Ballatori N, Smith HC. Ethanol increases apolipoprotein B mRNA editing in rat primary hepatocytes and McArdle cells. *Biochem. Biophys. Res. Commun.* 1998; **252**: 334–339.

38 Wehr H, Rodo M, Lieber CS, Baraona E. Acetaldehyde adducts and autoantibodies against VLDL and LDL in alcoholics. *J. Lipid Res.* 1993; **34**: 1237–1244.

39 Kervinen K, Horkko S, Beltz WF, Kesaniemi A. Modification of VLDL apoprotein B by acetaldehyde alters apoprotein B metabolism. *Alcohol* 1995; **12**: 189–194.

40 Hirano K, Yamashita S, Sakai N, Hiraoka H, Ueyama Y, Funahashi T, Matsuzawa Y. Low-density lipoproteins in hyperalphalipoproteinemic heavy alcohol drinkers have reduced affinity for the low-density lipoprotein receptor. *Clin. Biochem.* 1992; **25**: 357–362.

41 Seitz HK, Kuhn B, von Hodenberg E, Fiehn W, Conradt C, Simanowski UA. Increased messenger RNA levels for low-density lipoprotein receptor and 3-hydroxy-3-methylglutaryl coenzyme A reductase in rat liver after long-term ethanol ingestion. *Hepatology* 1994; **20**: 487–493.

42 Kesaniemi YA, Kervinen K, Miettinen TA. Acetaldehyde modification of low density lipoprotein accelerates its catabolism in man. *Eur. J. Clin. Invest.* 1987; **17**: 29–36.

43 Lecomte E, Herbeth B, Paille F, Steinmetz J, Artur Y, Siest G. Changes in serum apolipoprotein and lipoprotein profile induced by chronic alcohol consumption and withdrawal: determinant effect on heart disease? *Clin. Chem.* 1996; **42**: 1666–1675.

44 Hirano K, Matsuzawa Y, Sakai N, Hiraoka H, Nozaki S, Funahashi T, Yamashita S, Kubo M, Tarui S. Polydisperse low-density lipoproteins in hyperalphalipoproteinemic chronic alcohol drinkers in association with marked reduction of cholesteryl ester transfer protein activity. *Metab.* 1992; **41**: 1313–1318.

45 Ghosh P, Hale EA, Mayur K, Seddon J, Lakshman MR. Effects of chronic alcohol treatment on the synthesis, sialylation, and disposition of nascent apolipoprotein E by peritoneal macrophages of rats. *Am. J. Clin. Nutr.* 2000; **72**: 190–198.

46 Marmillot P, Rao MN, Liu QH, Lakshman MR. Desialylation of human apolipoprotein E decreases its binding to human high-density lipoprotein and its ability to deliver esterified cholesterol to the liver. *Metab.* 1999; **48**: 1184–1192.

47 Marmillot P, Rao MN, Liu QH, Chirtel SJ, Lakshman MR. Effect of dietary omega-3 fatty acids and chronic ethanol consumption on reverse cholesterol transport in rats. *Metab.* 2000; **49**: 508–512.

48 Lin RC, Miller BA. Effect of chronic alcohol ingestion on the binding of high density lipoproteins to rat hepatic membranes: involvement of apolipoprotein E. *Alcohol Clin. Exp. Res.* 1992; **16**: 1168–1173.

49 Santamarina-Fojo S, Lambert G, Hoeg JM, Brewer HB Jr. Lecithin-cholesterol acyltransferase: role in lipoprotein metabolism, reverse cholesterol transport and atherosclerosis. *Curr. Opin. Lipidol.* 2000; **11**: 267–275.

50 Gottrand F, Beghin L, Duhal N, Lacroix B, Bonte JP, Fruchart JC, Luc G. Moderate red wine consumption in healthy volunteers reduced plasma clearance of apolipoprotein AII. *Eur. J. Clin. Invest.* 1999; **29**: 387–394.

Chapter 16

Alcohol and polyunsaturated fatty acid metabolism in the cardiovascular system

John W. Karanian and Norman Salem

INTRODUCTION

The role of fatty acids in cardiovascular disease

Much evidence has accumulated from various lines of inquiry that indicates that the dietary fatty acid intake and lipid acyl composition of tissues is a determinant of many of the chronic diseases prominent in the Western World, notably cardiovascular disease. It has been appreciated since the 1950s that when dietary polyunsaturated fat intake is increased, a decrease in the total serum and lipoprotein cholesterol levels results [1]. Bang and Dyerberg, in their study of the Greenland Eskimos, a group in which CVD had an extremely low incidence, made the ground breaking inference that the high dietary intake of the long chain polyunsaturated fatty acids, eicosapentanoate and docosahexaenoate was responsible for this protection from disease [2]. More recently, several epidemiological studies have reported a relationship between dietary n-3 polyunsaturates and the risk of CVD [3–8]. For example, Dolechek *et al.* found an inverse relationship between alpha-linolenate and mortality from CVD, all CVD and on all cause mortality, however no relationships were found for linoleate [3]. They also observed an inverse relationship of fish oil fats with coronary heart disease, CVD, and all cause mortality. In agreement with these findings was the study by Siscovick *et al.* who observed that a level of fish fats equivalent to about one meal a week was associated with a 50% reduction in the risk of primary cardiac arrest [4]. The n-3 fatty acids have also been the subject of large secondary prevention trials. In the LYON Heart Study, deLorgeril *et al.* found that a diet enriched with alpha-linoleate was more effective than other diets in use for this purpose for the secondary prevention of coronary events and death [9]. Burr *et al.* in the DART trial, found a 29% reduction in overall mortality after 2 years when a large group of men advised to consume fish twice a week after surviving a heart attack [10]. Singh *et al.* reported a decline in coronary heart disease events in patients with suspected myocardial infarctions after one year of consuming either 2 g of long chain n-3 fatty acids or 2.9 g of alpha-linolenic acid per day [11]. A very large trial (GISSI-Prevenzionne) of 11,324 patients demonstrated that 850 mg of eicosapentaenoate/docosahexanoate per day led to a 20% reduction in total mortality over a 3.5 year follow-up period in patients with a history of CVD [12]. McLennan *et al.* found that fish oil fed marmoset monkeys were resistant to cardiac arrhythmias [13]. Billman *et al.* subsequently showed that dogs infused with a fish oil emulsion had a remarkable resistance to cardiac arrhythmias induced by compression of the left circumflex artery [14]. Kang and Leaf, in a series of publications (for review, see [15]), demonstrated that DHA had the highest efficacy in heart and neuronal cells in causing a reduction in electrical excitability; this is the basis for the protective effects of long chain polyunsaturates against arrhythmias. Lands *et al.* proposed the unifying concept that dietary supplementation with n-3 fatty acids leads to loss of cellular arachidonate and increases in eicosapentanoate and docosahexaenoate [16]. This then leads to a diminished eicosanoid response upon cellular stimulation due to the decreased efficacy of the n-3 eicosanoid analogues to the arachidonate-derived eicosanoids. Lands *et al.* suggested that the percentage of plasma phospholipid arachidonate is related to thromboxane generation and platelet activation and thus to the risk of cardiovascular deaths [16]. Harris, in his review, suggested that increased long chain n-3 fatty acid intake leads to decreases in plasma triglyceride levels due to decreased hepatic synthesis and secretion [17]. A recent meta-analysis of 17 studies involving over 46,000 men and 10,000 women suggested that the plasma triglycerides level is a risk factor for CVD that is independent of HDL-cholesterol [18]. In addition to the aforementioned studies, Knapp *et al.* found an anti-hypertensive effect of fish oil [19] and Christensen *et al.* a beneficial effect on heart rate variability [20]. It should be clear then that the balance of dietary fatty acids and the resulting tissue fatty acid composition are critical determinants of cardiovascular function and the predisposition to disease.

Fatty acid nomenclature

Essential fatty acids (EFA) are often defined metabolically; that is, they are the fatty acids that cannot be produced by *de novo* synthesis by a mammal. Both linoleic acid (LA) and alpha-linolenic acid (LNA) are the key essential fatty acids for mammals and must be supplied preformed in the diet. Plants have the enzymes necessary for total synthesis of these fats and provide for their origin in the food chain [21].

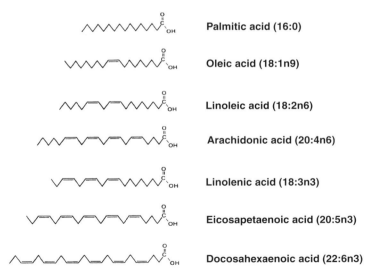

Palmitic acid (16:0)

Oleic acid (18:1n9)

Linoleic acid (18:2n6)

Arachidonic acid (20:4n6)

Linolenic acid (18:3n3)

Eicosapetaenoic acid (20:5n3)

Docosahexaenoic acid (22:6n3)

Figure 16.1 The structures of some essential and non-essential fatty acids commonly found in mammalian cells.

The structures of some of the most common fatty acids in biological organisms are presented in Figure 16.1. Fatty acids are characterized by their chain length, number of double bonds and the positions of their double bonds. A saturated fatty acid, like palmitate, contains no double bonds. An unsaturate like oleic acid, contains at least one double bond. A polyunsaturated fatty acid (PUFA), like linoleic acid contains two or more double bonds. Long chain polyunsaturates (LCP) are those fatty acids that are 20-carbons in length or more and contain multiple double bonds. Fatty acids are often abbreviated in the short-hand designation X:YnZ, where X is the number of carbons, Y is the number of double bonds, and Z represents the number of carbons counting from the methyl end of the molecule until the first double bond is encountered. Thus, linoleic acid is denoted as 18:2n6 and alpha-linolenic acid as 18:3n3. The principal LCPs in the n-6 and n-3 families are arachidonic acid (20:4n6, AA), and eicosapentaenoic acid (20:5n3, EPA) or docosahexaenoic acid (22:6n3, DHA), respectively (Figure 16.1). The fatty acids with the n-3 or n-6 structures are referred to as families because they are not metabolically inter-convertible in animals [21].

FATTY ACID COMPOSITION

Heart and smooth muscle

Significant effects of alcohol have been noted when 20-C and 22-C fatty acid distribution/content has been determined in heart [22], vascular smooth muscle [23] and platelet [24,25]. Reitz et al. [22] reported that both AA and DHA declined significantly in rat heart following alcohol in the drinking water for 1 month. Mice exposed to ethanol vapors for 10 d showed an increase in 18:2n6 (LA) and a decrease in DHA [26]. Acute inhalation was associated with a significant loss of heart DHA that was preventable by pretreatment with vitamin E. Cunnane et al. [27] have shown a loss in AA and DHA in hearts of hamsters given alcohol in their drinking water for one year.

Blood components

Reductions in AA have also been observed in rodent red blood cells [28–31], platelets [25,32] and serum [33] after alcohol administration. However, these results have also been inconsistent, since others have reported no effect [34] or an increase in AA [35]. Moreover, no effect of short-term alcohol administration on AA levels has been found in mouse red blood cells [35]. Interestingly, these effects of alcohol may be dependent on the duration of exposure, since longer-term alcohol administration (i.e., >21 days) has been shown in rat red blood cells [36] to result in reductions in AA. Consistent with this idea, the concentration of DHA was reduced in mouse blood following shorter-term (i.e., 7 day) alcohol administration [37].

Horrobin and Manku [38] have observed losses in both the plasma and red blood cell (RBC) PE level of AA and DHA in alcoholics. Similarly, subjects with alcoholic liver disease show losses in RBC LA, AA and DHA [39]. Glen et al. [40] reported a marked loss in all major RBC polyunsaturates with the exception of AA in a group of 123 alcoholics. Others have also noted significant declines in RBC AA and DHA in alcoholics [41,42]. In addition, the plasma of cirrhotic patients, of which half had an alcohol-related etiology, shows a decline in AA and DHA [43]. Withdrawing alcoholics also show less AA in certain platelet phospholipid pools such as phosphatidylcholine and phosphatidylinositol [24].

The diet as a source of fatty acids

It is well known that many alcoholics have a relatively poor diet (for general reviews, see [44–48]). For example, in a population of middle-aged Scottish men who consumed a mean alcohol intake of 66 g/d, it was shown that they had a lower intake of protein, fat, polyunsaturated fat and linoleic acid [49]. When the alcohol intake increases, there is a decrease in the amount of energy derived from macronutrients [50]. There is also a decrease in the intake and tissue concentration of many vitamins and minerals [51]. Alcoholism may also lead to nutritional deficiencies through decreased intestinal absorption, altered vitamin metabolism and reduced storage of ingested vitamins [52–54].

It may be hypothesized then, that a reduction in highly unsaturated PUFAs may also be found in the diets of alcoholics. As noted below, alcohol has direct effects on fatty acid anabolism and catabolism, and these may lead to a decrease in tissue PUFA levels. It may be surmised then that a reduction in dietary 18-carbon EFAs and their longer chain metabolites, as well as the antioxidant vitamins and minerals that help to protect them, will exacerbate the nutrient deficiencies caused by the direct actions of alcohol.

FATTY ACID METABOLISM

Fatty acid elongation/desaturation

Fatty acids can be interconverted through enzymatic reactions occurring primarily in the endoplasmaic reticulum that lead to an extension of the chain length, termed elongation, or introduction of double bonds, termed desaturation. Desaturation and elongation are often a concerted sequence of reactions that leads to LA or LNA being metabolized to their LCP forms, e.g., AA and DHA, respectively. The general pathway for the elongation/desaturation of the n-3 and n-6 families of essential fatty acids is presented in Figure 16.2.

It can readily be observed that LA is metabolized by desaturation to gamma-linolenic acid (18:3n6, GLA), elongated to dihommo-gamma-linolenic acid (20:3n6, DGLA) and then desaturated to AA, where metabolism often is terminated. However, metabolism may continue through elongation to docosatetraenoic acid (22:4n6, ETA), elongation to 24:4n6, desaturation to 24:5n6 and peroxisomal retroconversion to 22:5n6 (DPAn-6, [55]). Similarly, in the n-3 family, LNA is desaturated to 18:4n3, elongated to (blank weeded) 20:4n3, desaturated to 20:5n3 (EPA) and elongated to 22:5n3 (DPAn-3). The final desaturation reaction occurs in a manner analogous to that described above for the n-6 family as follows: 22:5n3 is elongated to 24:5n3, desaturated to 24:6n3 and then retroconverted to 22:6n3 (DHA).

Fatty acid metabolism in heart, blood cells and muscle

Although the primary site of essential fatty acid elongation/desaturation is in the liver and brain [56–58], organs and cells of the cardiovascular system may also participate in fatty acid metabolism. Heart cells in culture are known to possess the capability of performing elongation

ESSENTIAL FATTY ACID METABOLISM

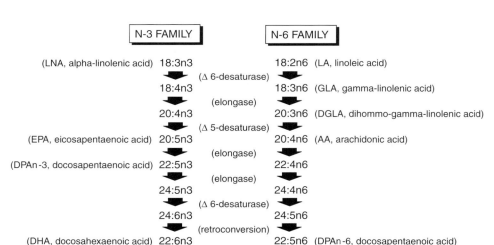

Figure 16.2 Metabolism of the n-3 and n-6 families of essential fatty acids.

and desaturation reactions [59] and also have a high level of mRNA for delta-5 desaturase [58]. Skeletal muscle and lung also contain mRNA for both delta-6 and delta-5 desaturase enzymes [57,58]. Erythrocytes and plasma are probably devoid of this activity although whole blood has been shown to incorporate radioactivity from ^{14}C-acetate into AA and DHA [60]. Leukocytes and platelets are able to incorporate radioactivity from acetate into complex lipids and fatty acids [61,62], but this activity represents primarily chain elongation and not desaturation reactions [63]. However, there is a report of apparent delta-6 and delta-5 desaturase activity in platelets [64]. Although the cardiovascular system is not known to be a major site for EFA metabolism, the level of activity and mRNA for the key desaturases in the heart in particular indicates that it participates in fatty acid anabolism.

Effects of alcohol on essential fatty acid metabolism

As established in a section above, alcohol lowers the levels of LCPs in many tissues. It has long been claimed that the mechanism underlying this change in fatty acid composition is the inhibitory action of alcohol on fatty acid desaturases [66]. This interpretation was based on a series of *in vitro* experiments in which it was shown that the addition of ethanol to a tissue homogenate or subcellular fraction led to a decrease in a radioactive EFA substrate conversion to its more unsaturated form [51,66,67]. For example, Nervi *et al.* demonstrated a decrease in both delta-6 and delta-5 desaturases in rat liver microsomes [68]. Wang and Reitz found a reduction in the delta-9, delta-6 and delta-5 desaturases in liver microsomes after animals were given either acute or chronic exposure to ethanol [69]. Nakamura *et al.* found a marked loss of delta-6 and delta-5 desaturase activity but no change in delta-9 desaturase activity in the minipig [70].

More recently, Pawlosky *et al.* were able to develop methods for the *in vivo* determination of overall fatty acid metabolism using the deuterated precursors deuterated-LA and deuterated-LNA [71]. This method does not measure single enzymatic steps but rather is the combination of elongation/desaturation rates coupled with the rates of transport and minus the catabolic processes at each stage; this is what is meant by overall accretion of labeled metabolites. It should be recognized though that overall accretion of LCPs is more closely related to the LCP composition of the tissue than is the measurement of desaturase activity in a liver homogenate or subcellular fraction *in vitro*. Pawlosky *et al.* found a *stimulation* of deuterated 18-carbon EFA incorporation into plasma AA and DHA in both cats [73] and rhesus monkeys [74] after chronic alcohol exposure. This is not consistent with the view that alcohol inhibits desaturases *in vivo*, in fact, a simpler explanation of the data may be that alcohol stimulates desaturases.

Pawlosky *et al.* proposed the hypothesis that alcohol, through a peroxidative challenge, caused a marked increase in EFA catabolism [72–74]. This was evidenced, for example, in the rhesus work by a large increase in plasma hydroxy-nonenal and an increase in isoprostanes [74]. The stimulation of EFA metabolism may thus be seen as an adaptive mechanism that attempts to maintain homeostasis in LCP composition during accelerated EFA catabolism. Clearly then, the rate of catabolism is dependent upon the degree of oxidative challenge from alcohol and this, in turn, is related to the dose, duration and frequency of alcohol consumption. In the rhesus studies of Pawlosky *et al.*, the loss of organ essential fatty acids coupled with a diet low in EFAs led to the development of liver fibrosis after 3 years of alcohol consumption [74]. This is significant, since higher levels of alcohol consumption in non-human primates have not led to liver fibrosis in several studies (for review, see [75]).

In support of the view that alcohol stimulates EFA metabolism are our recent metabolic studies of alcoholics (Salem N., unpublished). Alcoholics showed marked increases in the amount and enrichment of deuterium in plasma DHA when given an oral dose of deuterated-LNA. This study was performed on alcoholics during alcohol withdrawal and so is not directly comparable to studies where alcohol is present in the circulation. Nevertheless, the expected decline in deuterium enrichment of DHA was not observed, providing no support for the 'alcohol inhibits desaturase' hypothesis. Taken together with the two large animal studies reported above, it is likely that an intense alcohol challenge, as is the case for alcohol abusers, leads to stimulation of both EFA anabolism and catabolism.

Effects of alcohol on essential fatty acid catabolism

In support of the hypothesis that alcohol stimulates lipid degradation/peroxidation is a growing literature. Lands *et al.* have recently reviewed the literature concerning the alcohol-induced decline in various vitamins and antioxidants [51]. Alcohol may interact with Cytochrome P450 2E1 and produce hydroxy radicals that can react with proteins, lipids and nucleic acids [76,77]. Polyunsaturated fatty acids are susceptible to this attack and undergo reactions with molecular oxygen to generate hydroperoxy compounds as well as a variety of aldehydic compounds such as malonyldialdehyde (MDA) and the hydroxyalkenals, 4-hydroxynonenal (HNE) and 4-hydroxy-hexenal (HHE).

There have been several demonstrations that the *in vivo* level of aldehyde increases due to alcohol exposure [78–81]. For example, the plasma concentrations of HNE and HHE were increased, and markedly so in the case of HNE, in rhesus monkeys consuming alcohol [82]. Domestic cats also show a four-fold increase in brain HNE after six months of daily alcohol exposure [72]. In fetal liver mitochondria, HNE accumulates during alcohol exposure of the mother [83]. MDA increases in the bloodstream of humans following alcohol consumption

[82]. Aldehydes generated subsequent to alcohol consumption react in a covalent manner with proteins [84–86]. Aldehydes like HNE may interact synergistically with MDA in that the covalent reaction of HNE with BSA increases several-fold in the presence of MDA [87]. Also, lipid peroxidation and aldehyde formation is associated with a decrease in levels of anti-oxidants. For example, the production of MDA was linearly correlated with the alcohol-induced decrease in liver alpha-tocopherol and glutathione [88].

Another useful marker for *in vivo* lipid peroxidation is the generation of isoprostanes. These are non-enzymatically produced from PUFAs [89], typically from AA, as opposed to the eicosanoids that are enzymatically produced by enzymes like cyclooxygenase and lipoxygenase. For example, the isoprostane, 8-epi-F2-alpha has been used as an index of free radical mediated injury [90] and *in vivo* lipid peroxidation [91]. Isoprostane-like compounds have also been observed for DHA both *in vitro* [92] and *in vivo* in Alzheimer's brain [93]. The F2-isoprostanes have also been observed in Alzheimer's brain [94].

Alcohol consumption increases isoprostane concentration in rat and primate liver [95,96] and in rat plasma [97]. Pawlosky *et al.* correlated the level of 8-isoprostane F2-alpha with the amount of alcohol that individual rhesus monkeys consumed when allowed to drink on an ad libitum basis [74]. The alcohol consumption negatively correlated with plasma AA content indicating that AA catabolism was appreciable. Recently, several groups have reported increased isoprostanes in alcoholics [98–100].

EFFECT OF ALCOHOL ON EICOSANOID PRODUCTION AND CARDIOVASCULAR FUNCTION

Polyunsaturated fatty acids (PUFA) may also be metabolized to eicosanoids. These include potent biologically active compounds such as prostaglandins (PGs) and leukotrienes (LTs). These compounds are produced from 20- and 22-carbon polyunsaturates by cyclooxygenase (CO) or lipoxygenase (LO) enzymes [101,102] and are active in cardiovascular tissue such as platelets and smooth muscle. As depicted in Figure 16.3, acyl hydrolases such as phospholipase A_2 (PLA_2) release AA from phospholipids, which can then be metabolized by CO or LO to PGs and LTs, respectively. The activation of phospholipases and the resulting generation of non-esterified AA is considered to be one of the rate limiting steps in eicosanoid generation. Alcohol may increase phospholipase activity thus increasing the availability of precursor fatty acids (e.g., AA) for subsequent conversion to PGs or LTs by the PG/LT synthetase cascade of enzymes [103]. The reported fall in PG formation (summarized below) as substrate stores become depleted is consistent with this concept. The amounts of AA released or accumulated may also be dependent on the activity of the main catabolic enzymes, dehydrogenases, and the rate of PG release from the cell [103].

Prostaglandins such as prostacyclin (PGI_2) and thromboxane (TXA_2) are involved in cardiovascular homeostasis (Figure 16.3) and may play a role in the pathophysiology associated with alcohol consumption [104,105]. Alcohol abuse may lead to an increased incidence of hypertension, angina, myocardial infarct and stroke [106–108]. Conversely, moderate consumption of alcohol may produce qualitatively different effects in the cardiovascular system than does high consumption. Postmortem and epidemiologic data suggest that moderate consumption of alcohol protects against atherosclerosis-related cardiovascular disease [109–111]. Animal data that is consistent with these observations have demonstrated that moderate alcohol inhibited cholesterol- and saturated fatty acid-induced atherosclerosis in rabbits [112,113].

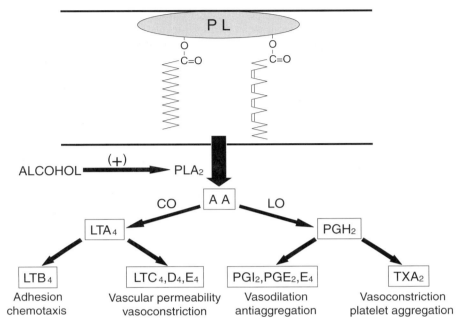

Figure 16.3 Schematic of arachidonic acid (AA) mobilization from membrane phospholipids and metabolism via cyclooxygenase (CO) enzymes to form prostaglandins (PG) and lipoxygenase (LO) enzymes to form leukotrienes (LT).

Effect of alcohol on eicosanoid metabolism

As summarized above, alcohol alters PUFA metabolism resulting in such effects as increased desaturase activity [72,73]. In addition, PG metabolism is also altered by alcohol resulting in enhanced conversion of PUFAs such as DGLA and AA to PGs [114,115]. Thus, alcohol stimulation of PUFA conversion to eicosanoids may initially result in an enhancement of the formation of PGs and LTs. Given that precursor stores are limited, this initial stimulation is likely to be followed by a decrease in eicosanoid formation as the available stores become depleted. Several studies have suggested that this alcohol-induced stimulation in eicosanoid production may contribute to the decrease in tissue polyunsaturated fatty acid levels associated with chronic alcohol exposure [105,116]. However, the effects of alcohol on fatty acid catabolism described above are expected to be of a greater magnitude and of greater relative importance in this regard.

Effect of alcohol on eicosanoid production and cardiovascular function

Horrobin and Manku [117] originally postulated that acute alcohol administration may increase the conversion of precursor fatty acids such as DGLA to 1-series PGs such as PGE_1, but that chronic exposure may cause PG output to decrease subsequent to partial depletion of the fatty acid precursor [117]. PGE_1 may exert its effects on cardiovascular function, albeit weak, via inhibition of platelet aggregation and decreased vascular smooth muscle tone. Pediconi *et al.* [118] reported a decrease in the basal levels of TXA_2 and PGI_2 metabolites (TXB_2 and 6-keto-$PGF_{1\alpha}$, respectively), which are capable of regulating platelet and vascular smooth muscle activity, in rat cortex after acute or chronic alcohol exposure. Conversely, it has been shown that alcohol exposure both *in vivo* [119] and *in vitro* [120] can stimulate PGI_2 and PGI_2-like production from rat aorta, respectively. Karanian *et al.* [121] described a stimulatory effect of alcohol on 6-keto-$PGF_{1\alpha}$ and TXB_2 production in rat aortic ring preparations, *in vitro*. Moreover, alcohol has been shown to stimulate PGI_2 release from cultured human endothelial cells [122]. The vasculature may be considered the most important producer of PGI_2 [123] a principal contributor to the maintenance of vascular tone and reactivity [124,125].

Effect of alcohol on vascular tone and platelet function

Data obtained from both humans and animals have demonstrated systemic administration of alcohol may induce vasoconstriction or biphasic effects on peripheral blood flow [126–129]. Short-term alcohol has also been shown to produce vasodilation and lower blood pressure, depending on dose [128, 130,131]. In addition, alcohol has been shown to either enhance or depress vascular smooth muscle contraction in response to PGs and catecholamines, depending on alcohol concentration and exposure time [132–134].

Furthermore, alcohol-induced changes in PG levels would be expected to alter platelet aggregability, thereby altering blood flow with associated changes in blood pressure and its reactivity [135]. In particular, an increase in the ratio of PGI_2 to TXA_2 can cause inhibition of platelet aggregation and reduced vascular tone. Acute alcohol administration by inhalation has been shown to increase the PGI_2/TXA_2 ratio four-fold, whereas chronic exposure has been shown to decrease the PGI_2/TXA_2 ratio [105]. Human studies have demonstrated impaired platelet function and hemostasis related to alcohol consumption [136,137]. Similarly, chronic alcohol administration has been shown to result in inhibition of both platelet aggregation and the release of TXA_2 [138]. These changes may be of pathophysiologic significance since the control of platelet aggregation at the aorta endothelial surface is considered important in limiting damage at atherosclerotic sites [139]. These changes in eicosanoid production are not specific to cyclooxygenase products alone since, for example, marked stimulation of platelet 12-lipoxygenase occurs after rats were exposed to 7 days of ethanol inhalation [116].

Mechanism of alcohol effect on eicosanoid production

The mechanism by which alcohol increases eicosanoid levels is not well understood, although several possibilities exist. For example, alcohol induces an increase in membrane disorder [140,141] and the activity of membrane enzymes is dependent on the physical state of the membrane [142,143]. More specifically, agents such as alcohol that alter acyl hydrolase activity (e.g., phospholipase A_2) induce changes in membrane physical properties including the introduction of free volume into the membrane bilayer [144–146]. In addition, alcohol alters hydrophobic interactions in the membrane [147], a common feature of stimuli, such as alcohol, that can cause synthesis and release of eicosanoids [103]. Studies of the modification of responses to alcohol by phospholipase inhibitors are consistent with a stimulatory effect of alcohol on PLA_2 activity. For example, mepacrine has been shown to block alcohol-induced PG release from isolated rat lung [115] indicating alcohol was acting through this mechanism. Thus, the observed stimulatory action of alcohol on eicosanoid production by vascular tissue probably occurs at least in part through an increase in substrate availability in the presence of alcohol.

The effects of alcohol on eicosanoid production and the cardiovascular system of mammals, in some cases, have produced conflicting results. This may be attributed in part to differences in the dose of alcohol, blood level or duration of exposure (e.g., unphysiologic levels), nutritional status, genetic predisposition, timing of measurements and the route of administration. More precise means of controlling alcohol exposure such as the cycling inhalation method [148,149] in combination with more physiological means such as the oral route [150,151] are required in order to better quantify alcohol exposure and effects.

CONCLUSIONS

Acutely, alcohol also leads to the stimulation of eicosanoid production with an increased PGI_2/TXA_2 resulting in decreased vascular tone and platelet aggregability. Chronic alcohol exposure, on the other hand, leads to a decrease in polyunsaturated fats, especially in the AA and DHA components of blood cells and vascular smooth muscle. This LCP decrease is likely caused by a potent stimulation of fatty acid catabolism as reflected in lipid peroxides, aldehydes and eicosanoids as well as isoprostanes. Chronic alcohol exposure also leads to a decreased eicosanoid production from platelets and smooth muscle resulting in a decreased PGI_2/TXA_2 ratio and increased vascular tone. The losses in membrane phospholipid LCPs, the increases in fatty acid catabolites and the alteration in eicosanoid balance may underlie, in part, the pathophysiology associated with alcoholism, including hypertension, angina, myocardial infarct and stroke.

REFERENCES

1 Keys A, Anderson JT, Grande F. 'Essential' fatty acids, degree of unsaturation, and effect of corn (maize) oil on the serum-cholesterol level in man. *Lancet* 1957; **i**: 66–68.

2 Dyerberg J, Bang HO. Haemostatic function and platelet polyunsaturated fatty acids in Eskimos. *Lancet* 1979; **i**: 433.

3 Dolecek TA. Epidemiological evidence of relationships between dietary polyunsaturated fatty acids and mortality in the multiple risk factor intervention trial. *Proc. Soc. Exper. Biol. Med.* 1992; **200**: 177–182.

4 Siscovick DS, Raghunathan TE, King I, Weinmann S, Wicklund KG, Albright J, Bovbjerg V, Arbogast P, Smith H, Kushi LH, Cobb LA, Copass MK, Psaty BM, Lemaitre R, Retzlaff B, Childs M, Knopp RH. Dietary intake and cell membrane levels of long-chain n-3 polyunsaturated fatty acids and the risk of primary cardiac arrest. *JAMA* 1995; **274**: 1363–1367.

5 Hirai A, Hamazaki T, Terano T, Nishikawa T, Tamura Y, Kumagai A. Eicosapentaenoic acid and platelet function in Japanese. *Lancet* 1980; **ii**: 1132.

6 Kromhout D, Bosschieter EB, Coulander CL. The inverse relation between fish consumption and 20-year mortality from coronary heart disease. *N. Engl. J. Med.* 1985; **312**: 1205.

7 Shekelle RB, Missell L, Paul O, Shryock AM, Stamler J. Letter to the editor. *N. Engl. J. Med.* 1985; **13**: 820.

8 Renaud S, Nordoy A. 'Small is beautiful': Alpha-linolenic acid and eicosapentaenoic acid in man. *Lancet* 1983; **i**: 1169.

9 de Lorgeril M, Renaud S, Mamelle N, Salen P, Martin J-L, Monjaud I, Guidollet J, Touboul P, Delaye J. Mediterranean alpha-linolenic acid-rich diet in secondary prevention of coronary heart disease. *Lancet* 1994; **343**: 1454–1459.

10 Burr ML, Fehily AM, Gilbert JF, Rogers S, Holliday RM, Sweetnam PM, Elwood PC, Deadman NM. Effects of changes in fat, fish and fibre intakes on death and myocardial reinfarction: Diet and reinfarction trial (DART). *Lancet* 1989; **2**: 757–761.

11 Singh RB, Niaz MA, Sharma JP, Kumar R, Rastogi V, Moshiri M. Randomized, double-blind, placebo-controlled trial of fish oil and mustard oil in patients with suspected acute myocardial infarction: The Indian experiment of infarct survival-4. *Cardiovasc. Drugs Ther.* 1997; **11**: 485–491.

12 Marchioli R. Dietary supplementation with n-3 polyunsaturated fatty acids and vitamin E after myocardial infarction: Results of the GISSI-Prevenzione trial. *Lancet* 1999; **354**: 447–455.

13 McLennan PL, Bridle TM, Abeywardena MY, Charnock JS. Dietary lipid modulation of ventricular fibrillation threshold in the marmoset monkey. *Am. Heart J.* 1992; **123**: 1555–1561.

14 Billman GE, Hallaq H, Leaf A. Prevention of ischemia-induced ventricular fibrillation by ω^3 fatty acids. *Proc. Natl. Acad. Sci. USA* 1994; **91**: 4427–4430.

15 Leaf A, Kang JX. Prevention of cardiac sudden death by N-3 fatty acids: A review of the evidence. *J. Intern. Med.* 1996; **240**: 5–12.

16 Lands WEM, Libelt B, Morris A, Kramer NC, Prewitt TE, Bowen P, Schmeisser D, Davidson MH, Burns JH. Maintenance of lower proportions of (n-6) eicosanoid precursors in phospholipids of human plasma in response to added dietary (n-3) fatty acids. *Biochim. Biophys. Acta* 1992; **1180**: 147–162.

17 Harris WS. Fish oils and plasma lipid and lipoprotein metabolism in humans: A critical review. *J. Lipid Res.* 1989; **30**: 785–807.

18 Hokanson JE, Austin MA. Plasma triglyceride level is a risk factor for cardiovascular disease independent of high-density lipoprotein cholesterol level: A metaanalysis of population-based prospective studies. *J. Cardiovascular Risk* 1996; **3**: 213–219.

19 Knapp HR, FitzGerald GA. The antihypertensive effects of fish oil: A controlled study of polyunsaturated fatty acid supplements in essential hypertension. *N. Engl. J. Med.* 1989; **320**: 1037–1043.

20 Christensen JH, Korup E, Aarøe J, Toft E, Møller J, Rasmussen K, Dyerberg J, Schmidt EB. Fish consumption, n-3 fatty acids in cell membranes, and heart rate variability in survivors of myocardial infarction with left ventricular dysfunction. *Am. J. Cardiology* 1997; **79**: 1670–1673.

21 Salem N Jr. In: *New Protective Roles for Selected Nutrients*, Spiller GA, Scala J. (Eds.), Alan R, Liss NY, 1989; 109–228.

22 Reitz RC, Helsabeck E, Mason DP. Effects of chronic alcohol ingestion on the fatty acid composition of the heart. *Lipids* 1973; **8**: 80–84.

23 Engler MM, Karanian JW, Salem N Jr. Ethanol inhalation and dietary n-6, n-3 and n-9 fatty acids in the rat: effect on platelet and aortic fatty acid composition. *Alcohol Clin. Exp. Res.* 1991; **15**: 483–488.

24 Neiman J, Curstedt T, Cronholm T. Composition of platelet phosphatidylinositol and phosphatidylcholine after ethanol withdrawal. *Thrombosis Research* 1987; **46**: 295–301.

25 Engler MM, Karanian JW, Salem N Jr. The effects of gamma-linolenic acid (18:3ω-6) on alcohol-induced changes in fatty acid composition, blood pressure and its reactivity. *Fed. Proc.* 1987; **46**: 1467.

26 Abu Murad CA, Littleton JM. Cardiac phospholipid composition during continuous administration of ethanol to mice: Effect of vitamin E. *Proc. BPS* March 29–30 1978; 374.

27 Cunnane SC, Huang Y-S, Horrobin DF. Dietary manipulation of ethanol preference in the Syrian Golden Hamster. *Pharmacology, Biochemistry and Behavior* 1986; **25**: 1285–1292.

28 Horrobin DF, Manku MS. Essential fatty acids in clinical medicine. *Nutrition and Health* 1983; **2**: 127–134.

29 Benedetti A, Birarelli AM, Brunelli E, Curatola G, Feretti G, Del Prete U, Jezequel AM, Orlandi F. Modification of lipid composition of erythrocyte membranes in chronic alcoholism. *Pharmacological Research Communications* 1987; **19**: 651–662.

30 Cunnane SC, McAdoo KR, Horrobin DF. Long-term ethanol consumption in the hamster: effects on tissue lipids, fatty acids and erythrocyte hemolysis. *Ann. Nutr. Metab.* 1987; **31**: 265–271.

31 Corbett R, Floch HH, Ménez J-F, Leonard BE. The effects of chronic ethanol administration on rat liver and erythrocyte lipid composition: modulatory role of evening primrose oil. *Alcohol Alcohol.* 1991; **26**: 459.

32 Nieman J, Nowak J, Benthin G, Numminen H, Hillbom M. Increased urinary excretion of a major thromboxane metabolite in early alcohol withdrawal. *Clin. Physiol.* 1994; **14**: 405–409.

33 Alling C, Liljequist S, Engel J. The effect of chronic ethanol administration on lipids and fatty acids in subcellular fractions of rat brain. *Med. Biol.* 1982; **60**: 149.

34 Alling A, Becker W, Jones AW, Änggärd E. Effects of chronic ethanol treatment on lipid composition and prostaglandins in rats fed essential fatty acid deficient diets. *Alcohol Clin. Exp. Res.* 1984; **8**: 238.

35 La Droitte P, Lamboeuf Y, Saint Blanquat G. Membrane fatty acid changes and ethanol tolerance in rat and mouse. *Life Sci.* 1984; **35**: 1221.

36 La Droitte P, Lamboeuf Y, Saint-Blanquat G. Lipid composition of the synaptosome and erythrocyte membranes during chronic ethanol-treatment and withdrawal in the rat. *Biochem. Pharmacol.* 1984; **33**: 615.

37 Wing DR, Harvey DJ, Hughes J, Dunbar PG, McPherson KA, Paton WDM. Effects of chronic ethanol administration on the composition of membrane lipids in the mouse. *Biochem. Pharmacol.* 1982; **31**: 3431.

38 Horrobin D, Manku M. In: *Nutrition and Health*, Vol. 2, Academic, Berkhamsted, UK, 1983.

39 Driss F, Gueguen M, Delamaire D, Durand F, Darcet PH. Abnormalities of erythrocyte deformability and membrane lipid composition in alcoholic liver disease. *Clin. Hemorheol.* 1985; **5**: 245–250.

40 Glen AIM, Glen EMT, MacDonell LEF, Skinner FK. In: *Omega-6 Essential Fatty Acids: Pathophysiology and Roles in Clinical Medicine*, Liss, New York, 1990.

41 Gatti P, Viani P, Cervato G, Testolin G, Simonetti P, Cestaro B. Effects of alcohol abuse: studies on human erythrocyte susceptibility to lipid peroxidation. *Biochem. Mol. Biol. Int.* 1993; **30**: 807–817.

42 Adachi J, Hojo K, Ueno Y, Naito T, Ninomiya I, Imamichi H, Tatsuno Y. Identification of cholesta-3, 5-dien-7-one by gas chromatography-mass spectrometry in the erthrocyte membrane of alcoholic patients. *Alcohol Clin. Exp. Res.* 1996; **20**: 51A–55A.

43 Gonzales J, Periago J, Gil A, Cabre E, Abad-Lacruz A, Gassull MA, Sanchez de Medina F. Malnutrition-related polyunsaturated fatty acid changes in plasma lipid fractions of cirrhotic patients. *Metabolism* 1992; **41**: 954–960.

44 Goldsmith RH, Iber FL, Miller PA. Nutritional status of alcoholics of different socioeconomic class. *J. Am. Coll. Nutr.* 1983; **2**: 215.

45 Mezey E. Interaction between alcohol and nutrition in the pathogenesis of alcoholic liver disease. *Semin. Liver Dis.* 1991; **11**: 340.

46 Morgan MY. Alcohol and nutrition. *Br. Med. Bull.* 1982; **38**: 21.

47 Neville JN, Eagles JA, Samson G, Olson RE. Nutritional status of alcoholics. *Am. J. Clin. Nutr.* 1968; **21**: 1329.

48 World MJ, Ryle PR, Thomson AD. Alcoholic malnutrition and the small intestine. *Alcohol & Alcoholism* 1985; **20**: 89.

49 Thomson M, Fulton M, Elton RA, Brown S, Wood DA, Oliver MF. Alcohol consumption and nutrient intake in middle-aged Scottish men. *Am. J. Clin. Nutr.* 1988; **47**: 139.

50 Hillers VN, Massey LK. Interrelationships of moderate and high alcohol consumption with diet and health status. *Am. J. Clin. Nutr.* 1985; **41**: 356.

51 Lands WEM, Pawlosky RJ, Salem N Jr. In: *Antioxidant Status, Diet, Nutrition, and Health*, Papas AM (Ed), CRC Press, Boca Raton, Florida, 1998.

52 Marsano L. Alcohol and malnutrition. *Alcohol Health & Res. World* 1993; **17**: 284.

53 Mezey E. Metabolic effects of alcohol. *Federation Proc.* 1985; **44**: 134.

54 Somogyi JC, Kopp PM. Relation between chronic alcoholism, drug addiction, and nutrition with special reference to the thiamine status. *Bibl. Nutr. Dieta.* 1981; **30**: 131.

55 Voss A, Reinhart M, Sankarappa S, Sprecher H. The metabolism of 7,10,13,16,19-docosapentaenoic acid to 4,7,10,13,16,19-docosahexaenoic acid in rat liver is independent of a 4-desaturase. *J. Biol. Chem.* 1991; **266**: 19995–20000.

56 Naughton JM. Supply of polyenoic fatty acids to the mammalian brain: the ease of conversion of the short-chain essential fatty acids to their longer chain polyunsaturated metabolites in liver, brain, placenta, and blood. *Int. J. Biochem.* 1980; **13**: 21–32.

57 Cho HP, Nakamura MT, Clarke SD. Cloning, expression, and nutritional regulation of the mammalian Δ-6 desaturase. *J. Biol. Chem.* 1999; **274**: 471–477.

58 Cho HP, Nakamura MT, Clarke SD. Cloning, expression, and fatty acid regulation of the human Δ-5 desaturase. *J. Biol. Chem.* 1999; **274**: 37335–37339.

59 Haggerty DF, Gerschenson LE, Harary I, Mead JF. The metabolism of linoleic acid in mammalian cells in culture. *Biochemical Biophysical Research Communications* 1965; **21**: 568–574.

60 Leupold F, Kremer G. Biosynthesis of polyenoic fatty acids in human whole blood. *Nature* 1961; **191**: 805–806.

61 Deykin D. The subcellular distribution of platelet lipids labeled by acetate-1-C. *J. Lipid. Res.* 1971; **12**: 9–11.

62 Marks PA, Gellhorn A, Kidson C. Lipid synthesis in human leukocytes, platelets, and erythrocytes. *J. Biol. Chem.* 1960; **235**: 2579–2583.

63 Majerus PW, Lastra R. Fatty acid biosynthesis in human leukocytes. *J. Clin. Inv.* 1967; **46**: 1596–1602.

64 Schoene N. Metabolism of linoleic and arachidonic acids in human. *Fed. Proc.* 1973; **32**: 919.

65 Reitz RC. Dietary fatty acids and alcohol: effects on cellular membranes. *Alcohol & Alcoholism* 1993; **28**: 59–71.

66 Salem N Jr, Ward G. In: *Alcohol, Cell Membranes, and Signal Transduction in Brain*, Alling C. (Ed.), Plenum Press, New York, 1993.

67 Salem N Jr, Olsson NU. In: *Handbook of Essential Fatty Acid Biology: Biochemistry, Physiology, and Behavioral Neurobiology*, Yehuda S, Mostofsky DI. (Eds.), Humana Press Inc., Totowa, NJ, 1997.

68 Nervi AM, Peluffo RO, Brenner RR, Leikin AI. Effect of ethanol administration on fatty acid desaturation. *Lipids* 1980; **15**: 263–268.

69 Wang D, Reitz R. Ethanol ingestion and polyunsaturated fatty acids: Effects on the acyl-CoA desaturases. *Alcohol Clin. Exp. Res.* 1983; **7**: 220–226.

70 Nakamura M, Tang AB, Villaneuva J, Halsted CH, Phinney SD. Selective reductions of delta6 and delta5 desaturase activities but not delta9 desaturase in minipigs chronically fed ethanol. *J. Clin. Inv.* 1994; **93**: 450–454.

71 Pawlosky RJ, Sprecher HW, Salem N Jr. High sensitivity negative ion GC-MS method for detection of desaturated and chain-elongated products of deuterated linoleic and linolenic acids. *J. Lipid Res.* 1992; **33**: 1711–1717.

72 Pawlosky RJ, Gupta S, Salem N Jr. In: *Essential Fatty Acids and Eicosanoids: Invited Papers from the Fourth International Congress*, Riemersma RA, Armstrong R, Kelley RW, Wilson R. (Eds.), AOCS Press, Champaign, Illinois, 1998.

73 Pawlosky RJ, Salem N Jr. Alcohol consumption in Rhesus monkeys depletes tissues of polyunsaturated fatty acids and alters essential fatty acid metabolism. *Alcoholism: Clin. Exp. Res.* 1999; **23**: 311–317.

74 Pawlosky RJ, Flynn BM, Salem N Jr. The effects of low dietary levels of polyunsaturates on alcohol-induced liver disease in Rhesus monkeys. *Hepatology* 1997; **26**: 1386–1392.

75 Derr RF. A trail of alcoholic liver disease research: A quest which proved ethanol-nutrient synergism. *Biochem. Arch.* 1993; **9**: 175–195.

76 French SW, Wong K, Jui L, Albano E, Hagbjork A-L, Ingleman-Sundberg M. Effect of ethanol on cytochrome P450 2E1 (CYP2E1). Lipid peroxidation and serum protein adduct formation in relation to liver pathology pathogenesis. *Exper. Mol. Path.* 1993; **58**: 61–75.

77 Morimoto M, Hagbjork A-L, Nanji AA, Ingelman-Sundberg M, Lindors KO, Fu PC, Albano E, French SW. Role of cytochrome P4502E1 in alcoholic liver disease pathogenesis. *Alcohol* 1993; **10**: 459–464.

78 Albano E, Poli G, Tomasi A, Goria-Gatti L, Dianzani MU. In: *Medical, Biochemical and Chemical Aspects of Free Radicals*, Hayashi O, Niki E, Kondo M, Yoshikawa T. (Eds.), Elsevier Amsterdam, The Netherlands, 1988.

79 Hageman JJ, Bast A, Vermeulen NP. Monitoring of oxidative free radical damage *in vivo*: analytical aspects. *Chem.–Biol. Interactions* 1992; **82**: 243.

80 Tsuchida H, Miura T, Mitzutami K, Aibara K. Fluorescent substances in mouse and human serum as a parameter of *in vivo* lipid peroxidation. *Biochim. Biophys. Acta* 1985; **834**: 196.

81 Uchida K, Szweda LI, Chae H-Z, Stadtman ER. Immunochemical detection of 4-hydroxynonenal protein adducts in oxidized hepatocytes. *Proc. Natl. Acad. Sci. USA* 1993; **90**: 8742.

82 Vendemeiale G, Altomare E, Grattagliano I, Albano O. Increased plasma levels of glutathione and malondialdehyde after acute ethanol ingestion in humans. *J. Hepatology* 1989; **9**: 359.

83 Chen JJ, Schenker S, Henderson GI. 4-hydroxynonenal levels are enhanced in fetal liver mitochondria by *in utero* ethanol exposure. *Hepatology* 1997; **25**: 142.

84 Esterbauer H. Cytotoxicity and genotoxicity of lipid-oxidation products. *Am. J. Clin. Nutr.* 1993; **57**(s): 779s.

85 Esterbauer H, Schaur RJ, Zollner H. Chemistry and biochemistry of 4-hydroxynonenal malonaldehyde and related aldehydes. *Free Rad. Biol. Med.* 1990; **11**: 81.

86 Uchida K, Stadtman ER. Modification of histidine residues in proteins by reaction with 4-hydroxynonenal. *Proc. Natl. Acad. Sci. USA* 1992; **89**: 4544.

87 Tuma DJ, Thiele GM, Xu D, Klassen LW, Sorrell MF. Acetaldehyde and malondialdehyde react together to generate distinct adducts in the liver during long-term ethanol administration. *Hepatology* 1996; **23**: 872–880.

88 Reitz RC, Wang L, Schilling RJ, Starich GH, Bergstrom JD, Thompson JA. Effects of ethanol ingestion on the unsaturated fatty acids from various tissues. *Prog. Lipid Res.* 1981; **20**: 209.

89 Morrow JD, Awad JA, Boss HJ, Blair IA, Roberts LJ. Non-cycloxygenase-derived prostanoids (F2-isoprostanes) are formed *in situ* on phospholipids. *Proc. Natl. Acad. Sci. USA* 1992; **89**: 10721–10725.

90 Delanty N, Reilly D, Pratico D, Fitzgerald DJ, Lawson JA, Fitzderald GA. 8-epi PGF2-alpha: specific analysis of an isoeicosanoid as an index of oxidant stress *in vivo*. *Br. J. Clin. Pharmacol.* 1996; **42**: 15–19.

91 Praticò D, Barry OP, Lawson JA, Adiyaman M, Hwang S-W, Khanapure SP, Iuliano L, Rokach J, FitzGerald GA. IPF$_2\alpha$-I: An index of lipid peroxidation in humans. *Proc. Natl. Acad. Sci. USA* 1998; **95**: 3449–3454.

92 Nrooz-Zadeh J, Liu ECL, Anggard EE, Halliwell B. F4-isoprostanes: A novel class of prostanoids formed during peroxidation of docosahexaenoic acid (DHA). *Biochem. Biophys. Res. Commun.* 1998; **242**: 338.

93 Roberts LJ II, Montine TH, Markesbery WR, Tapper AR, Hardy P, Chemtob S, Dettbarn WB, Morrow JD. Formation of isoprostane-like compounds (neuroprostanes) *in vivo* from docosahexaenoic acid. *J. Biol. Chem.* 1998; **273**: 13605–13612.

94 Montine TJ, Markesbery WR, Morrow JD, Roberts LJ II. Cerebrospinal fluid F_2-isoprostane levels are increased in Alzheimer's Disease. *Ann. Neurol.* 1998; **44**: 410–413.

95 Lieber C, Leo MA, Aleynik SI, Aleynik MK, DeCarli LM. Polyenylphosphatidylcholine decreases alcohol-induced oxidative stress in the baboon. *Alcoholism: Clin. Exp. Res.* 1997; **21**: 375–379.

96 Marley R, Harry D, Anand R, Bimbi F, Davies S, Moore K. 8-isoprostaglandin F2-alpha, a product of lipid peroxidation, increases portal pressure in normal and cirrhotic rats. *Gastroenterology* 1997; **112**: 208–213.

97 Nanji AA, Khwaja S, Tahan SR, Hossein Sadrzadeh SM. Plasma levels of a novel noncyclooxygenase-derived prostanoid (8-isoprostane) correlate with severity of liver injury in experimental alcoholic liver disease. *J. Pharm. Exp. Ther.* 1993; **269**: 1280–1285.

98 Aleynik SI, Leo MA, Aleynik MK, Lieber CS. Increased circulating products of lipid peroxidation in patients with alcoholic liver disease. *Alcoholism: Clin. Exper. Res.* 1998; **22**: 192–196.

99 Meagher EA, Barry OP, Burke A, Lucey MR, Lawson JA, Rokach J, FitzGerald GA. Alcohol-induced generation of lipid peroxidation products in humans. *J. Clin. Inv.* 1999; **104**: 805–813.

100 Hill DB, Awad JA. Increased Urinary F_2-isoprostane excretion in alcoholic liver disease. *Free Rad. Biol. & Med.* 1999; **26**: 656–660.

101 Anggard E. In: *Recent Developments in Alcoholism*, Vol. 3, Galanter M. (Ed.), Plenum Press, New York, 1985.

102 Karanian JW, Kim H-Y, Salem N Jr. In: *Cardiovascular Disease 2*, Gallo LL. (Ed.), Plenum Press, New York, 1995.

103 Piper P, Vane JR. The release of prostaglandins from lung and other tissues. *Ann. NY. Acad. Sci.* 1971; **180**: 363–365.

104 Horrobin DF. A biochemical basis for alcoholism and alcohol-induced damage including the fetal alcohol syndrome and cirrhosis: interference with essential fatty acid and prostaglandin metabolism. *Med. Hypothesis* 1980; **6**: 929–942.

105 Karanian JW, Salem N Jr. In: *Cardiovascular Disease*, Gallo LG. (Ed.), Plenum Publishing Corp., NY, 1987.

106 Klatsky AL, Friedman GD, Sieglaub AB. Alcohol consumption before myocardial infarction. *Ann. Intern. Med.* 1974; **81**: 294.

107 Klatsky AL, Friedman GD, Sieglaub AB. Alcohol consumption and blood pressure. *N. Engl. J. Med.* 1977; **296**: 1194.

108 Taylor JR. Alcohol and strokes. *N. Engl. J. Med.* 1982; **306**: 1111.

109 Laporte RE, Cresanta JL, Kuller LH. The relationship of alcohol consumption to atherosclerotic heart disease. *Prev. Med.* 1980; **9**: 22–40.

110 Gruchow HW, Hoffman RO, Anderson AJ, Barboriak JJ. Effects of drinking patterns on the relationship between alcohol and coronary occlusion. *Atherosclerosis* 1982; **43**: 393–399.

111 Doll R. Prospects for prevention. *Br. J. Med.* 1983; **286**: 445–453.

112 Goto Y, Kikuchi M, Abe K, Nagahashi Y, Ohiva S, Kudo M. The effect of ethanol on the onset of experimental atherosclerosis. *Tohuku J. Exp. Med.* 1974; **114**: 35–40.

113 Renaud S, Marzain R, McGregor L, Baudier F. Dietary fats on platelet functions in relation to atherosclerosis and coronary heart disease. *Haemostasis* 1979; **8**: 234–239.

114 Retrosen J, Mandio D, Segarnick D. Ethanol and prostaglandin E_1: Biochemical and behavioral interactions. *Life Sci.* 1980; **26**: 1867–1876.

115 Thomas M, Boura ALA, Vijayakumar R. Prostaglandin release by aliphatic alcohols from the rat isolated lung. *Clin. Exp. Pharmacol.* 1980; **7**: 373–380.

116 Salem N Jr. Alcohol, fatty acids, and diet. *Alcohol Heath & Research World* 1989; **13**: 211–218.

117 Horrobin DF, Manku MS. Possible role of prostaglandin E_1 in affective disorders and in alcoholism. *Br. Med. J.* 1980; **280**: 1363–1366.

118 Pediconi M, Colombo C, Galli C. Effects of acute and chronic ethanol administration on thromboxane and prostacyclin levels and release in rat brain cortex. *Prostaglandins* 1985; **30**: 313–322.

119 Pennington SN, Woody DG, Rumbley RA. Ethanol-induced changes in the oxidative metabolism of arachidonic acid. *Prostaglandins Leukotrienes Med.* 1982; **19**: 151–156.

120 Adolphs MJP, Elliot GR. The stimulation by ethanol of rat aorta ring prostacyclin-like synthesis is related to the age of the animal. *Agents Actions* 1982; **11**: 217–224.

121 Karanian JW, Stojanov M, Salem N Jr. The effect of ethanol on prostacyclin and thromboxane A_2 synthesis in rat aortic rings *in vitro*. *Prostaglandins Leukotrienes Med.* 1985; **20**: 175–186.

122 Landolfi R, Steiner M. Ethanol raises prostacyclin *in vivo* and *in vitro*. *Blood* 1984; **64**: 679–684.

123 MacIntyre DE, Pearson JD, Gordon JL. Localization and stimulation of prostaglandin production in vascular cells. *Nature* 1978; **271**: 549–551.

124 Vane JR, Williams TC. The contribution of prostaglandin production to contractions of isolated uterus of the rat. *Br. J. Pharmacol.* 1974; **48**: 628–633.

125 Willis AL, Davison P, Ramwell PW. Inhibition of intestinal tone, motility and prostaglandin biosynthesis by 5,8,11,14-eicosatetraynoic acid. *Prostaglandins* 1974; **5**: 355–360.

126 Fewings JD, Hanna MJD, Walsh JD, Whelan RF. The effects of ethylalcohol on the blood vessels of the hand and forearm in man. *Br. J. Pharmacol.* 1966; **27**: 93–106.

127 Goldman M, Saperstein LA, Murphy S, Moore J. Alcohol and regional blood flow in brains of rats. *Proc. Soc. Exp. Biol. Med.* 1973; **144**: 983–988.

128 Nakano J, Prancan AV. Effects of adrenergic blockade on cardiovascular responses to ethanol and acetaldehyde. *Arch. Int. Pharmacodyn.* 1972; **196**: 259–268.

129 Altura BM, Altura BT, Carella A. Ethanol produces coronary vasospasm: Evidence for a direct action of ethanol on vascular muscle. *Br. J. Pharmacol.* 1983; **78**: 260–262.

130 Altura BM, Ogunkoya A, Gebrewold A, Altura BT. Effects of ethanol on terminal arterioles and muscular venules: Direct observations on the microcirculation. *J. Cardiovasc. Pharmacol.* 1979; **1**: 97–113.

131 Friedman HS, Matsuzaki S, Choe S-S, Ferwando MA, Celis A, Zaman Q, Lieber CS. Demonstration of dissimilar acute haemodynamic effects of ethanol and acetaldehyde. *Cardiovasc. Res.* 1979; **13**: 479–487.

132 Edgarian H, Altura BM. Ethanol and contraction of venous smooth muscle. *Anesthesiology* 1976; **44**: 311–317.

133 Karanian JW, Stojanov M, Yergey J, Salem N Jr. In: *Challenging Frontiers for Prostaglandin Research*, Katori M, Yamamoto S, Hayaishi O. (Eds.), Gendai-Iryosha, *Tokyo*, 1985.

134 Karanian JW, D'Souza N, Salem N Jr. The effect of chronic alcohol inhalation on blood pressure and the pressor response to noradrenaline and the thromboxane-mimic U46619. *Life Sci.* 1986; **39**: 1245–1255.

135 Manku MS, Oka M, Horrobin DF. Alcohol consumption and coronary heart disease. *Lancet* 1979; **1**: 1404.

136 Hwang DH. Ethanol inhibits the formation of endoperoxide metabolites in human platelets. *Prostaglandins Med.* 1981; **7**: 511–516.

137 Bengmark S, Doransson G, Idvall J, Zoucas E. Myocardial function and lipid metabolsim in the chronic alcoholic animal. *Haemostasis* 1980; **43**: 203–207.

138 Mikhailidas DP, Jeremy JY, Barradas MA, Green N, Dandona P. Effect of ethanol on vascular PGI_2 synthesis, platelet aggregation and platelet TXA_2 release. *Br. Med. J.* 1983; **287**: 1495–1498.

139 Moncada S, Higgs EA, Vane JA. Human arterial and venous tissues generate prostacyclin (prostaglandin X), a potent inhibitor of platelet aggregation. *Lancet* 1977; **1**: 16–19.

140 Chin JH, Goldstein DB, Parsons LM. Fluidity and lipid composition of mouse biomembranes during adaptation to ethanol. *Alcohol Clin. Exp. Res.* 1977; **3**: 47–49.

141 Chin JH, Goldstein DB. Drug tolerance in biomembranes: A spin label study of the effects of ethanol. *Science* 1979; **196**: 684–685.

142 Franks F, Eagland D. Influence of hydration on protein structure. *Crit. Rev. Biochem.* 1975; **3**: 165–172.

143 Rimon G, Hanski E, Braun S, Levitski A. Mode of coupling between hormone receptors and adenylate cyclase elucidated by modulation of membrane fluidity. *Nature* 1978; **276**: 394–396.

144 Mitchell DC, Lawrence JTR, Litman BJ. Primary alcohols modulate the activation of the G protein-coupled receptor rhodopsin by a lipid-mediated mechanism. *J. Biol. Chem.* 1996; **271**: 19033–19036.

145 Liu MS, Glosh S, Yang Y. Change in membrane lipid fluidity induced by phospholipase A_2 activation: A mechanism of exdotoxic shock. *Life Sci.* 1983; **33**: 1995–2002.

146 Jain MK, Cordes EH. Phospholipases I: Effect of n-alkanols on the rate of enzymatic hydrolysis of egg phosphatidylcholine. *J. Membr. Biol.* 1973; **14**: 101–118.

147 Seeman P. The membrane actions of anesthetics and tranquilizers. *Pharmacol. Rev.* 1972; **24**: 583–592.

148 Karanian JW, Yergey JL, Lister RL, Linnoila M, Salem N Jr. Characterization of an automated apparatus for precise control of inhalation chamber ethanol vapor and blood ethanol concentration. *Alcoholism Clin. Exp. Res.* 1986; **10**: 16–22.

149 Salem N Jr, Reyzer M, Karanian J. Losses of arachidonic acid in rat liver after alcohol inhalation. *Lipids* 1996; **31**: S153–S156.

150 Tsukamoto H, Towner SJ, Ciofalo LM, French SW. Ethanol-induced liver fibrosis in rats fed high fat diet. *Hepatology* 1986; **6**: 814–822.

151 Pawlosky RJ, Salem N Jr. Ethanol exposure causes a decrease in docosahexaenoic acid and an increase in docosapentaenoic acid in feline brains and retinas. *Am. J. Clin. Nutr.* 1995; **61**: 1284–1289.

Chapter 17

Alcohol and heart muscle proteins: with special reference to measurement of protein synthesis *in vivo*

*V.R. Preedy, M.J. Dunn, R. Hunter, D. Mantle,
S. Worrall, P.J. Richardson*

INTRODUCTION

The ingestion of alcohol in excessive quantities causes both metabolic and functional abnormalities in the heart, including diastolic dysfunction, atrial fibrillation, myofibrillary disarray and raised cardiac enzyme activities [1–5]. Left ventricular hypertrophy or cardiomegaly may be present. As an approximation, alcoholic cardiomyopathy (ACM) may be associated with an alcohol consumption of 80 g ethanol/day, with a duration of continuous exposure in excess of 10 years or more, or a cumulative ethanol ingestion of 250 kg. Cumulative alcohol intake correlates inversely with cardiac ejection fraction and directly with left ventricular mass [4]. In the latter study of some 52 alcoholic subjects, regression analysis of the author's data showed that ejection fractions of 55% or less were obtained when the total cumulative ethanol intake was approximately 1400 kg of ethanol (assuming that average body weight was 70 kg [4]). The proposition that cumulative (as opposed to immediate) intake of alcohol is important in the genesis of alcoholic cardiomyopathy is supported by observations showing that this disease entity is uncommon in subjects under 40 years of age [6,7]. However, a pre-clinical form of alcoholic cardiomyopathy may be apparent only after stress or additional pathophysiological stimuli in some subjects [6,7].

There is a considerable divergence in subject sensitivity to alcohol, suggestive of a genetic element for alcoholic cardiomyopathy. However, many studies have employed different criteria either to define ACM, or have studied heart muscle in patients with different levels of alcohol intake. To give just two examples of such study-variability, patients have been investigated with mean cumulative intakes of 500 kg alcohol [8] or 2030 kg [9] (also reviewed in [10]). In another study, cumulative intakes ranged from 350 to 2800 kg ethanol [4]. These disparities suggest that in order to study the detailed pathogenesis of ACM, more consistency in investigative processes is needed, which has led to the development of suitable animal models of alcohol-induced heart muscle damage.

HISTOLOGICAL FEATURES OF ALCOHOL INDUCED CARDIOMYOPATHY IN CLINICAL STUDIES

Histological features of alcoholic cardiomyopathy have been described in detail in previous studies (see for example, [4,11–15]). Changes include fibrosis and increased lipid deposits (with inflammation in some samples). Mitochondrial and sarcolemmal abnormalities have been described, though most pertinent to this chapter are the perturbations in myofibrillary architecture (also reviewed in [10]). At the light microscopic level, in alcoholic cardiomyopathy there are considerable size variations between the myofibrils, with concomitant loss of cross striations, destruction, vacuolization and oedema [15,16]. At the electron microscopic level, degenerative changes are apparent with disruption, fragmentation or loss of the myofibrils, loss of structural arrangement, dissolution and rearrangement of the filamentous structures [11–14]. Although many of the histological features of dilated cardiomyopathy and alcoholic cardiomyopathy are traditionally thought to be indistinguishable [14], subtle differences have been described [9]. Thus, in dilated cardiomyopathy the degree of myocyte hypertrophy, fibrosis and nuclear alterations is greater than for corresponding measurements in myocytes from alcoholics [9]. The differences between these two disorders may result from specific and distinct etiological pathways.

HISTOLOGICAL FEATURES IN THE RAT MODEL

Similar histochemical changes to those seen clinically above can be reproduced in animal models, including myofibrillary lysis, separation and disintegration, with scattered foci of lesions (fibrosis) and loss of parallel array [17–19]. The severity of these lesions worsen with increasing alcohol intake [20]. Overall, there are clear indications that the contractile apparatus is perturbed via experimental alcohol feeding. In the chronic alcoholic feeding model (using the Lieber-DeCarli feeding regimen), left ventricle weights are increased at 4–11 months, though no changes are seen at 2 months [21]. These changes are accompanied by functional defects, such as reduced cardiac output [21]. The model employing 6 weeks alcohol feeding in a pair-feeding regimen represents a transient phase in the development of the cardiomyopathy, and hence provides a suitable means of studying the pathogenesis of the disease process. The concepts of pair-feeding in chronic alcohol dosing studies have been described elsewhere [22,23].

MEASURING CHANGES IN PROTEIN SYNTHESIS *IN VIVO*

Changes in cardiac protein levels occur as a result of perturbations in protein synthesis and/or degradation. Rates of protein synthesis can be determined using labeled amino acids via measurement of the rate of their incorporation into cardiac proteins. This necessitates characterization of time-course changes in the specific radioactivities of the precursor, i.e., the amino acyl tRNA (S_{tRNA}), and the product, i.e., the labeled amino acids in the tissue protein [24]. Whilst measuring the specific radioactivity of the protein-bound amino acid presents few practical problems, determining the specific radioactivity of S_{tRNA} is more difficult to quantify on a routine basis. This is because tRNA is extremely labile and occurs in low abundance, such that techniques have been devised to approximate S_{tRNA} or determine its value indirectly. Frequently, S_{tRNA} is represented by either:

(i)   the specific radioactivities of the free amino acid in the intracellular pool (measured as the specific radioactivity of the free amino acid in the acid supernatants of heart homogenates, i.e., S_i), or;

(ii) the specific radioactivity of the free amino acid in the extracellular pool (measured as the specific radioactivity of the free amino acid in the acid supernatant of the plasma, i.e., S_p).

In animal studies, there are three methods for measuring protein synthesis *in vivo*, two of which are reliable and in current use. In the pulse tracer injection method, the isotope is injected in small quantities. Figure 17.1 shows that immediately after the pulse injection of the tracer isotope in small laboratory animals, there are complex changes in both S_i and S_p, which makes it difficult to define these curves especially in the initial phase of the radio-labeling period (Phase a). More subtle changes occur in the aftermath of the initial injection period (Phase b) compared to the more dynamic Phase a. However, accurate assessment of protein synthesis necessitates quantifying the area under the entire curve for either S_i or S_p during the radiolabeling period. This involves sacrifice of a large number of animals to characterize the curves for S_i and S_p. As a consequence of the practical constraints inherent in the method, the pulse injection technique is considered unreliable.

The 'constant infusion' method facilitates the measurement of protein synthesis rates in single rats. In this method, a tracer amount of amino acid is infused over a few hours (usually between 3–6 hours) in rats. The specific radioactivities rise to a plateau in Phase a, whereas the specific radioactivities of both S_i and S_p attain steady state values in the latter period of Phase b. The disadvantage of this method is that there are large differences between S_i and S_p for tissues with high turnover rates (such as liver and intestine). Furthermore, animals have to be immobilized for up to 3–6 hours, which precludes the use of this method in acute studies. Because of the complex time-course changes in protein turnover and its possible influence on S_i and S_p, the derived value of the fractional synthesis rate (k_s) may be in error. This is because, calculation of k_s depends on the final S_i and S_p values and the cumulative incorporation of label into proteins, occurring over the 3–6 hour infusion period. For example, we have shown that the rates of muscle protein synthesis in rats measured in the morning (09:00–12:00 hours) are higher than those in the afternoon (15:00–18:00 hours) [25]. This is not easily discernible with the *constant infusion* method [25].

In the *flooding dose* technique, now considered the 'gold standard' method for measuring protein synthesis, the radio-label is injected with a large amount of 'cold' amino acid. With this method there are small decreases in both S_i and S_p, which can in practice be considered to be linear over short labeling periods, such as 10 minutes. In the heart, the changes in S_i are quite small (approx. 5%) over 10 mins, and rats are killed at one time-point only. Thus, the features of both Phase a and Phase b are identical. The *flooding dose* method overcomes many of the practical limitations inherent in the *constant infusion* method. For example, in tissues with high protein turnover rates, the differences between S_i and S_p are minimized with the *flooding dose* method in contrast to the large differences between S_i and S_p noted above. The *flooding dose* method has been employed in over 600 studies to date, and investigation of heart muscle protein changes include the effects of running, growth hormone, alcohol, intrauterine growth retardation and IGF-I dosage [26–31].

In the *flooding dose* method, animals are injected intravenously with phenylalanine (0.150 mmol per 100 g body weight) and sacrificed after 10 minutes [32]. Phenylalanine is chosen as this amino acid is (i) not considered to be a regulator of protein synthesis; (ii) it is very soluble; (iii) it occurs in very low concentrations in the intracellular pool, thereby facilitating the flooding phenomena and rapid equilibration between subcellular compartments; (iv) its specific radioactivity can be determined by test-tube techniques. Some studies have injected the labeled isotope intraperitoneally, but this is not recommended as ethanol affects the partitioning of phenylalanine between extracellular and intracellular compartments of free amino acid pools [33]. After intravenous injection and allowing a suitable radio-labeling period (usually 10 minutes) fractional rates of cardiac protein synthesis (i.e., percentage of the cardiac protein pool renewed each day, i.e., k_s, % per day)

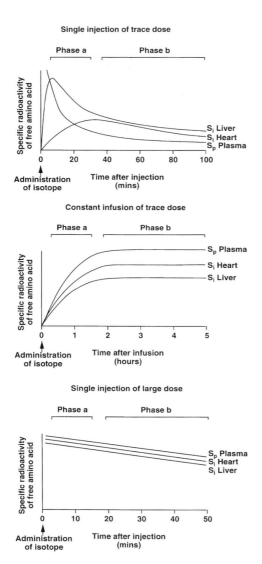

Figure 17.1 Changes in precursor specific radioactivities in different methods for measuring protein synthesis *in vivo*. The three methods of measuring protein synthesis are (top) pulse injection of a tracer amount of amino acid, (middle) constant infusion of a tracer amino acids and (bottom) injection of a flooding dose of amino acid. Phase (a) and (b) are arbitrary assigned periods of each method. For a fuller explanation see text. Adapted from works of P.J. Garlick.

are calculated from the formula: $k_s = (S_b \times 100) / (S_i \times t)$ [32]. Where, S_b is the specific radioactivity of the labeled phenylalanine in cardiac protein; S_i is the specific radioactivity of the free amino acid in the intracellular pool; t is the labeling period, in units of a day, i.e., for a 10-min labeling period, 0.00694 days [32].

CHANGES IN CARDIAC PROTEIN SYNTHESIS IN ANIMAL MODELS

Acute ethanol toxicity reduces cardiac protein synthesis *in vivo* [34]; the greatest decreases in protein synthesis occur after 24 hours when all circulating ethanol has disappeared (Figure 17.2). The atria and ventricles appear equally susceptible to ethanol-induced perturbations in protein synthesis [27]. Hypertension exacerbates these regional effects of ethanol on cardiac myofibrillary protein synthesis [27,35]. It seems that synthesis of the major protein fractions is decreased, including the myofibrillary and mitochondrial proteins (Table 17.1; [35–37]).

Acetaldehyde is a potent inhibitor of myocardial protein synthesis. Thus, when ethanol-dosed rats are pre-treated with cyanamide (an inhibitor of acetaldehyde dehydrogenase which elevates endogenous acetaldehyde levels), the depression is approximately 80% compared to the approximately 15–20% depression in k_s seen with alcohol alone (Figure 17.3; [10,37,38]). Cardiac ATP content remains unaltered compared to saline or ethanol-injected rats, even when ethanol-dosed rats are pre-treated with cyanamide (Figure 17.3; [38]). Circulating cardiac Troponin-T, a marker of cardiac damage, increases at 2.5 hours after an acute dose of alcohol and this effect is exacerbated with cyanamide pretreatment (Figure 17.3; [39]).

The precise mechanism whereby alcohol decreases protein synthesis is still unclear, as there are many steps leading to the synthesis of new proteins. Alcohol reduces the ability of the sarcoplasmic reticulum to gain and store Ca^{2+}, resulting in increased intracellular calcium

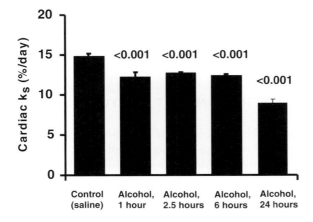

Figure 17.2 Cardiac protein synthesis in response to acute alcohol. Rats were injected i.p. with 0.15 mol/l saline (NaCl); or ethanol (75 mmol/kg body weight, i.p). All data are means ± SEM of 6–8 observations. From [73].

Table 17.1 Rate of protein synthesis in various fractions of the rat heart

| Protein Fraction | Ventricular k_s (%/day) | | | |
	Control	Ethanol	Difference as % from control	p
Total	22.4 ± 1.5	17.8 ± 1.3	-21	<0.01
Subsarcolemmal mitochondria	16.9 ± 1.1	13.0 ± 0.8	-23	<0.01
Intermyofibrillary mitochondria	10.9 ± 0.5	18.1 ± 0.5	-26	<0.01
Nuclear fraction	12.9 ± 1.0	10.3 ± 0.6	-20	<0.05

Male Wistar rats were injected with either 0.15 mol/l NaCl or isovolumetric solutions of ethanol (75 mmol/kg body weight, i.p.) 2.5 hours prior to the measurement of protein synthesis with a *flooding dose* of L-[4-^{3}H]phenylalanine. All data are mean $\pm$ SEM of 6–7 observations in each group. Differences between means were assessed by Student's t test, using 2-tailed tables. Significance was indicated when $p < 0.05$. From [36].

levels leading to metabolic derangements such as mitochondrial dysfunction, reductions in protein synthesis, increased proteolysis and defective energy-coupling [40–48]. Increases in intracellular proteolysis may derange subcellular organelles and/or cardiac architecture and indirectly influence k_s [49]. Of additional importance is a study showing that calcium channel blockade prevents coronary artery constriction due to alcohol; this has particular relevance as the rise in circulating cardiac troponin-T in alcohol dosed rats may be an ischaemic related event [50]. Unfortunately, investigations into alcohol and cardiac calcium homeostasis have mainly been carried out *in vitro*, and there are no studies on the relationship between cardiac protein synthesis and calcium homeostasis *in vivo*. However, both acute and chronic treatment with the dihydropyridine calcium channel (L-type voltage dependent) antagonist amlodipine fails to alter changes in protein synthesis induced by alcohol (Table 17.2). It is possible that alcohol acts directly on a discrete component of protein synthesis in the myocardium, a supposition supported by studies in perfused heart showing that alcohol and acetaldehyde (albeit, using supraphysiological concentrations) can reduce cardiac protein synthesis *in vitro* [51].

CHANGES IN CARDIAC PROTEIN CONTENT *IN VIVO*

Changes in tissue protein content can be considered at either the total protein or the individual protein levels. Analysis of whole tissue protein content takes no account of the potentially complex changes occurring in diseased tissue in which individual protein levels may be increased, decreased, or unaltered. Unfortunately, many studies using the flooding dose technique described above have analyzed whole tissue proteins or crude protein fractions such as the myofibrillary (also termed contractile protein fraction), sarcoplasmic (also termed soluble or 33,000 g fraction) and stromal fractions (also termed the insoluble or collagen fraction), which can be separated using differential solubility and high speed centrifugation techniques [52–60]. Using these techniques, we have shown

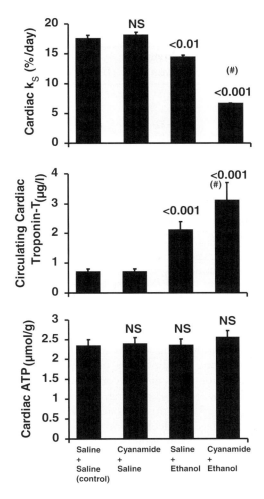

Figure 17.3 Cardiac protein synthesis, ATP and plasma troponin-T in rats treated with alcohol. Data are mean ± SEM of 4–9 observations in each group. Ethanol (75 mmol/kg body weight; i.p.) was given with or without cyanamide pretreatment (0.5 mmol/kg body weight; i.p.). Rats were killed 2.5 hours after ethanol dosing. *p* values over histograms pertain to differences from saline plus saline controls. (#) Difference in ks between saline plus ethanol and cyanamide plus ethanol, *p* < 0.01. Data from various studies of the authors and [73].

that the protein content of the total (composite mixture of sarcoplasmic, myofibrillary and stromal proteins) and myofibrillary protein fractions decrease in response to chronic alcohol feeding [56]. Using one-dimensional sodium dodecyl sulphate polyacrylamide gel electrophoresis (SDS-PAGE), we have shown that the reductions in total and myofibrillary proteins are accompanied by a marked reduction in myosin heavy chain content [61]. Recently, however, the approach of proteomic analysis has been developed and applied to the investigation of the effects of chronic ethanol feeding. In this method, individual proteins in whole tissues or organs (particularly in small laboratory animals) are extracted,

Table 17.2 The chronic effect of amlodipine treatment and alcohol on LV total and protein fraction synthesis rates

		Difference as % from control (1)	Statistical Significance (p)
Ventricular total k_s (%/day)			
1 Control (saline)	10.7 ± 0.7		
2 Alcohol	8.4 ± 0.6	−22	< 0.01
3 Amlodipine + Saline	9.6 ± 0.4	−10	NS
4 Amlodipine + Alcohol	8.0 ± 0.6	−25	< 0.01
Differences between 3 and 4, −17 %, p < 0.05			
Ventricular k_{RNA} (mg protein/day/ mg RNA)			
1 Control (saline)	12.3 ± 0.8		
2 Alcohol	9.6 ± 0.7	−23	< 0.01
3 Amlodipine + Saline	11.0 ± 0.6	−11	NS
4 Amlodipine + Alcohol	9.0 ± 0.6	−27	< 0.001
Differences between 3 and 4, −18 %, p < 0.05			

Male Wistar rats were treated with either tap water or amlodipine 10 mg/day/kg body weight for 30 days followed by an acute i.p. dose of either saline 0.15 mol/l (NaCl) or ethanol 75 mmol/kg body weight. All data are mean ± SEM of 7–8 observations. Differences were assessed by Student's t-test for unpaired samples using the pooled estimate of variance [73].

separated and identified [62–69]. After an initial (first-dimensional) separation by isoelectric focusing (IEF), a second-dimensional separation using sodium dodecyl sulphate polyacrylamide gel electrophoresis under denaturing conditions is employed. Individual proteins can be tentatively identified after appropriate staining; confirmation of protein identity is carried out by either immunoblotting, microsequencing, amino acid composition or mass spectrometry (reviewed in [70–72]). Using this approach, it has been shown that the protein profile of rat heart is altered by feeding alcohol for 6 weeks [38]. Over 400 proteins have been detected in rat heart and expressed in terms of relative abundance, 7% of these proteins are significantly increased whilst 3% are reduced after 6 weeks chronic alcohol exposure *in vivo* [38]. Heat Shock Proteins (HSP) 60 and 70, actin, desmin and myosin light chain 2 are decreased whereas creatine kinase is increased [38]. The latter findings are compatible with separate studies showing that cardiac creatine kinase activity is increased in rats fed alcohol for 6 weeks, albeit in the presence of hypertension [73]. In contrast, there is little or no change in total or subcellular protein content of the heart in response to acute (for example, 2.5 hours) ethanol dosage. The identities of the other proteins altered following chronic alcohol dosage (and the possibility that acute ethanol dosage affects the levels of yet undefined proteins), remains to be elucidated, although further studies are continuing in this area.

ROLE OF ACETALDEHYDE-PROTEIN ADDUCTS AND FREE RADICALS

It is important to emphasize that changes in the heart protein content in response to alcohol exposure may arise via a number of mechanisms including:

I. Perturbations in DNA structure and function (via free radical damage or adduct formation);

II. Changes (increases and decreases) in mRNA level;

III. Protein adduct formation;

IV. Free radical induced protein damage;

V. Increased or decreased protease activities.

The liver is the main site of alcohol-derived acetaldehyde production, an extremely reactive metabolite. Acetaldehyde binds with proteins to form protein-adducts which may induce auto-immunogenic responses (as identified by raised serum antibodies) or render the affected protein functionally inoperative [74–82]. In rats subjected to 6 weeks ethanol feeding, ELISA showed increased amounts of reduced- and unreduced-acetaldehyde protein adducts as well as malondialdehyde-acetaldehyde protein adducts (Worrall S, Richardson PJ, Preedy VR, unpublished). However, there was no evidence of increased malondialdehyde and α-hydroxyethyl-protein adducts in hearts of ethanol fed rats compared to pair-fed controls (Worrall S, Richardson PJ, Preedy VR unpublished).

The increase in malondialdehyde-acetaldehyde protein adducts supports previous suggestions that alcohol induces cardiac lipid peroxidation [83,84] concomitant with endogenous cardiac-derived acetaldehyde formation, possibly via alcohol dehydrogenase (ADH) or cytochrome P450 actions. However, although the activity of cardiac alcohol dehydrogenase is low, catalase may also generate acetaldehyde [85–88]. The importance of these studies relates to the observation that malondialdehyde-acetaldehyde adducts are cytotoxic, inducing the release of TNF-alpha and up-regulating ICAM-1 in endothelial cells *in vitro* [89].

Reactive oxygen free radical species may play a prominent role in alcohol-induced heart muscle damage. Cardiac tissue from chronic alcohol misusers shows increased '*age pigments*' indicative of damage by reactive oxygen species [90]. Involvement of reactive oxygen species damage is also implicated by studies showing that in alcohol-fed rats, the resulting shift in fatty acid profile is inhibited by dietary alpha-tocopherol, a potent anti-oxidant [91]. The decrease in cardiac enzyme activities such as creatine kinase after acute ethanol-dosage is also ascribed to damage resulting from reactive oxygen species [92]. In addition, hydroxyl radicals change the conformational properties of the contractile proteins, as determined by electrophoretic analysis [93]. In acute alcohol toxicity, increases and subsequent oxidation of circulating catecholamines may induce myocardial damage via production of superoxide free radicals [94].

Acetaldehyde may induce myocardial ischaemia and coronary vasospasm [50]. Elevations in circulating cardiac troponin-T occur after 2.5–6 hours in response to acute ethanol dosage in rats, suggestive of a membrane-mediated event [10,95]. We have recently examined the effects of cyanamide, propranolol, and the xanthine oxidase inhibitors allopurinol and oxypurinol on plasma cardiac troponin-T (Patel VB, Sherwood R, Richardson PJ, Preedy VR, unpublished observations). Propranolol pre-treatment reduced the alcohol-induced increase in plasma troponin-T. This may be due to the well-described beta-receptor blocking properties of propranolol or because it also has xanthine oxidase inhibiting properties [96]. However, pre-treatment with the xanthine oxidase inhibitors allopurinol and oxypurinol was unable to reduce elevated troponin-T, suggesting that the raised cardiac troponin-T levels in alcohol affected hearts may be due to beta-receptor stimulation suggestive of elevated catecholamines in alcohol-dosage. Whether this may involve increased free radical formation and/or impairment of antioxidant status remains to be

Table 17.3 The acute effect of alcohol and propranolol on protein synthesis rates

		Difference as % from control (1)	Statistical Significance (p)
Ventricular total k_s (%/day)			
1 Saline + Saline	17.6 ± 0.6		
2 Saline + Alcohol	14.4 ± 0.4	−18	< 0.01
3 Propranolol + Saline	18.9 ± 1.2	+8	NS
4 Propranolol + Alcohol	13.7 ± 0.8	−22	< 0.01
5 Propranolol (×10) + Saline	16.9 ± 0.7	−4	NS
6 Propranolol (×10) + Alcohol	14.5 ± 1.7	−18	< 0.01
Differences between 3 and 4, − 28%, $p < 0.001$; 5 vs. 6, −14%, $p < 0.05$			
Ventricular k_{RNA} (mg protein/day/mg RNA)			
1 Saline + Saline	12.8 ± 0.2		
2 Saline + Alcohol	10.7 ± 0.3	−18	< 0.01
3 Propranolol + Saline	13.8 ± 0.6	+8	NS
4 Propranolol + Alcohol	10.0 ± 0.5	−22	< 0.001
5 Propranolol (×10) + Saline	13.4 ± 0.4	−4	NS
6 Propranolol (×10) + Alcohol	11.6 ± 0.4	−18	< 0.01
Differences between 3 and 4, −28%, $p < 0.001$; 5 vs. 6, −13%, $p < 0.025$			

Male Wistar rats approximately 150 g body weight were injected i.p. with either 0.15 mol/l saline (NaCl); ethanol 75 mmol/kg body weight; propranolol 5 mg kg body weight or the higher dose of propranolol (×10) 50 mg/kg body weight. All data are mean ± SEM of 6–8 observations. Differences were assessed by Student's t-test for unpaired samples using the pooled estimate of variance. From [73].

determined [94]. Despite the fact that ethanol-induced increases in troponin-T can be prevented by propranolol, this agent does not prevent the ethanol-induced reduction in cardiac protein synthesis, suggestive of a complex aetiology in the pathogenesis of alcohol-induced heart damage (Table 17.3; [73]).

In conclusion, alcohol affects the heart in a variety of ways, changing both composition and protein synthesis. Presently, however, there are no published studies on the effects of free radical damage to cardiac enzymes such as those involved in proteolysis, or studies showing how cardiac myofibrillary enzymes are altered by acetaldehyde.

ACKNOWLEDGMENTS

Financial support from the British Heart Foundation, The Medical Research Council and the JRC is acknowledged.

ABBREVIATIONS

ACM   alcoholic cardiomyopathy
ROS   reactive oxygen species
S_i specific radioactivity of the free amino acid in the intracellular pool
S_p specific radioactivity of the free amino acid in the extracellular pool

REFERENCES

1 Spodick DH, Pigott VM, Chirife R. Preclinical cardiac malfunction in chronic alcoholism. Comparison with matched normal controls and with alcoholic cardiomyopathy. *N. Engl. J. Med.* 1972; **287**: 677–680.

2 Wu CF, Sudhaker M, Ghazanfar J, Ahmed SS, Regan TJ. Preclinical cardiomyopathy in chronic alcoholics: a sex difference. *Am. Heart J.* 1976; **91**: 281–286.

3 Richardson PJ, Wodak AD, Atkinson L, Saunders JB, Jewitt DE. Relation between alcohol intake, myocardial enzyme activity, and myocardial function in dilated cardiomyopathy. Evidence for the concept of alcohol induced heart muscle disease. *Br. Heart J.* 1986; **56**: 165–170.

4 Urbano Marquez A, Estruch R, Navarro Lopez F, Grau JM, Mont L, Rubin E. The effects of alcoholism on skeletal and cardiac muscle. *N. Engl. J. Med.* 1989; **320**: 409–415.

5 Kupari M, Koskinen P, Suokas A, Ventila M. Left ventricular filling impairment in asymptomatic chronic alcoholics. *Am. J. Cardiol.* 1990; **66**: 1473–1477.

6 Bertolet BD, Freund G, Martin CA, Perchalski DL, Williams CM, Pepine CJ. Unrecognized left ventricular dysfunction in an apparently healthy alcohol abuse population. *Drug Alcohol Depend.* 1991; **28**: 113–119.

7 Cerqueira MD, Harp GD, Ritchie JL, Stratton JR, Walker RD. Rarity of preclinical alcoholic cardiomyopathy in chronic alcoholics less than 40 years of age. *Am. J. Cardiol.* 1991; **67**: 183–187.

8 Gillet C, Juilliere Y, Pirollet P, Aubin HJ, Thouvenin A, Danchin N, Cherrier F, Paille F. Alcohol consumption and biological markers for alcoholism in idiopathic dilated cardiomyopathy: a case-controlled study. *Alcohol Alcohol.* 1992; **27**: 353–358.

9 Teragaki M, Takeuchi K, Takeda T. Clinical and histologic features of alcohol drinkers with congestive heart failure. *Am. Heart J.* 1993; **125**: 808–817.

10 Richardson PJ, Patel VB, Preedy VR. Alcohol and the myocardium. *Novartis. Found Symp.* 1998; **216**: 35–45; discussion 45–50.

11 Hibbs RG, Ferrans VJ, Black WC, Weilbaecher DG, Walsh JJ, Burch GE. Alcoholic cardiomyopathy. An electron microscopy study. *Am. Heart J.* 1965; **69**: 766–769.

12 Alexander CS. Idiopathic heart disease. II. Electron microscopic examination of myocardial biospy in alcoholic heart disease. *Am. J. Med.* 1966; **41**: 229–234.

13 Alexander CS. Electron microscopic observations in alcoholic heart disease. *Brit. Heart J.* 1967; **29**: 200–206.

14 Bulloch RT, Pearce MB, Murphy ML, Jenkins BJ, Davis JL. Myocardial lesions in idiopathic and alcoholic cardiomyopathy. Study by ventricular septal biopsy. *Am. J. Cardiol.* 1972; **29**: 15–25.

15 Klein H, Harmjanz D. Effect of ethanol infusion on the ultrastructure of human myocardium. *Postgrad. Med. J.* 1975; **51**: 325–329.

16 Ferrans VJ, Hibbs RG, Weilbaecher DG, Black WC, Walsh JJ, Burch GE. Alcoholic cardiomyopathy. A histochemical study. *Am. Heart J.* 1965; **69**: 748–765.

17 Burch GE, Colcolough HL, Harb JM, Tsui CY. The effect of ingestion of ethyl alcohol, wine and beer on the myocardium of mice. *Am. J. Cardiol.* 1971; **27**: 522–528.

18 Czarnecki CM, Schaffer SW, Evanson OA. Ultrastructural features of ethanol-induced cardiomyopathy in turkey poults. *Comp. Biochem. Physiol. A.* 1985; **82**: 939–943.

19 Capasso JM, Li P, Guideri G, Anversa P. Left ventricular dysfunction induced by chronic alcohol ingestion in rats. *Am. J. Physiol.* 1991; **261**: H212–H219.

20 Segel LD, Rendig SV, Choquet Y, Chacko K, Amsterdam EA, Mason DT. Effects of chronic graded ethanol consumption on the metabolism, ultrastructure, and mechanical function of the rat heart. *Cardiovasc. Res.* 1975; **9**: 649–663.

21 Segel LD. The development of alcohol-induced cardiac dysfunction in the rat. *Alcohol Alcohol.* 1988; **23**: 391–401.

22   Preedy VR, Duane P, Peters TJ. Biological effects of chronic ethanol consumption: a reappraisal of the Lieber-De Carli liquid-diet model with reference to skeletal muscle. *Alcohol Alcohol.* 1988; **23**: 151–154.

23   Preedy VR, McIntosh A, Bonner AB, Peters TJ. Ethanol dosage regimens in studies of ethanol toxicity: influence of nutrition and surgical interventions. *Addict. Biol.* 1996; **1**: 255–262.

24   Garlick PJ, McNurlan MA, Essen P, Wernerman J. Measurement of tissue protein synthesis rates *in vivo*: a critical analysis of contrasting methods. *Am. J. Physiol.* 1994; **266**: E287–E297.

25   Preedy VR, Garlick PJ. The influence of restraint and infusion on rates of muscle protein synthesis in the rat. Effect of altered respiratory function. *Biochem. J.* 1988; **251**: 577–580.

26   Bates PC, Aston R, Holder AT. Growth hormone control of tissue protein metabolism in dwarf mice: enhancement by a monoclonal antibody. *J. Endocrinol.* 1992; **132**: 369–375.

27   Siddiq T, Richardson PJ, Morton J, Smith B, Sherwood RA, Marway JS, Preedy, VR. Rates of protein synthesis in different regions of the normotensive and hypertrophied heart in response to acute alcohol toxicity. *Alcohol Alcohol.* 1993; **28**: 297–310.

28   Henriksen EJ, Munoz KA, Aannestad AT, Tischler ME. Cardiac protein content and synthesis *in vivo* after voluntary running or head-down suspension. *J. Appl. Physiol.* 1994; **76**: 2814–2819.

29   Burrin DG, Davis TA, Ebner S, Schoknecht PA, Fiorotto ML, Reeds PJ. Colostrum enhances the nutritional stimulation of vital organ protein synthesis in neonatal pigs. *J. Nutr.* 1997; **127**: 1284–1289.

30   Davis TA, Fiorotto ML, Burrin DG, Pond WG, Nguyen HV. Intrauterine growth restriction does not alter response of protein synthesis to feeding in newborn pigs. *Am. J. Physiol.* 1997; **272**: E877–E84.

31   Czerwinski SM, Cate JM, Francis G, Tomas F, Brocht DM, McMurtry JP. The effect of insulin-like growth factor-I (IGF-I) on protein turnover in the meat-type chicken (*Gallus domesticus*). *Comp. Biochem. Physiol.* 1998; **119**: 75–80.

32   Garlick PJ, McNurlan MA, Preedy VR. A rapid and convenient technique for measuring the rate of protein synthesis in tissues by injection of [3H]phenylalanine. *Biochem. J.* 1980; **192**: 719–723.

33   Preedy VR, Peters TJ. Changes in protein, RNA and DNA and rates of protein synthesis in muscle-containing tissues of the mature rat in response to ethanol feeding: a comparative study of heart, small intestine and gastrocnemius muscle. *Alcohol Alcohol.* 1990; **25**: 489–498.

34   Preedy VR, Peters TJ. The acute and chronic effects of ethanol on cardiac muscle protein synthesis in the rat *in vivo*. *Alcohol* 1990; **7**: 97–102.

35   Siddiq T, Sandhu G, Richardson PJ, Preedy VR. Effects of acute ethanol on ventricular myo-fibrillary protein synthesis *in vivo* in normotensive and hypertensive rats. *Addict. Biol.* 1997; **2**: 87–93.

36   Siddiq T, Salisbury JR, Richardson PJ, Preedy VR. Synthesis of ventricular mitochondrial proteins *in vivo*: effect of acute ethanol toxicity. *Alcoholism: Clin. Exp. Res.* 1993; **17**: 894–899.

37   Siddiq T, Richardson PJ, Mitchell WD, Teare J, Preedy VR. Ethanol-induced inhibition of ventricular protein synthesis *in vivo* and the possible role of acetaldehyde. *Cell. Biochem. Funct.* 1993; **11**: 45–54.

38   Patel VB, Corbett JM, Dunn MJ, Winrow VR, Portmann B, Richardson PJ, Preedy VR. Protein profiling in cardiac tissue in response to the chronic effects of alcohol. *Electrophoresis* 1997; **18**: 2788–2794.

39   Patel VB, Sherwood RA, Richardson PJ, Preedy VR. Cardiac troponin-T as a marker for heart muscle damage following acute alcohol administration: prevention by propranolol. *Eur. Heart. J.* 1996; Supplement 17: p. 939.

40   Auffermann W, Wu S, Parmley WW, Higgins CB, Wikman Coffelt J. Reversibility of chronic alcohol cardiac depression: 31P magnetic resonance spectroscopy in hamsters. *Magn. Reson. Med.* 1989; **9**: 343–352.

41   Thomas AP, Sass EJ, Tun Kirchmann TT, Rubin E. Ethanol inhibits electrically-induced calcium transients in isolated rat cardiac myocytes. *J. Mol. Cell. Cardiol.* 1989; **21**: 555–565.

42   Martinez JL, Penna M. Influences of changes in calcium concentration and verapamil on the cardiac depressant effect of ethanol in cat papillary muscle. *Gen. Pharmacol.* 1992; **23**: 1051–1056.

43 Kojima S, Wu ST, Wikman Coffelt J, Parmley WW. Acute effects of ethanol on cardiac function and intracellular calcium in perfused rat heart. *Cardiovasc. Res.* 1993; **27**: 811–816.

44 Guppy LJ, Littleton JM. Binding characteristics of the calcium channel antagonist [3H]-nitrendipine in tissues from ethanol-dependent rats. *Alcohol Alcohol.* 1994; **29**: 283–293.

45 Guppy LJ, Crabbe JC, Littleton JM. Time course and genetic variation in the regulation of calcium channel antagonist binding sites in rodent tissues during the induction of ethanol physical dependence and withdrawal. *Alcohol Alcohol.* 1995; **30**: 607–615.

46 Brown RA, Filipovich P, Walsh MF, Sowers JR. Influence of sex, diabetes and ethanol on intrinsic contractile performance of isolated rat myocardium. *Basic. Res. Cardiol.* 1996; **91**: 353–360.

47 Brown RA, Sundareson AM, Lee MM, Savage AO. Differential effects of chronic calcium channel blocker treatment on the inotropic response of diabetic rat myocardium to acute ethanol exposure. *Life Sci.* 1996; **59**: 835–847.

48 Horton JW, White DJ. Cardiac contractile and sarcoplasmic reticulum function after acute ethanol consumption. *J. Surg. Res.* 1996; **64**: 132–138.

49 Lewis SE, Anderson P, Goldspink DF. The effects of calcium on protein turnover in skeletal muscles of the rat. *Biochem. J.* 1982; **204**: 257–264.

50 Ando H, Abe H, Hisanou R. Ethanol-induced myocardial ischemia: close relation between blood acetaldehyde level and myocardial ischemia. *Clin. Cardiol.* 1993; **16**: 443–446.

51 Schreiber SS, Evans CD, Oratz M, Rothschild MA. Ethanol and cardiac protein synthesis. *Adv. Myocardiol.* 1985; **5**: 123–135.

52 Preedy VR, Garlick PJ. Protein synthesis in skeletal muscle of the perfused rat hemicorpus compared with rates in the intact animal. *Biochem. J.* 1983; **214**: 433–442.

53 Preedy VR, Peters TJ. Acute effects of ethanol on protein synthesis in different muscles and muscle protein fractions of the rat. *Clin. Sci.* 1988; **74**: 461–466.

54 Preedy VR, Garlick PJ. Inhibition of protein synthesis by glucagon in different rat muscles and protein fractions *in vivo* and in the perfused rat hemicorpus. *Biochem. J.* 1988; **251**: 727–732.

55 Preedy VR, Sugden PH. The effects of fasting or hypoxia on rates of protein synthesis *in vivo* in subcellular fractions of rat heart and gastrocnemius muscle. *Biochem. J.* 1989; **257**: 519–527.

56 Preedy VR, Peters TJ. Synthesis of subcellular protein fractions in the rat heart *in vivo* in response to chronic ethanol feeding. *Cardiovasc. Res.* 1989; **23**: 730–736.

57 Preedy VR, Peters TJ. The effect of chronic ethanol ingestion on synthesis and degradation of soluble, contractile and stromal protein fractions of skeletal muscles from immature and mature rats. *Biochem. J.* 1989; **259**: 261–266.

58 Preedy VR, Peters TJ. Changes in protein, RNA and DNA and rates of protein synthesis in muscle-containing tissues of the mature rat in response to ethanol feeding: a comparative study of heart, small intestine and gastrocnemius muscle. *Alcohol Alcohol.* 1990; **25**: 489–498.

59 Preedy VR, Gove CD, Panos MZ, Sherwood R, Portmann B, Williams R, Peters TJ. Liver histology, blood biochemistry and RNA, DNA and subcellular protein composition of various skeletal muscles of rats with experimental cirrhosis: implications for alcoholic muscle disease. *Alcohol Alcohol.* 1990; **25**: 641–649.

60 Preedy VR, Macallan DC, Griffin GE, Cook EB, Palmer TN, Peters TJ. Total contractile protein contents and gene expression in skeletal muscle in response to chronic ethanol consumption in the rat. *Alcohol* 1997; **14**: 545–549.

61 Sandhu GS, Patel VB, Corbett JM, Dunn MJ, Richardson PJ, Preedy VR. Altered myosin heavy chain in hearts of ethanol exposed rats. *Biochem. Soc. Trans.* 1996; **24**: 261S.

62 Sutton CW, Pemberton KS, Cottrell JS, Corbett JM, Wheeler CH, Dunn MJ, Pappin DJ. Identification of myocardial proteins from two-dimensional gels by peptide mass fingerprinting. *Electrophoresis* 1995; **16**: 308–316.

63 Wheeler CH, Berry SL, Wilkins MR, Corbett JM, Ou K, Gooley AA, Humphery Smith I, Williams KL, Dunn MJ. Characterisation of proteins from two-dimensional electrophoresis gels

by matrix-assisted laser desorption mass spectrometry and amino acid compositional analysis. *Electrophoresis* 1996; **17**: 580–587.

64 Dunn MJ, Corbett JM, Wheeler CH. HSC-2DPAGE and the two-dimensional gel electrophoresis database of dog heart proteins. *Electrophoresis* 1997; **18**: 2795–2802.

65 Evans G, Wheeler CH, Corbett JM, Dunn MJ. Construction of HSC-2DPAGE: a two-dimensional gel electrophoresis database of heart proteins. *Electrophoresis* 1997; **18**: 471–479.

66 Sutton CW, Wheeler CH, Sally U, Corbett JM, Cottrell JS, Dunn MJ. The analysis of myocardial proteins by infrared and ultraviolet laser desorption mass spectrometry. *Electrophoresis* 1997; **18**: 424–431.

67 Corbett JM, Why HJ, Wheeler CH, Richardson PJ, Archard LC, Yacoub MH, Dunn MJ. Cardiac protein abnormalities in dilated cardiomyopathy detected by two-dimensional polyacrylamide gel electrophoresis. *Electrophoresis* 1998; **19**: 2031–2042.

68 Heinke MY, Wheeler CH, Yan JX, Amin V, Chang D, Einstein R, Dunn MJ, dos Remedios CG. Changes in myocardial protein expression in pacing-induced canine heart failure. *Electrophoresis* 1999; **20**: 2086–2093.

69 Weekes J, Wheeler CH, Yan JX, Weil J, Eschenhagen T, Scholtysik G, Dunn MJ. Bovine dilated cardiomyopathy: proteomic analysis of an animal model of human dilated cardiomyopathy. *Electrophoresis* 1999; **20**: 898–906.

70 Wilkins MR, Williams KL, Appel RD, Hochstrasser DF. Proteome research: new frontiers in functional genomics. Heidelberg: Springer-Verlag, 1997.

71 Rabilloud T. Proteome research: two-dimensional gel electrophoresis and identification methods. Heidelberg: Springer-Verlag, 2000.

72 Dunn MJ. Studying heart disease using the proteomic approach. *Drug Discovery Today* 2000; **5**: 76.

73 Patel VB. Biochemical investigations into experimental alcoholic cardiomyopathy and hypertension. PhD Thesis, University of London, 1997.

74 Hoerner M, Behrens UJ, Worner T, Lieber CS. Humoral immune response to acetaldehyde adducts in alcoholic patients. *Res. Commun. Chem. Pathol. Pharmacol.* 1986; **54**: 3–12.

75 Lin RC, Smith RS, Lumeng L. Detection of a protein-acetaldehyde adduct in the liver of rats fed alcohol chronically. *J. Clin. Invest.* 1988; **81**: 615–619.

76 Worrall S, de Jersey J, Shanley BC, Wilce PA. Antibodies to acetaldehyde-modified epitopes: Presence in alcoholic, nonalcoholic liver disease and control subjects. *Alcohol Alcohol.* 1990; **25**: 509–517.

77 Niemela O, Juvonen T, Parkkila S. Immunohistochemical demonstration of acetaldehyde-modified epitopes in human liver after alcohol consumption. *J. Clin. Invest.* 1991; **87**: 1367–1374.

78 Worrall S, de Jersey J, Shanley BC, Wilce PA. Detection of stable acetaldehyde-modified proteins in ethanol-fed rats. *Alcohol Alcohol.* 1991; **26**: 437–444.

79 Worrall S, de Jersey J, Shanley BC, Wilce PA. Antibodies to acetaldehyde-modified epitopes: An elevated immunoglobulin A response in alcoholics. *Eur. J. Clin. Invest.* 1991; **21**: 90–95.

80 Clot P, Bellomo G, Tabone M, Arico S, Albano E. Detection of antibodies against proteins modified by hydroxyethyl free radicals in patients with alcoholic cirrhosis. *Gastroenterology* 1995; **108**: 201–207.

81 Sotomayor RE, Washington MC. Formation of etheno and oxoethyl adducts in liver DNA from rats exposed subchronically to urethane in drinking water and ethanol. *Cancer Lett.* 1996; **100**: 155–161.

82 Worrall S, de Jersey J, Wilce PA, Seppa K, Hurme L, Sillanaukee P. Relationship between alcohol intake and immunoglobulin A immunoreactivity with acetaldehyde-modified bovine serum albumin. *Alcoholism: Clini. Exp. Res.* 1996; **20**: 836–840.

83 Antonenkov VD, Pirozhkov SV, Popova SV, Panchenko LF. Effect of chronic ethanol, catalase inhibitor 3-amino-1,2,4-triazole and clofibrate treatment on lipid peroxidation in rat myocardium. *Int. J. Biochem.* 1989; **21**: 1313–1318.

84 Coudray C, Boucher F, Richard MJ, Arnaud J, De Leiris J, Favier A. Zinc deficiency, ethanol, and myocardial ischemia affect lipoperoxidation in rats. *Biol. Trace. Elem. Res.* 1991; **30**: 103–118.

85 Holmes RS, Courtney YR, VandeBerg JL. Alcohol dehydrogenase isozymes in baboons: tissue distribution, catalytic properties, and variant phenotypes in liver, kidney, stomach, and testis. *Alcoholism: Clin. Exp. Res.* 1986; **10**: 623–630.

86 Julia P, Farres J, Pares X. Characterization of three isoenzymes of rat alcohol dehydrogenase. Tissue distribution and physical and enzymatic properties. *Eur. J. Biochem.* 1987; **162**: 179–189.

87 Soffia F, Penna M. Ethanol metabolism by rat heart homogenates. *Alcohol* 1987; **4**: 45–48.

88 Felder MR, Watson G, Huff MO, Ceci JD. Mechanism of induction of mouse kidney alcohol dehydrogenase by androgen. Androgen-induced stimulation of transcription of the Adh-1 gene. *J. Biol. Chem.* 1988; **263**: 14531–14537.

89 Hill GE, Miller JA, Baxter BT, Klassen LW, Duryee MJ, Tuma DJ, Thiele GM. Association of malondialdehyde-acetaldehyde (MAA) adducted proteins with atherosclerotic-induced vascular inflammatory injury. *Atherosclerosis* 1998; **141**: 107–116.

90 Jaatinen P, Saukko P, Hervonen A. Chronic ethanol exposure increases lipopigment accumulation in human heart. *Alcohol Alcohol.* 1993; **28**: 559–569.

91 Pirozhkov SV, Eskelson CD, Watson RR, Hunter GC, Piotrowski JJ, Bernhard V. Effect of chronic consumption of ethanol and vitamin E on fatty acid composition and lipid peroxidation in rat heart tissue. *Alcohol* 1992; **9**: 329–334.

92 Hininger I, Ribiere C, Nordmann R. Disturbances in myocardial creatine kinase following ethanol administration to rats – trials of prevention by allopurinol, desferrioxamine and propranolol. *Alcohol Alcohol.* 1991; **26**: 303–307.

93 Robert V, Ayoub S, Berson G. Effects of hydroxyl radicals on ATPase and protein structure of myofibrils from rat heart. *Am. J. Physiol.* 1991; **261**: H1785–H1790.

94 Rupp H, Dhalla KS, Dhalla NS. Mechanisms of cardiac cell damage due to catecholamines: significance of drugs regulating central sympathetic outflow. *J. Cardiovasc. Pharmacol.* 1994; **24** (Suppl. 1): S16–S24.

95 Patel VB, Sherwood R, Why H, Poyser K, Richardson PJ, Preedy VR. The acute and chronic effects of alcohol toxicity upon rat plasma troponin-T levels. *Alcohol Alcohol.* 1995; **30**: 525.

96 Hininger I, Ribiere C, Nordmann R. Disturbances in myocardial creatine kinase following ethanol administration to rats – trials of prevention by allopurinol, desferrioxamine and propranolol. *Alcohol Alcohol.* 1991; **26**: 303–307.

Chapter 18

Cocaethylene: immunologic, hepatic and cardiac effects

Albert D. Arvallo and Ronald R. Watson

Alcohol, the most consumed drug in the world, is often not recognized as a drug or addictive by the public and the media, because of its legal use and acceptance. The public, on the other hand, recognizes cocaine as an addictive drug with traumatic effects on its users. Some users of cocaine begin to mix cocaine with alcohol as together they extend the euphoric sensation. Cocaine plus concomitant ethanol use results in cocaethylene, a compound synthesized *in vivo* and only identified in 1979 [2]. It also has been named in the literature as ethylcocaine, ethylbenzoylecgonine, and benzoylecgonine ethyl ester [2]. Therefore, we will review effects of combined alcohol plus cocaine use as well as cocaethylene in use by 4.5% of 18–25 year olds in the USA in 1988 model studies. In 1990, an NIAAA Survey reported that 5.3 million Americans had used cocaine concurrently (during the same period of time) with alcohol, and 4.6 million simultaneously (on the same occasion) with alcohol [10]. It is interesting to note that 90% of cocaine users take ethanol concomitantly. Ethanol enhances and prolongs the euphoric effects of cocaine and lessens the dysphoria associated with cessation of cocaine use [9]. This, therefore, is the rational for using ethanol simultaneously with cocaine. Despite its prevalence, very little research has been aimed at identifying the possible underlying biological consequences resulting from the addictive drugs [5]. How do they affect key organ systems like the heart and liver?

Ethanol and cocaine have opposite pharmacologic effects. Ethanol is a central nervous system depressant. Low amounts of alcoholic beverages increase sociability, while higher levels impair cognitive ability and depress sensorimotor function. The acute *in vivo* cardiovascular response to moderate levels of ethanol intake involves sympathetic activation, probably due to peripheral vasodilatation, and usually results in an increase in heart rate and maintained or elevated cardiac output [3]. Cardiac arrhythmia seems to be more prevalent. Delbridge *et al.*'s recent findings report identifying ethanol at 0.05%(v/v) as a modulator of cardiac contractility. Kinetic analyses indicate that the mechanism of action involves disturbance of sarcoplasmic reticulum function and this may contribute to arrhythmogenic vulnerability – especially in an *in vivo* context of heightened compensatory sympathetic drive [3]. The study goes on to state that the stabilizing effects of ethanol on intracellular Ca^{2+} stores may be the cellular basis for the arrhythmogenic response to acute ethanol exposure – a response which is more evident in the normal than in the myopathic myocardium [3].

Cocaine is a sympathomimetic agent with stimulant and local anesthetic properties [15]. The pathophysiology of cocaine-related myocardial ischemia and infarction is probably multifactorial and is due to one or a combination of (1) increased myocardial oxygen demand in the setting of limited or fixed supply; (2) marked coronary arterial vasoconstriction; and

(3) enhanced platelet aggregation and thrombus formation [11]. In eight healthy cocaine addicts receiving intravenous cocaine (0.325 mg/kg or 0.650 mg/kg), it was noted that pulse and mean arterial pressure peaked 5 min post-cocaine injection and maximal response was sustained for a further 15 min and 35 min afterwards, respectively. Cocaine administration had no significant effect on peripheral oxygen saturation, and no clinically significant abnormalities of rhythm or conduction were seen on the electrocardiogram. These doses and method of single-dose intravenous cocaine administration, and our procedures for cardiovascular monitoring, appear relatively safe for laboratory studies of healthy cocaine addicts with no pre-existing cardiovascular disease. Cocaine-taking resulted in a small but statistically insignificant improvement in learning on the Digit Symbol Substitution Task [7].

The effects of individual and concurrent use of alcohol and cocaine have been studied extensively, yet much less is known about cocaethylene production and value in the effects of dual drug use. Although, the mechanism by which the combination of cocaine and ethanol may be particularly deleterious to the cardiovascular system is unknown, Pitt et al. propose two hypotheses: (1) It may markedly increase the determinants of myocardial oxygen demand and simultaneously diminish supply, leading to a marked supply:demand imbalance. In human volunteers, the use of both drugs produces a greater increase in heart rate than either substance alone; (2) The concomitant ingestion of cocaine and ethanol and may lead to the production of a metabolite which induces marked coronary arterial vasoconstriction, leading to myocardial ischemia, infarction, and/or sudden death [11]. Animal studies indicate that the combination of ethanol with cocaine increases the lethality of cocaine [15]. Morishima et al.'s findings correspond with studies reported by other investigators in conscious and anesthetized rats and monkeys in which cocaethylene produced effects similar to those of cocaine at approximately equivalent doses [8]. Whether cocaethylene induces coronary arterial vasoconstriction in humans is unknown [11]. Incoming patients received into a hospital emergency department in a lower-income area were drug screened with no standard criteria for benzoylecgonine ester (BE). If positive for BE or cocaethylene, the patient was considered positive for cocaine use. Patients positive for drugs in addition to BE and ethanol, except for acetaminophen or salicylate, were excluded. The

Table 18.1 Symptoms reported by cocaine and alcohol concomitantly using patients

Cocaine and Ethanol	Cocaine Only
• Higher incidence of confusion • Lower Glasgow Coma Scale (GCS) • Lower BUN and Ph • Non trauma patient heart rate higher • More often intubated and admitted to Intensive Care Units • Higher mean number of care days • Myocardial Infarction confirmed on 2 non-trauma patients • Cardiac arrhythmia in 15 patients hospitalized	• Higher incidence of chest pain • Lower incidence of back and extremity pain • Higher body temperature and a higher incidence of hallucinations • Myocardial Infarction conformed on 2 non-trauma patients • Cardiac arrhythmia in 15 patients • Non trauma patients heart rate lower • Respiratory failure • Muscle spasms, convulsions, and coma • Gastrointestinal complication • Greater mean total Creatine Kinase

modified from [10]

incidence of trauma was increased twofold in the cocaine and alcohol using group compared with the cocaine group (50% vs. 22%, $p > 0.001$). The cocaine/alcohol group had a higher incidence of violent trauma than the cocaine patients did (37% vs. 17%, $p > 0.001$) [15]. There were no differences with regard to frequency of laboratory tests, or the results of determinations of WBC count, hemoglobin, serum potassium, or blood glucose.

The combination of cocaine plus alcohol use increases the heart rate 1.5–5 times more than with either substance alone and produces a slight increase in blood pressure [15]. In this same study, 91% of patients that tested positive for BE and ethanol were positive for cocaine in the serum or cocaethylene in the urine or serum. This indicates simultaneous use of cocaine and ethanol (unpublished data). Concurrent abuse of cocaine and ethanol is very high. A 1995 study estimated that 60–80% of cocaine users consume ethanol simultaneously [4], and concluded:

1   Combined alcohol and cocaine use is the rule;
2   The Drug Abuse Warning Network has identified cocaine plus alcohol combination as the most prominent substance abuse pattern among individuals presenting themselves to emergency rooms with abuse problems;
3   With alcohol plus cocaine use, users can ameliorate the unpleasant physical and psychological sequel of cocaine ingestion primarily paranoia and agitation;
4   Combined abuse of cocaine and alcohol results in alteration of the metabolic profile of cocaine and the formation of the pharmacologically active metabolite, cocaethylene [4].

In a more in depth report, nearly half of patients who tested positive for cocaethylene cited trauma as the primary reason for reporting to the emergency [12]. Also 60% of the postmortem human tissue examined had cocaethylene. This led to the speculation that cocaethylene was, at least in part, responsible for the dramatic increase in the risk for sudden death in persons combining cocaine and ethanol [12]. Although, the mechanisms mediating the increased incidence of sudden death of the combined abuse of cocaine and alcohol are not identified, the formation of cocaethylene and the inhibition of cocaine metabolism are implicated [4].

Studying the immune system and hepatotoxic effects of cocaine and cocaethylene during HIV infection among intravenous cocaine users shows that simultaneous administration of ethanol and cocaine potentiated the immunosuppressive effects of cocaine in mice [10]. Yet, this depended on the dose and the duration of administration. For example heroin addicts were given cocaine in small amounts which increased the depressed percentage of E-rosette forming T cells more than heroin alone. The study indicates that a 0.6 mg/kg dose of cocaine produced a three-to-four-fold increase in natural killer cell activity in peripheral blood, and an increase in circulating natural killer cells. A similar effect on NK cell activity was also demonstrated in mice chronically treated with cocaine. Studies on isolated human T-Lymphocytes showed that cocaine *in vitro* acts as an up-regulator of CD2 antigen expression, suppressing the phytohemagglutinin (PHA)-induced proliferation of T cells [10]. Cocaine also causes thrombocytopenia and the immune abnormalities observed included antiplatelet antibodies of the IgG and IgM type, disturbances in serum compliment levels and extensive circulating immune complexes [10]. With cocaethylene in mice there are also variable immunological effects. Just as there were opposite results depending on the doses and duration of ethanol and cocaine, the results shown with coca-ethylene alone produced a significant inhibition of gamma-interferon, tumor necrosis factor, and also interleukin-2 formation by isolated splenocytes with a dose of 20 mg/kg injected twice daily. Administration of ethanol with cocaethylene simultaneously resulted in a stronger decreased immunological effect [10]. Research was done on conscious dogs to check for the effects of ethanol and cocaethylene pharmacokinetics. Preliminary studies indicate that the dog does not form detectable quantities of cocaethylene after co-admin-istration of cocaine and intravenous ethanol [9], while it was formed when cocaine and ethanol were consumed simultaneously in humans, monkeys, and mice. Formation of cocaethylene resulted from transesterification of cocaine by hepatic carboxylesterases in the liver. Lab studies of human liver extracts indicate that inhibition of hepatic carboxyl-esterase mediated metabolism of cocaine to benzoylecgonine in the presence of ethanol [9]. It was thought that ethanol may have contributed to the decrease in cocaine metabol-ism; it is possible that cocaethylene inhibited cocaine's metabolism. Early lab studies showed no significant plasma concentrations of cocaethylene detected in the dogs when cocaine is given with intravenous ethanol. Interestingly enough, researchers were not able to detect cocaethylene in measurable quantities (725 ng/ml) in the plasma of Sprague-Dawley rats after a single dose administration of cocaine and alcohol in doses similar to the doses used in the current study (unpublished observation) [4]. Not to find cocaethylene in the blood plasma in the dog was unexpected, as smaller doses of co-administered cocaine and cocaethylene given to human subjects have been shown to result in measur-able cocaethylene plasma concentrations [14]. Further studies must be done in species that resemble humans to determine the pathways and significance of the cocaine and cocaethylene combination. Studies on microsomial fractions on rats, Beagle dogs, and humans suggest that large interspecies differences in hepatic carboxylesterase activity may exist [14].

The *in vivo* studies of dogs and humans show that cocaethylene formation is greater in humans, which is in contrast to our *in vitro* incubation studies in hepatic microsomes that clearly demonstrate much greater cocaethylene in the dog than human microsomial pre-parations. Hepatic drug metabolism, *in vitro*, has successfully predicted *in vivo* metabolism of drugs. However, cocaine is subject to extra hepatic hydrolysis in the plasma and possibly other sites are not present in hepatic microsomal preparations. Therefore, interspecies differences in extra hepatic cocaine metabolism could affect the correlation between *in vitro* and *in vivo* metabolism [14].

The toxicity from combined cocaine plus ethanol use is not due to enhanced sensitivity to alcohol in cocaine abusers. The blunt response to alcohol in limbic regions and in cortical regions connected to limbic areas could result from a decreased sensitivity of reward circuits in cocaine abusers [16]. In rats, cocaethylene exposure during the brain growth spurt period causes teratogenic effects slowing brain growth. Cocaethylene is a neuro-teratogen as indicated by altered concentrations of catecholamines and indoleamines in developing brains. There was a region-specific alteration in neurotransmitter levels in response to six days of cocaethylene exposure. It also seems that cocaethylene is more similar to ethanol than cocaine in terms of neuroteratogeneis [2]. Sobel and others studied the interaction of cocaethylene and cocaine and of cocaethylene and alcohol on schedule-controlled responding in rats [13]. Their statement concerning blood levels was indicative that they do not know the contribution of cocaethylene to the effects of cocaine and alcohol consumed concurrently. It is their contention that blood levels of cocaine, ethanol and cocaethylene must be directly and concurrently determined when cocaine and alcohol are co-administered to begin to unravel the interaction of cocaine and alcohol. It was thought that the doses of cocaethylene and cocaine and/or of coca-ethylene and alcohol may have contributed to the greater effects produced by concurrent use of cocaine and alcohol. Other research mentioned measured cocaine and cocaethylene concentration in postmortem human cerebral cortex and showed that combined use of cocaine and ethanol increased the risk of death 18-fold [14].

In the first primate study, the effects of intravenously administered cocaine on extra-cellular dopamine in the primate were compared to the effects to those of cocaethylene [6]. Here, numerous biochemical and pharmacological differences between primates, rodents and dogs that make it important to study primates if immediate extensions to clinical research studies are to be made. The results suggest that the reported differences in potency between cocaine and cocaethylene at producing euphoria in clinical research studies may be due to decreased potency of cocaethylene at blocking 5-HT and/or nor-epinephrine uptake [6]. Both cocaethylene and cocaine are equipotent and were found to increase extracellular dopamine in the caudate nucleus. Cocaethylene retains similar activity to cocaine, including inhibition of the dopamine transporter [14]. When a pleas-urable event is occurring, it is accompanied by large increase in the amounts of dopamine released in the nucleus accumbens by neurons. In the normal communication process, dopamine is released by a neuron into a synapse (the small gap between two neurons) where it binds with specialized proteins (called dopamine receptors) on the neighboring neuron, thereby sending a signal to that neuron. Drugs of abuse interfere with this normal communication process. Cocaine, for example, blocks the removal of dopamine from the synapse, resulting in an accumulation of dopamine. This buildup of dopamine cause con-tinuous stimulation of receiving neurons probably resulting in the euphoria commonly reported by cocaine abusers [1]. In most case studies, the potentiality of cocaine and cocaethylene seem to point to equal potency *in vitro* experiments, by analyzing organs, or *in vivo* by measuring blood plasma and the drug concentrations. As yet, there are discrep-ancies as to when the potency of cocaine plus ethanol was stronger than cocaethylene effects compared to cocaine or ethanol alone as various researches indicates. But it seems that when cocaine is abused with alcohol, cocaine effects and toxicity can be increased further because of the formation of cocaethylene. In the organs of 60% of the addicts seeking medical attention in emergency rooms or human postmortem specimens, the compound cocaethylene has been found. We still need to investigate the factors that affect the inhibition of cocaine metabolism by ethanol or that affect the fraction of cocaine dose metabolized to cocaethylene. We also need to know how to determine how changes in the cocaine metabolic profile and the formation of cocaethylene are reflected in the pharmacological effects [4].

ACKNOWLEDGMENTS

Research supported by grant R25RR10163 (for Albert D. Arvallo) and an NIDA supple-ment to HL63667. Thanks to Andrew Morrison for his editing and Manny Villa, Christo-pher Soto and Donna Sider for their assistance. A special thanks to Mrs. Angelina Arvallo and Dr. R.R. Watson for all the moral support.

REFERENCES

1 Cocaine Abuse and Addiction. 1999. National Institute on Drug Abuse. p. 1 of 4.

2 Chen W-JA, West JR. Cocaethylene exposure during the brain growth spurt period: Brain growth restrictions and neurochemisty studies. *Develop. Brain Res.* 1997; **100**: 220–229.

3 Delbridge LM, Connell PJ, Harris PJ, Morgan TO. Ethanol effects on cardiomyocyte contractility. *Clinical Sci.* 2000; **98**: 401–407.

4 Hedaya MA, Pan W-J. Cocaine and alcohol interactions in naive and alcohol-pretreated rats. *Drug Metabol. Disposi.* 1996; **24**: 807–812.

5 Horowitz JM, Bhatti E, Devi BG, Torres G. Behavior and drug measurements in long-evans and Sprague-Dawley rats after ethanol-cocaine exposure. *Pharmacol. Biochem. and Behav.* 1998; **62**: 329–337.

6 Iyer RN, Nobiletti JB, Jatlow PI, Bradberry CW. Cocaine and coaethylene: effects on extracellular dopamine in the primate. *Psychopharmacol.* 1995; **120**: 150–155.

7 Johnson B, Overton D, Wells L, Kenny P, Abramson D, Dhother S, Chen Y, Bordnick P. Effects of acute intravenous cocaine on cardiovascular function, human learning, and performance in cocaine addicts. *Psychiatry Res.* 1998; **77**: 35–42.

8 Morishima HMD, Whittington RMD, Iso AMD, Cooper TBMA. The comparative toxicity of cocaine and its metabolites in conscious rats. *Anesthesiol.* 1999; **90**: 1684–1690.

9 Parker RB, Williams CL, Laizure SC, Mandrell TD, Labranche GS. Effects of ethanol and cocaethylene on cocaine pharmacokinetics in conscious dogs. *Drug Metabol. Disposit.* 1996; **24**: 850–853.

10 Pirozhkov SV, Watson RRP. Immunomodulalting and hepatotoxic effects of cocaine and coaerthylene: enhancement by simultaneous ethanol administration. *Alcologia* 1993; **5**: 113–116.

11 Pitts WR, Lange RA, Cigarroa JE, David HL. Cocaine-induced myocardial ischemia and infarction: pathophysiol, recognition, and management. *Progress in Cardiovascular Diseases* 1997; **40**: 65–75.

12 Signs SAP, Dickey-White HIM, Schechter MDP, Kulics ATP. The formation of cocaethylene and clinical presentation of ED patients testing positive for the use of cocaine and ethanol. *Amer. Emergen. Med.* 1996; **14**: 665–670.

13 Sobel BF, Hutchinnson AC, Diamond HF, Etkind SA, Ziervogel SD, Ferrari CM, Riley AL. Assessment of cocaethylene lethality in long-evans female and male rats. *Neurotoxicol. Teratol.* 1997; **20**: 459–463.

14 Song N, Parker RB, Laizure CS. Cocaethylene formation in rat, dog, and human hepatic microsomes. *Life Sci.* 1999; **64**: 2101–2108.

15 Vanek VWM, Howard I Dickey-White M, Signs SAP, Buss TP, Kulics ATP. Concurrent use of cocaine and alcohol by patients treated in the emergency department. *Ann. Emergen. Med.* 1996; **28**: 508–514.

16 Volkow ND, Wang G-J, Fowler JS, Franceschi D, Thanos PK, Wong C, Gatley SJ, Ding YS, Molina P, Schlyer D, Alexoff D, Hitzemann R, Pappas N. Cocaine abusers show a blunted response to alcohol intoxication in limbic brain regions. *Life Sci.* 1999; **66**: 161–167.

Chapter 19

Cardiotoxicity of cocaine use by humans and rodents: synergisms of concomitant cocaine plus alcohol exposure

David Solkoff and Ronald R. Watson

COCAINE CARDIOTOXICITY

As cocaine abuse has become widespread, the number of cocaine related cardiovascular events, such as angina pectoris, myocardial ischemia and infarction, cardiac myopathy, left ventricular hypertrophy, and sudden death has increased substantially [1–15]. These occur in young subjects, a significant percentage of whom had no evidence of atherosclerotic coronary artery disease on subsequent angiography [10,11,18–21]. Twice as many men as women experience cocaine related cardiac ischemic events, at least partly caused by a greater frequency of cocaine use in men. The concomitant use of cigarettes and/or ethanol is pervasive, with up to 75% of cocaine users admitting to each. Although myocardial ischemia, infarction, and sudden death are most likely to occur in chronic cocaine users, they have been reported in first time users as well. These events can occur from any route of administration and with a large or small amount of the drug [3,4,8,9,20–29]. It is thought that the pathophysiology of cocaine-related myocardial ischemia and infarction is most likely multidimensional, and that it is caused by individual and/or combined conditions including increased myocardial oxygen demand in the setting of limited or fixed supply, marked coronary artery vasoconstriction, and enhanced platelet aggregation and thrombus formation [1].

These hypotheses are supported by a variety of previous studies. In humans, the intracoronary infusion of cocaine in amounts sufficient to achieve a high drug concentration in coronary sinus blood causes a deterioration of left ventricular systolic and diastolic performance [30]. Even a small amount (2 mg/kg)of cocaine causes 'inappropriate' coronary arterial vasoconstriction, meaning that myocardial oxygen supply fell in the setting of increased demand [31]. Cocaine-induced thrombosis is an important mechanism in the development of myocardial infarction in the presence of normal or diseased coronary arteries [32]. Autopsies following cocaine-related deaths have complete thrombotic occlusions of normal and atherosclerotic coronary arteries [8,12,25,33]. Coronary artery thrombosis and subsequent ischemia in these cases may be attributed to alterations in platelet and endothelial cell functions [34]. Endothelial damage may occur at the site of vascular spasm resulting in thrombus formation, and cocaine may cause coronary artery thrombosis by initiating coronary artery spasm [18,35,36]. *In vitro* studies have demonstrated that cocaine activates platelets, increases platelet aggregation, and potentiates platelet thromboxane production [37–39]. The idea that cocaine exerts pro-coagulant effects is further supported by findings of combined protein C and antithrombin III depletion in patients with cocaine-related arterial thromboses [40]. Levels of both anticoagulants returned to normal following discontinuation of cocaine use. Similarly, cocaine users have increased risk of developing upper extremity deep vein thrombosis (Paget-Schroetter syndrome) [41].

Cocaine causes central and peripheral adrenergic stimulation by blocking the presynaptic reuptake of norepinephrine and dopamine, thus increasing their postsynaptic concentrations [42]. The coronary arteries have both α and β-adrenergic receptors. Stimulation of α-adrenergic receptors causes vascular smooth muscle contraction, while β-adrenergic stimulation induces the opposite. The cardiovascular effects of cocaine are partially mediated by α-adrenergic stimulation, since they were reversed by phentolamine, an α-adrenergic antagonist [31].

Some researchers have advocated the use of β-adrenergic blocking agents in patients with acute cocaine ingestion [43,44]. Indeed, previous studies have shown that β-adrenergic receptor antagonists such as propranolol have been effective at lessening the pressor, positive inotropic, and heart rate responses to cocaine intoxication [43,45–50]. However, since β-adrenergic stimulation causes coronary vasodilation, β-adrenergic blockade may allow for unopposed α-adrenergically mediated coronary arterial vasoconstriction. This hypothesis has been vindicated in a previous study demonstrating that cocaine increases myocardial oxygen demand while simultaneously reducing supply, as reflected by a decrease in coronary sinus blood flow and coronary arterial diameter. The study went on to describe how the cocaine-induced fall in myocardial oxygen supply is actually *exacerbated* by propranolol. Therefore, β-adrenergic blockade may actually increase the magnitude of cocaine-related myocardial ischemia, and thus should not be used in patients with cocaine intoxication. We hypothesize, vis a vis the treatment of cocaine intoxication in humans, it is more important to reverse the vasoconstriction than it is to decrease heart rate, i.e., slow the heart down.

A significant amount of patients suffering from cocaine-associated angina pectoris or myocardial infarction report the onset of symptoms several hours after drug administration, when the blood concentration of cocaine is low or undetectable [3,51]. This delay in experiencing symptoms may be caused not by the cocaine itself, but by the drug's major metabolites, benzoylecgonine and ethyl methyl ecgonine [52].

Further study of the cardiotoxic effects of cocaine in humans, indicate that patients with atherosclerotic coronary artery disease are probably at increased risk of having an ischemic event in response to cocaine when compared against patients not suffering such malady. This may occur because diseased coronary arterial segments usually exhibit pronounced endothelial dysfunction such as greatly impaired or absent production of endothelium-derived relaxing factors [53,54].

CONCOMMITANT COCAINE AND ETHANOL CONSUMPTION

A survey conducted in 1991, found that 9 million people in the US abuse cocaine and ethanol simultaneously [55]. The combined use of cocaine and ethanol appears to be associated with increased morbidity and mortality over either drug alone. Their simultaneous use increased the risk of drug-induced sudden death 18-fold [56]. Deaths due to drug overdose involving the use of ethanol were associated with cocaine blood concentrations that were lower than those measured in subjects dying of cocaine overdose alone (900 vs. 2,800 mg/L, respectively) [57]. This is suggestive of an additive or synergistic effect of ethanol on cocaine-induced catastrophic events [57]. Several hypotheses have been proposed to account for this synergistic effect. Since the combined use of both drugs in human volunteers produces a greater increase in heart rate than either substance alone, the combination may do more than either of its individual constituents to substantially increase the determinants of myocardial oxygen demand while at the same time reducing supply, thus leading to a marked supply:demand imbalance [58,59]. While alcohol has been reported to induce coronary vasodilation, it has the proven ability to cause intense vasoconstriction as well, thus compounding the deleterious vasoconstriction caused by cocaine [60–65]. Another possible explanation for the synergistic cardiotoxic effects of the ethanol + cocaine combination may be found in the study of cocaethylene, a unique metabolite that is formed by hepatic transesterification after the concomitant ingestion of cocaine and ethanol. Cocaethylene is thought by some investigators to induce marked coronary arterial vasoconstriction leading to myocardial ischemia, as well as infarction and/or sudden death. Like cocaine, it blocks dopamine reuptake at the synaptic cleft. This compound is often detected in subjects who were determined to have died of cocaine-ethanol toxicity. Furthermore, in experimental animals, cocaethylene is more lethal than cocaine [66–68].

Regarding the management of cocaine-induced myocardial ischemia and infarction, recent evidence indicates that in addition to avoiding the use of β-blockers in patients with cocaine-related chest pain (since β-adrenergic blockade may potentiate cocaine-induced vasoconstriction by allowing unopposed α-adrenergic stimulation), the α-adrenergic blocker phentolamine should not be used either, since it usually causes a substantial fall in systemic arterial pressure [1,31,69].

The present drugs of choice for the management of cocaine-associated chest pain are nitroglycerin and verapamil, since they reverse the cocaine-induced increase in systemic arterial pressure and coronary arterial vasoconstriction. Nitroglycerin causes direct vasodilation of diseased and nondiseased coronary arterial segments [70]. It has been shown to eliminate the coronary vasoconstrictor response to α-adrenergic stimulation caused by smoking and exercise [12,34,71]. Nitroglycerin, administered in a dose sufficient to reduce mean systemic arterial pressure 10–15%, effectively alleviates cocaine induced coronary arterial vasoconstriction [72]. Since cocaine may cause vasoconstriction by altering calcium transport in vascular smooth muscle, in addition to α-adrenergic stimulation, the calcium channel blocker verapamil is also recommended for the treatment of cocaine-associated chest pain [73,74]. Verapamil is thought to work because it may directly block the cocaine-induced increase in calcium concentration within vascular smooth muscle cells, thereby preventing vasoconstriction. It may also block cocaine's adrenergically mediated vasoconstrictor effects, since the cocaine-induced release of catecholamines from the presynaptic terminal is calcium dependent. Studies in experimental animals have shown that calcium antagonists attenuate the cocaine-induced elevation of circulating catecholamines [75,76]. Calcium antagonists have also been shown to bind vascular α-adrenergic receptors [77,78], thus potentially preventing the cocaine-induced effects of catecholamines by blocking postsynaptic adrenergic receptors.

It has proved a difficult task to determine the long-term cardiovascular consequences of cocaine use. One such study that attempted to ascertain this information was The Coronary Artery Risk Development in Young Adults(CARDIA)study [[79]. The purpose of this study was to identify the distribution of coronary heart disease risk factors (including illicit drug use) among a randomly sampled, biethnic cohort of men and women (3,848 persons,

20–32 years of age) of varied socioeconomic status in 1987, and then to evaluate the relationship between lifetime cocaine use in 1987 and cardiovascular disease risk factors 5 years later. The longitudinal design, the cardiovascular focus of CARDIA, and the inclusion of essentially healthy individuals at baseline, provided a unique opportunity to assess the cardiotoxicity of chronic cocaine use. Results of the CARDIA study indicate that lifetime cocaine use experience in 1987, after adjustment for age, ethnicity, daily alcohol intake, cigarettes smoked per day, body mass index, sum of skinfolds, physical activity, and other illicit drug use, was not related to blood pressure, blood pressure difference, heart rate, or hypertension prevalence in cross-sectional analysis in either men or women. Regarding the long-term, multivariate relationships between lifetime cocaine use experience in 1987 and blood pressure, blood pressure difference, and heart rate in 1992, the data from CARDIA indicates that no relationship is evident between lifetime cocaine use experience and blood pressure in men or women. Results of the CARDIA study thus suggest that lifetime cocaine use among Black and White men and women aged 20–32 years is not associated with higher blood pressure, higher heart rate, or increased prevalence hypertension cross-sectionally in 1987 or 5 years later. Therefore, cocaine-induced cardiovascular events or cardiac myopathy in this age group may not be strongly related to changes in cardiovascular disease risk factors, but may instead be related to cardiotoxicity only via its acute effects [14,15,80]. It should be noted however that the cocaine use data found in the CARDIA study was based on self-reported substance use, whose validity and reliability is open to question. Also, it may be that the 5-year evaluation period was insufficient to detect important cocaine-related changes in the studied cardiovascular disease risk factors.

CARDIOVASCULAR EFFECTS OF COCAINE USING RAT AND MOUSE MODELS

The rat model continues to be one of the primary models of choice for the study of the cardiovascular effects of cocaine. Recently, the rat model has been utilized to study the acute and chronic effects of cocaine self-administration behavior on cardiovascular function [81]. When rats were self-administered injections of cocaine 0.5 mg/kg there was a significant increase in blood pressure. Tolerance developed to this effect within 3 daily sessions. During saline-substitution sessions, a significant ($p < 0.05$) decrease in blood pressure and heart rate was observed. When the injected doses of cocaine were increased (1.0, 2.0, and 4.0 mg/kg per injection)a dramatic increase in blood pressure or heart rate was not produced despite a substantial cumulative cocaine intake(20–27 mg/kg). It has thus been hypothesized that operant-conditioned behavior and/or the direct reinforcing effects of cocaine modulate the cardiovascular effects of cocaine. The results of the just described study are in agreement with previous reports of acute tolerance to cardiovascular actions of cocaine in humans and rats [82,83].

The rat model is also being used to increase understanding of the pharmacodynamic action of cocaine. The cardiovascular and behavioral effects of cocaine may be intricately connected with respect to their mechanisms of origination [84]. Recent behavioral and cardiovascular data indicate that cocaine elicits two distinct and temporally separable effects in conscious rats [84]. The first involves a sodium-channel-independent, monoamine effect of a rapid onset. This consists of a brief and intense behavioral arousal associated with rapid and large increases in blood pressure and heart rate, i.e., abrupt hemodynamic stimulation. The second effect appears to be a dopamine-mediated response of a slower onset, whereby cocaine exerts an inhibitory effect on dopamine reuptake in the brain. This is manifested by prolonged and parallel increases in blood pressure, heart rate, and locomotion.

The rat model has also been used to study cocaine's alterations in myocardial cell structure. Several studies have indicated that cocaine is directly toxic to myocardial cells. Cocaine altered cellular structure, producing intracellular vacuolization and pseudopodia in cultured cardiomyocytes [85]. These morphological alterations occurred as early as 1 h after exposure to cocaine, and were followed by a clear indicator of cytotoxicity, that being substantial leakage of lactate dehydrogenase after 24 h of treatment [85]. In rats chronically treated with cocaine, alterations of cardiac mitochondria were observed, such as mitochondrial swelling, and disruption of intramitochondrial cristae [86]. Furthermore, a recent study conducted in order to evaluate the effect of cocaine on mitochondrial function in cultured rat myocardial cells showed that cocaine may exert cardiotoxic effects by compromising cardiac mitochondrial function since not only was cellular ATP found to be decreased by cocaine, but cocaine was also shown to dissipate the membrane potential (the driving force behind oxidative phosphorylation) in a dose and time dependent manner [87].

The alteration of cardiac gene expression in cocaine-induced cardiomyopathy has recently been investigated using a rat model [88]. Specifically, the effects of acute as well as prolonged administration of cocaine were studied with respect to the transcription of atrial natriuretic factor (ANF) mRNAs as a marker of acute mechanical overload [89–91]. Acute and prolonged dosing with cocaine was also investigated with respect to the encoding of myosin heavy chain mRNAs as markers of prolonged mechanical overload [90,92–94]. Additionally, the study also sought to determine the effect of acute and prolonged administration of cocaine in terms of the transcription of type I and III procollagens as markers of active fibrosis [91,95]. The study found that acute injection of cocaine induced ANF gene expression. Cocaine treatment during 28 days resulted in left ventricular hypertrophy (+20% after 24 days) with normal blood pressure, associated with an accumulation of mRNAs encoding ANF and type I and III collagens (+66% and +55%). This chronic treatment also induced a shift in myosin heavy chain gene expression(−40% and +50%). Results further showed that plasma levels of triiodothyronine and thyroxine were lowered. Thus cocaine activates markers of both hemodynamic overload and fibrosis. Such an activation may result from direct and/or indirect effects of the drug such as myocardial ischemia, mechanical overload, and/or hypothyroidism.

In contrast to the rat model, use of the mouse to study cardiotoxic effects of cocaine is practically nonexistent. A review of the biomedical sciences literature indicates that only one study has even remotely attempted to specifically ascertain cocaine-induced cardiovascular changes in non-fetal, non-embryonic mice.

That study sought to determine the effect of cocaine on heart rate in four different inbred mouse strains [96]. At the highest dose studied(15 mg/kg), cocaine actually induced a small decrease only in the heart rate of the C3H mice. This is in agreement with other studies that at high doses, cocaine's anesthetic effects on the heart predominate, resulting in a reduction in heart function (see mechanisms review, if needed). This study noted that the strain of mice (among the 4 tested)found to be most resistant to cocaine-induced changes in heart rate was C57BL/6I.

ACKNOWLEDGMENT

Supported by NIDA supplement to grant HL63667.

REFERENCES

1 Pitts WR, Lange RA, Cigarroa JE, Hillis LD. Cocaine-induced myocardial ischemia and infarction: Pathophysiology, recognition, and management. *Prog. Cardiovasc. Dis.* 1997; **40**(1): 65–76.

2 Kloner RA, Hale S, Alker K, Rezkalla S. The effects of acute and chronic cocaine use on the heart. *Circulation.* 1992; **85**: 407–419.

3 Isner JM, Estes NA, Thompson PD *et al.* Acute cardiac events temporally related to cocaine abuse. *N. Engl. J. Med.* 1986; **315**: 1438–1443.

4 Cregler LL, Mark H. Medical complications of cocaine abuse. *N. Engl. J. Med.* 1986; **315**: 1495–1500.

5 Goldfrank LR, Hoffman RS. The cardiovascular effects of cocaine. *Ann. Emerg. Med.* 1991; **20**: 165–175.

6 Lange RA, Willard JE. The cardiovascular effects of cocaine. *Heart Dis. Stroke* 1993; **2**: 136–141.

7 Coleman DL, Ross TF, Naughton JL. Myocardial ischemia and infarction related to recreational cocaine use. *West. J. Med.* 1982; **136**: 444–446.

8 Kossowsky WA, Lyon AF. Cocaine and acute myocardial infarction: A probable connection. *Chest* 1984; **86**: 729–731.

9 Schachne JS, Roberts BH, Thompson PD. Coronary artery spasm and myocardial infarction associated with cocaine use. *N. Engl. J. Med.* 1984; **310**: 1665–1666.

10 Howard RE, Hueter DC, Davis GJ. Acute myocardial infarction following cocaine abuse in a young woman with normal coronary arteries. *JAMA* 1985; **254**: 95–96.

11 Pasternack PF, Colvin SB, Baumann FG. Cocaine-induced angina pectoris and acute myocardial infarction in patients younger than 40 years. *Am. J. Cardiol.* 1985; **55**: 847.

12 Simpson RW, Edwards WD. Pathogenesis of cocaine-induced ischemic heart disease. *Arch. Path. Lab. Med.* 1986; **110**: 479–484.

13 Cigarroa CG, Boehere JD, Brickner ME, Eichorn EJ, Grayburn PA. Exaggerated pressor response to treadmill exercise in chronic cocaine abusers with left ventricular hypertrophy. *Circulation* 1992; **86**: 226–231.

14 Ruttenber AJ, Sweeney PA, Mendlein JM, Wetli CV. Preliminary findings of an epidemiologic study of cocaine-related deaths, Dade County, Florida, 1978–85. In: Schober S, Schade C (Eds.). The Epidemiology of Cocaine Use and Abuse. Rockville, Md: National Institute on Drug Abuse. *Research Monograph* 1991; **110**: 95–112.

15 Hoegerman GS, Lewis CE, Flack JM *et al.* Lack of association of recreational cocaine and alcohol use with left ventricular mass in young adults. *J. Am. Coll. Cardiol.* 1995; **25**: 895–900.

16 Isner JM, Chokshi SK. Cocaine-induced myocardial infarction: Clinical observations and pathogenetic considerations. *NIDA Res. Monogr.* 1991; **108**: 121–130.

17 Zimmerman FH, Gustafson GM, Kemp HG Jr. Recurrent myocardial infarction associated with cocaine abuse in a young man with normal coronary arteries: Evidence for coronary artery spasm culminating in thrombosis. *J. Am. Coll. Cardiol.* 1987; **9**: 964–968.

18 Hadjimilitiades S, Covalesky V, Manno BV *et al.* Coronary arteriographic findings in cocaine abuse-induced myocardial infarction. *Cathet. Cardiovasc. Diagn.* 1988; **14**: 33–36.

19 Minor RL, Scott BD, Brown DD *et al.* Cocaine-induced myocardial infarction in patients with normal coronary arteries. *Ann. Intern. Med.* 1991; **115**: 797–806.

20 Mittleman RE, Wetli CV. Death caused by recreational cocaine use: An update. *JAMA* 1984; **252**: 1889–1893.

21 Wilkins CE, Mathur VS, Ty RC, Hall RJ. Myocardial infarction associated with cocaine abuse. *Texas Heart Inst. J.* 1985; **12**: 385–387.

22 Weiss RJ. Recurrent myocardial infarction caused by cocaine abuse. *Am. Heart J.* 1986; **111**: 793.

23 Gould L, Gopalaswamy C, Patel C, Betzu R. Cocaine-induced myocardial infarction. *N.Y. State J. Med.* 1985; **85**: 660–661.

24 Smith III HW, Liberman HA, Brody SL *et al.* Acute myocardial infarction temporally related to cocaine use: Clinical, angiographic, and pathophysiologic observations. *Ann. Intern. Med.* 1987; **107**: 13–18.

25 Virmani R, Robinowitz M, Smialek JE, Smyth DF. Cardiovascular effects of cocaine: An autopsy study of 40 patients. *Am. Heart J.* 1988; **115**: 1068–1074.

26 Stenberg RG, Winniford MD, Hillis LD. Simultaneous acute thrombosis of two major coronary arteries following intravenous cocaine use. *Arch. Pathol. Lab. Med.* 1989; **113**: 521–524.

27 Brody SL, Slovis CM, Wrenn KD. Cocaine-related medical problems: Consecutive series of 233 patients. *Am. J. Med.* 1990; **88**: 325–331.

28 Majid PA, Patel B, Kim HS *et al.* An angiographic and histologic study of cocaine-induced chest pain. *Am. J. Cardiol.* 1990; **65**: 812–814.

29 Mathias DW. Cocaine-associated myocardial ischemia. *Am. J. Med.* 1986; **81**: 675–678.

30 Pitts WR, Vongpatanasin W, Cigarroa JE, Hillis LD, Lange RA. Effects of the intracoronary infusion of cocaine on left ventricular systolic and diastolic function in humans. *Circulation* 1998; **97**: 1270–1273.

31 Lange RA, Cigarroa RG, Yancy CW *et al.* Cocaine-induced coronary artery vasoconstriction. *N. Engl. J. Med.* 1989; **321**: 1557–1562.

32 Mouhaffel AH, Madu EC, Satmary WA, Fraker TD Jr. (1995) Cardiovascular complications of cocaine. *Chest* 1995; **107**: 1426–1434.

33 Mittleman RE, Wetli CV. Cocaine and sudden 'natural' death. *J. Forensic Sci.* 1987; **32**: 11–19.

34 Laposata EA. Cocaine-induced heart disease: Mechanisms and pathology. *J. Thorac. Imaging* 1991; **6**: 68–75.

35 Vincent GM, Anderson JL, Marshall HW. Coronary spasm producing coronary thrombosis and myocardial infarction. *N. Engl. J. Med.* 1983; **300**: 220–223.

36 Gertz SD, Uretsky G, Wajnberg RS *et al.* Endothelial cell damage and thrombus formation after partial arterial constriction: Relevance to the role of coronary artery spasm in the pathogenesis of myocardial infarction. *Circulation* 1981; **63**: 476–486.

37 Zucker MB. Platelet function. In: Williams WJ, Butler E, Erslev AJ *et al.* (Eds.). *Hematology.* 4th ed. New York: McGraw-Hill. 1983; p. 1179.

38 Folts JD, Bonebrake FC. The effects of cigarette smoke and nicotine on platelet thrombus formation in stenosed dog coronary arteries. *Circulation* 1982; **65**: 465–470.

39 Tonga G, Tempesta E, Tonga AR *et al.* Platelet responsiveness and biosynthesis of thromboxane and prostacyclin in response to *in vitro* cocaine treatment. *Haemostasis* 1985; **15**: 100–107.

40 Chokshi SK, Rongione A, Miller G *et al.* Cocaine and cardiovascular disease: The leading edge. *Cardiology* 1989; **111**: 1–11.

41 Lisse JR, Davis CP, Thumond-Anterle M. Cocaine abuse and deep venous thrombosis. *Ann. Intern. Med.* 1989; **110**: 571–572.

42 Catterall W, Mackie K. Local anesthetics. In: Hardman JG, Gilman AG, Limbird LE (Eds.). *Goodman and Gilman's Pharmacologic Basis of Therapeutics.* 9th ed. New York: McGraw-Hill. 1996; pp. 331–338.

43 Rappolt RT, Gay GR, Inaba DS. Propranolol: A specific antagonist to cocaine. *Clin. Toxicol.* 1977; **10**: 265–271.

44 Rappolt RT Sr. Gay GR, Soman M, Kobernick M. Treatment plan for acute and chronic adrenergic poisoning crisis utilizing sympatholytic effects of the B_1–B_2 receptor site blocker propranolol (inderal) in concert with diazepam and urine acidification. *Clin. Toxicol.* 1979; **14**: 55–69.

45 Branch CA, Knuepfer MM. Adrenergic mechanisms underlying cardiac and vascular responses to cocaine in conscious rats. *J. Pharmacol. Exp. Ther.* 1992; **263**: 742–751.

46 Gay GR. Clinical management of acute and chronic cocaine poisoning. *Ann. Emerg. Med.* 1982; **11**: 562–572.

47 Pollan S, Tadjziechy M. Esmolol in the management of epinephrine and cocaine-induced cardiovascular toxicity. *Anesth. Analg.* 1989; **69**: 663–667.

48 Schindler CW, Tella SR, Goldberg SR. Adrenoreceptor mechanisms in the cardiovascular effects of cocaine in conscious squirrel monkeys. *Life Sci.* 1992; **51**: 653–660.

49 Stambler BS, Komamura K, Shara T *et al.* Acute intravenous cocaine causes transient depression followed by enhanced left ventricular function in conscious dogs. *Circulation* 1993; **87**: 1687–1697.

50 Tella SR, Korupolu GR, Schindler CW *et al.* Pathophysiological and pharmacological mechanisms of acute cocaine toxicity in conscious rats. *J. Pharmacol. Exp. Ther.* 1992; **262**: 936–946.

51 Amin M, Gabelman G, Karpel J, Buttrick P. Acute myocardial infarction and chest pain symptoms after cocaine use. *Am. J. Cardiol.* 1990; **66**: 1434–1437.

52 Brogan WC, Lange RA, Glamann DB, Hillis LD. Recurrent coronary vasoconstriction caused by intranasal cocaine: Possible role for metabolites. *Ann. Intern. Med.* 1992; **116**: 556–561.

53 Flores ED, Lange RA, Cigarroa RG, Hillis LD. Effect of cocaine on coronary artery dimensions in atherosclerotic coronary artery disease: Enhanced vasoconstriction at sites of significant stenoses. *J. Am. Coll. Cardiol.* 1990; **16**: 74–79.

54 Vanhoutte PM, Shimokawa H. Endothelium-derived relaxing factor and coronary vasospasm. *Circulation* 1989; **80**: 1–9.

55 Grant BF, Harford TC. Concurrent and simultaneous use of alcohol with cocaine: Results of national survey. *Drug Alcohol Depend.* 1990; **25**: 97–109.

56 Rose S, Hearn WL, Hime GW *et al.* Cocaine and cocaethylene concentrations in human postmortem cerebral cortex. *Neuroscience* 1990; **16**: 14.

57 Escobedo LG, Ruttenber AJ, Agocs MM *et al.* Emerging patterns of cocaine use and the epidemic of cocaine overdose deaths in Dade County, Florida. *Arch. Path. Lab. Med.* 1991; **115**: 900–905.

58 Foltin RW, Fischmann MW. Ethanol and cocaine interactions in humans: Cardiovascular consequences. *Pharmacol. Biochem. Behav.* 1988; **31**: 877–883.

59 Farre M, De La Torre R, Llorente M *et al.* Alcohol and cocaine interactions in humans. *J. Pharmacol. Exp. Ther.* 1993; **266**: 1364–1373.

60 Altura BM, Altura BT, Carella A. Ethanol produces coronary vasospasm: Evidence for a direct action of ethanol on vascular smooth muscle. *Br. J. Pharmacol.* 1983; **78**: 260–262.

61 Hayes SN, Bove AA. Ethanol causes epicardial coronary artery vasoconstriction in the intact dog. *Circulation* 1988; **78**: 165–170.

62 Pescio S, Macho P, Penna M, Domenech RJ. Changes in total and transmural coronary blood flow induced by ethanol. *Cardiovasc. Res.* 1983; **17**: 604–607.

63 Abel FL. Direct effects of ethanol on myocardial performance and coronary resistance. *J. Pharmacol. Exp. Ther.* 1980; **212**: 28–33.

64 Ganz V. The acute effect of alcohol on the circulation and on the oxygen metabolism of the heart. *Am. Heart. J.* 1963; **66**: 494–497.

65 Lasker N, Sherrod TR, Kilam KF. Alcohol on the coronary circulation of the dog. *J. Pharmacol. Exp. Ther.* 1955; **113**: 414–420.

66 Hearn WL, Flynn DD, Hime GW *et al.* Cocaethylene: A unique cocaine metabolite displays high affinity for the dopamine transporter. *J. Neurochem.* 1991; **56**: 698–701.

67 Dean RA, Chridtian CD, Sample RHB, Bosron WF. Human liver cocaine esterases: Ethanol-mediated formation of ethylcocaine. *FASEB J.* 1991; **5**: 2735–2739.

68 Hearn WL, Rose S, Wagner J *et al.* Cocaethylene is more potent than cocaine in mediating lethality. *Pharmacol. Biochem. Behav.* 1991; **39**: 531–533.

69 Lange RA, Cigarroa RG, Flores ED *et al.* Potentiation of cocaine-induced coronary vasoconstriction by β-adrenergic blockade. *Ann. Intern. Med.* 1990; **112**: 897–903.

70 Brown BG, Bolson E, Peterson RB *et al*. The mechanisms of nitroglycerin action: Stenosis vasodilation as a major component of the drug response. *Circulation* 1981; **64**: 1089–1097.

71 Winniford MD, Jansen DE, Reynolds GA *et al*. Cigarette smoking-induced coronary vasoconstriction in atherosclerotic coronary artery disease: Prevention by calcium antagonists and nitroglycerin. *Am. J. Cardiol.* 1987; **59**: 203–207.

72 Brogan III WC, Lange RA, Kim AS *et al*. Alleviation of cocaine-induced coronary vasoconstriction by nitroglycerin. *J. Am. Coll. Cardiol.* 1991; **18**: 581–586.

73 Egashira K, Morgan KG, Morgan JP. Effects of cocaine on excitation-contraction coupling of aortic smooth muscle from the ferret. *J. Clin. Invest.* 1991; **87**: 1322–1328.

74 Negus BH, Willard JE, Hillis LD *et al*. Alleviation of cocaine-induced coronary vasoconstriction with intravenous verapamil. *Am. J. Cardiol.* 1994; **73**: 510–513.

75 Trouve R, Nahas GG, Manger WM *et al*. Interactions of nimodipine and cocaine on endogenous catecholamines in the squirrel monkey. *Proc. Soc. Exp. Biol. Med.* 1990; **193**: 171–175.

76 Trouve R, Nahas GG, Manger WM. Catecholamines, cocaine toxicity, and their antidotes in the rat. *Proc. Soc. Exp. Biol. Med.* 1991; **196**: 184–187.

77 Knight DR, Vatner SF. Calcium channel blockers induce preferential coronary vasodilation by an α-1 mechanism. *Am. J. Physiol.* 1987; H604–H613.

78 Van Zwieten PA, Van Meel JCA, Timermans P. Pharmacology of calcium entry blockers: Interaction with vascular α-adrenoreceptors, *Hypertension* 1987; **5**(Suppl. II): 118.

79 Braun BL, Murray DM, Sidney S. Lifetime cocaine use and cardiovascular characteristics among young adults: The CARDIA study. *Am. J. Pub. Health* 1997; **87**(4): 629–634.

80 Tazelaar HD, Karch SB, Stephens BG, Billingham ME. Cocaine and the heart. *Hum. Pathol.* 1987; **18**: 195–199.

81 Ambrosio E, Tella SR, Goldberg SR, Schindler CW, Erzouki H, Elmer GI. Cardiovascular effects of cocaine during operant cocaine self-administration. *Eur. J. Pharmacol.* 1996; **315**: 43–51.

82 Fischman MW, Schuster CR, Javaid J, Hatano Y, Davis J. Acute tolerance to the cardiovascular and subjective effects of cocaine. *J. Pharmacol. Exp. Ther.* 1985; **235**: 677–682.

83 Smith TL, Callahan M, Williams D, Dworkin SI. Tachyphylaxis in cardiovascular responses to cocaine in conscious rats. *J. Cardiol. Pharmacol.* 1993; **21**: 272–278.

84 Tella SR. Possible novel pharmacodynamic action of cocaine: Cardiovascular and behavioral evidence. *Pharmacol. Biochem. Behav.* 1996; **54**(2): 343–354.

85 Welder AA, Grammas P, Melchert RB. Cellular mechanisms of cocaine cardiotoxicity. *Toxicol. Lett.* 1993; **69**: 227–238.

86 Maillet M, Chriarasini D, Nahas G. Myocardial damage induced by cocaine administration of a week's duration in the rat. *Adv. Biosci.* 1991; **80**: 187.

87 Yuan C, Acosta D Jr. Cocaine-induced mitochondrial dysfunction in primary cultures of rat cardiomyocytes. *Toxicology* 1996; **112**: 1–10.

88 Besse S, Assayag P, Latour C, Janmot C, Robert V, Delcayre C, Nahas G, Swynghedauw B. Molecular characteristics of cocaine-induced cardiomyopathy in rats. *Eur. J. Pharmacol.* 1997; **338**: 123–129.

89 Mercadier JJ, Samuel JL, Michel JB, Zongazo MA, de la Bastie D, Lompre AM, Wisnewsky C, Rappaport L, Levy B, Schwartz K. Atrial natriuretic factor gene expression in rat ventricle during experimental hypertension. *Am. J. Physiol.* 1989; **257**: H979–H987.

90 Feldman AM, Weinberg EO, Ray PE, Lorell BH. Selective changes in cardiac gene expression during compensated hypertrophy and the transition to cardiac decompensation in rats with chronic aortic banding. *Circ. Res.* 1993; **73**: 184–192.

91 Robert V, Ven Thiem N, Cheav SL, Mouas C, Swynghedauw B, Delcayre C. Increased cardiac types I and III collagen mRNAs in aldosterone-salt hypertension. *Hypertension* 1994; **24**: 30–36.

92 Lompre AM, Schwartz K, d'Albis A, Lacombe G, Thiem NV, Swynghedauw B. Myosin isoenzyme redistribution in chronic heart overload. *Nature* 1979; **282**: 105–107.

93 Izumo S, Lompre AM, Matsuoka R, Koren G, Schwartz K, Nadal-Ginard B, Mahdavi V. Myosin heavy chain messenger RNA and protein isoform transitions during cardiac hypertrophy: Interaction between hemodynamic and thyroid hormone-induced signals. *J. Clin. Invest.* 1987; **79**: 970–977.

94 Besse S, Assayag P, Delcayre C, Carre F, Cheav SL, Lecarpentier Y, Swynghedauw B. Normal and hypertrophied senescent rat heart: Mechanical and molecular characteristics. *Am. J. Physiol.* 1993; **265**: H183–H190.

95 Bhambi B, Eghbali M. Effect of norepinephrine on myocardial collagen gene expression and response of cardiac fibroblasts after norepinephrine treatment. *Am. J. Pathol.* 1991; **139**: 1131–1142.

96 Ruth JA, Ullman EA, Collins AC. An analysis of cocaine effects on locomotor activities and heart rate in four inbred mouse strains. *Pharmacol. Biochem. Behav.* 1988; **29**: 157–162.

Chapter 20

Mechanisms of cocaine cardiotoxicity

David Solkoff and Ronald R. Watson

Cocaine abuse induces coronary vasospasm [1–5], myocardial infarction [6–8], hypertension [9,10], stroke [7,11], and fatal cardiac rhythm disorders, including ventricular fibrillation [12–15]. Chronic cocaine abuse has also been shown to cause dilated cardiomyopathy [16,17], and left ventricular hypertrophy in normotensive cocaine users [18–20]. It is only since modern electrocardiographic techniques have come into widespread use that the effect of cocaine on cardiac rhythm has been effectively studied. These techniques were the first to demonstrate that cocaine produced severe intractable ventricular arrhythmias that resulted in death during routine nasal surgery [21].

Cocaine functions as a strong cardiac stimulant that potentiates the actions of the sympathetic nervous system by inhibiting both peripheral and central neuronal catecholamine uptake [22–24]. The resulting changes in cardiac autonomic neural balance may significantly contribute to the formation of arrhythmias, since increased sympathetic activity reduces cardiac electrical stability, thus exposing the heart to ventricular fibrillation [25,26]. Therefore parasympathetic activation may oppose these sympathetic effects and thereby protect against cocaine induced malignant arrhythmias [22,23]. Also, high doses of cocaine have caused significant reductions in heart rate variability, which serves as a marker of cardiac vagal tone [27,28]. These changes were shown to be increasingly pronounced during myocardial ischemia, when cocaine exacerbated the autonomic response to a coronary artery occlusion [29]. Post cocaine, myocardial ischemia elicited a significantly enhanced tachycardia, resulting from both enhanced sympathetic activation and an increased withdrawal of parasympathetic tone. Thus cocaine-induced changes in autonomic control of the heart play a critical role in the development of ventricular fibrillation during myocardial ischemia.

The previously mentioned cocaine-induced accumulation of catecholamines can hyperactivate α- and β-adrenergic receptors, thus provoking coronary vasospasm (myocardial infarction and ischemia), increased contractile force resulting in increased metabolic demand and cardiac arrhythmias [1]. β-Adrenergic receptor antagonists have been shown to lessen many of the hemodynamic effects of cocaine [30–33]. Therapeutic doses of propranolol blunt the pressor, positive inotropic, and heart rate responses to cocaine intoxication [34–36]. Propranolol has also reduced the number of cardiac arrhythmias induced by programmed electrical stimulation after intravenous cocaine [37]. However, propranolol failed to alter the toxic actions of high doses of cocaine [38]. Furthermore, propranolol increased, rather than reduced, the fatal effects of large doses of cocaine [33,39]. The conflicting data suggest that additional mechanisms are needed to fully explain the arrhythmogenic action of cocaine.

In the myocardium, there are a large number of α-adrenergic receptors [40]. Activation of these receptors increases cardiac myocyte calcium levels, triggers a delayed after-depolarization, and induces ventricular arrhythmias [40,41]. Therefore, cocaine-linked increases in catecholamines, which activate α-adrenergic receptors, may cause ventricular arrhythmias. This hypothesis has received support from a study showing that prazosin, an α_1-adrenergic receptor antagonist, significantly lessened the incidence of malignant arrhythmias induced by a cocaine, exercise, plus ischemia test [42]. In the same study WB4101, an α_{1A}-adrenergic receptor antagonist, prevented cocaine-provoked arrhythmias. Other studies have shown that paradoxically, the non-selective α-adrenergic receptor antagonist phentolamine augmented, rather than suppressed, the cardiotoxic properties of cocaine [33,43–44]. When examined wholistically, these data infer that cocaine-induced activation of adrenergic receptors may be responsible for the disruption in cardiac electrical stability that results in ventricular fibrillation and induction of malignant arrhythmias.

The previously discussed hyperactivation of α- and β-adrenergic post-synaptic receptors by cocaine-released catecholamines causes increases in intracellular second messengers. These intracellular factors may be responsible for the cellular events that trigger arrhythmias. Adenylate cyclase is activated when myocardial β-adrenergic receptors are stimulated, and this results in elevated cyclic adenosine monophosphate (cAMP) levels. This has the effect of increasing calcium entry and calcium release from cytosolic stores [45,46]. Similarly, α-adrenergic receptors activate the inositol triphosphate second messenger cascade, which also increases cytosolic calcium [45,47]. α_{1A}-adrenrgic receptor stimulates the breakdown of phosphoinositides via a pertussin toxin-sensitive G protein, thus stimulating calcium influx [48]. It has therefore been postulated that α- and β-adrenergic receptor stimulation acts synergistically to increase calcium entry and cytosolic calcium levels. This mechanism represents the end of the pathway that begins with a cocaine-mediated elevation in catecholamine release, and finishes with ventricular fibrillation.

Cardiac arrhythmias result from abnormalities in impulse conduction, impulse generation, or both. Previous studies have shown that these abnormalities may be caused by alterations in cellular calcium [49–50]. They have also demonstrated that cocaine raises intracellular calcium levels [51], and that it also stimulates the release of calcium from the sarcoplasmic reticulum [52]. Furthermore, Kimura et al. [53] have described cocaine's ability to prolong action-potential duration and to induce after-depolarization, thus triggering extrasystoles in isolated feline cardiomyocytes. They demonstrated that these oscillatory after-potentials were enhanced by catecholamines and suppressed by the calcium channel antagonist verapamil. When compared against those who suffered drug-related deaths not involving cocaine, the heart of individuals who experienced acute fatal cocaine cardiotoxicity displayed myocardial contraction bands more frequently. These pathological changes are thought to indicate abnormalities in calcium homeostasis [49,54]. Thus, it has been hypothesized that interventions resulting in a reduction of elevated cytosolic calcium levels may protect against cocaine-linked ventricular fibrillation. Experimental evidence supporting this hypothesis includes a study which found that cocaine-induced ventricular fibrillation was prevented in 8 of 12 animals treated with the intracellular calcium-specific chelator BAPTA-AM [43]. The drug also significantly lessened both the pressor and inotropic response to cocaine. Similarly, a number of organic (verapamil, nifedipine, diltiazem, and flunarizine) and inorganic (magnesium) calcium channel antagonists eliminated cocaine-provoked ventricular fibrillation [55]. These antagonists, by suppressing the cocaine-induced accumulation of cytosolic calcium, may prevent oscillatory changes in membrane potential, thus preventing the trigger for malignant arrhythmias.

In addition to its sympathomimetic actions, cocaine has potent local anasthetic properties [22,23]. Cocaine blocks sodium channels, thus inhibiting action-potential generation and conduction in both nerve and cardiac tissue. Cocaine causes depression of Purkinje cell automaticity as well as depressed phase 0 of the cardiac action potential (the rapid upstroke due to sodium influx) [56]. Cocaine blocks a calcium dependent potassium channel thereby delaying repolarization [57]. When tested on intact animal preparations in a dose dependent manner, cocaine has been reported to increase QRS duration, prolong P-R interval, and increase the H-V interval on *His* bundle recordings [29,58–60]. For high doses of cocaine, conduction block and asystole have also been reported [15,61]. Similarly, cocaine inhibits potassium channels thus prolonging repolarization of isolated cardiac tissue [62], lengthening the duration of QT interval in intact animals [29,60]. The resulting conduction delays and inhomogeneities of repolarization may contribute to the formation of arrhythmias [63]. This inhomogeneity exists when excitability in one area of the heart returns before adjacent areas have repolarized fully. Therefore, the tissue that has remained in a depolarized state longer than the surrounding tissue may act to reexcite the fully repolarized regions and generate a premature impulse. This inhomogeneity of repolarization has been reported for a variety of local anesthetics [64] and plays an important role in the induction of ventricular fibrillation [63]. These observations suggest that the local anesthetic properties of cocaine may also contribute to the formation of malignant arrhythmias. With respect to the heart, the local anesthetic effects of cocaine are quite obvious following the administration of large doses of the drug.

These local anesthetic properties may also negatively affect cardiac mechanical function. High doses of cocaine can exert a direct depression of myocardial performance thereby contributing to its cardiovascular mortality [65]. Fraker *et al.* [66] found significant reductions in regional left ventricular ejection fraction (as measured by two-dimensional echocardiography) following the administration of a large dose of cocaine (4 mg/kg) to either conscious or pentobarbitol anesthetized instrumented dogs. Similar studies have shown that cocaine infusions caused significant declines in the index of contractility known as left ventricular dP/dT [65,67]. This depression was partly normalized by nifedipine, a potent coronary vasodilator, suggesting that the declines in mechanical function may partially result from cocaine-induced reductions in coronary perfusion.

In addition to its actions on cardiac muscle, cocaine can indirectly affect cardiac electrophysiological and mechanical properties by influencing the coronary vasculature. In approximately one-third of the patients studied (myocardial infarction cases resulting from the recreational use of cocaine) the infarction victims possessed normal coronary vessels. The investigators concluded that the cocaine-induced myocardial infarction in these individuals probably involved adrenergically mediated increases in myocardial oxygen consumption and vasoconstriction of the coronary vessels. Thus, the increased release of catecholamines during cocaine intoxication, and the resulting activation of α-adrenergic receptors located on coronary vascular smooth muscle, may be responsible for a powerful vasoconstriction. Many of the fatal consequences of cocaine, including ventricular arrhythmias, may therefore arise secondarily from the resulting myocardial ischemia and infarction. Several previous studies further demonstrate the coronary vasoconstrictive effects of cocaine [68–74]. Cocaine produces a dose-dependent vasoconstriction of the coronary vasculature in intact dogs and conscious rats. These actions were prevented by calcium channel antagonists [67], and α-adrenergic receptor blockade [71,72]. Vascular actions of cocaine may create an imbalance between myocardial oxygen supply (coronary vasoconstriction) and oxygen demand (increased heart rate, arterial pressure, and inotropic state), thus increasing the likelihood of ischemic events and the associated reduction in cardiac electrical stability and mechanical performance. It is interesting to note that the deleterious effects of cocaine on myocardial oxygen supply and demand are exacerbated by concomitant cigarette smoking [75]. This combination markedly increases the metabolic requirement of the heart for oxygen but simultaneously decreases the diameter of diseased coronary arterial segments. As to whether ethanol exacerbates the cardiotoxic properties of cocaine, it has been reported that the combination of intranasal cocaine and intravenous ethanol causes an increase in the determinants of myocardial oxygen demand. At the same time, however, it also increases epicardial coronary arterial diameter [76].

ACKNOWLEDGMENT

Supported by NIDA supplements to grant HL63667.

REFERENCES

1 Billman G. Cocaine: A review of its toxic actions on cardiac function. *Crit. Rev. Toxicol.* 1995; **25**: 113–132.

2 Ascher EK, Stauffer JCE, Gaasch WH. Coronary artery spasm, cardiac arrest, transient electrocardiographic Q waves, and stunned myocardium in cocaine-associated acute myocardial infarction. *Am. J. Cardiol.* 1988; **61**: 939–941.

3 Brogan WC, Lange RA, Kim AS *et al.* Alleviation of cocaine-induced coronary vasoconstriction by nitroglycerin. *J. Am. Coll. Cardiol.* 1991; **18**: 581–585.

4 Lange RA, Cigarro RG, Yancy CW Jr. *et al.* Cocaine-induced coronary artery vasoconstriction. *N. Eng. J. Med.* 1989; **321**: 1557–1568.

5 Mathias DW. Cocaine-associated myocardial ischemia: Review of clinical and angiographic findings. *Am. J. Med.* 1986; **81**: 675–678.

6 Cregler LL, Mark H. Relation of acute myocardial infarction to cocaine abuse. *Am. J. Cardiol.* 1985; **56**: 794.

7 Isner JM, Estes M, Thompson PD *et al.* Acute cardiac events temporally related to cocaine abuse. *N. Eng. J. Med.* 1986; **315**: 1438–1443.

8 Milnor RL Jr., Scott BD, Brown DD *et al.* Cocaine-induced myocardial infarction in patients with normal coronary arteries. *Ann. Int. Med.* 1991; **115**: 797–806.

9 Resnick RB, Kestenbaum RS, Schwartz LK. Acute systemic effects of cocaine in man: A controlled study by intranasal and intravenous routes. *Science* 1977; **195**: 696–698.

10 Wilkerson RD. Cardiovascular effects of cocaine in conscious dogs: Importance of fully functional autonomic and central nervous systems. *J. Pharmacol. Exp. Ther.* 1988; **246**: 466–471.

11 Levine SR, Washington JM, Kieran SN *et al.* Crack cocaine-associated stroke. *Neurology* 1987; **37**: 1849–1953.

12 Benchimol A, Bartall H, Desser KB. Accelerated ventricular rhythm and cocaine abuse. *Ann. Intern. Med.* 1978; **88**: 519–520.

13 Billman GE, Hoskins RS. Cocaine-induced ventricular fibrillation protection afforded by the calcium antagonist verapamil. *FASEB J.* 1988; **2**: 2990–2995.

14 Lathers CM, Tyau LSY, Spino MM *et al.* Cocaine-induced seizures, arrhythmias, and sudden death. *J. Clin. Pharmacol.* 1988; **28**: 584–593.

15 Nanji AA, Filipenko JD. Asystole and ventricular fibrillation associated with cocaine intoxication. *Chest* 1984; **85**: 132–138.

16 Hogya PT, Wolfson AB. Chronic cocaine abuse associated with dilated cardiomyopathy. *Am. J. Emerg. Med.* 1990; **8**: 203–204.

17 Weiner RS, Lockhart JT, Schwartz RG. Dilated cardiomyopathy and cocaine abuse: Report of two cases. *Am. J. Med.* 1986; **81**: 699–701.

18 Brickner ME, Willard JE, Eichhorn EJ *et al.* Left ventricular hypertrophy associated with chronic cocaine abuse. *Circulation* 1991; **84**: 1130–1135.

19 Chakko S, Fernandez A, Mellman TA *et al.* Cardiac manifestations of cocaine abuse: A cross-sectional study of asymptomatic men with a history of long-term abuse of crack cocaine. *J. Am. Coll. Cardiol.* 1992; **20**: 1168–1174.

20 Om A, Ellahham S, Vetrovec GW *et al.* Left ventricular hypertrophy in normotensive cocaine users. *Am. Heart J.* 1993; **125**: 1441–1443.

21 Young D, Glauber JJ. Electrocardiographic changes resulting from acute cocaine toxicity. *Am. Heart J.* 1947; **34**: 272–279.

22 Billman GE. Mechanisms responsible for the cardiotoxic effects of cocaine. *FASEB J.* 1990a; **4**: 2469–2475.

23 Billman GE. The effect of carbachol and cyclic GMP on susceptibility to ventricular fibrillation. *FASEB J.* 1990b; **4**: 1668–1673.

24 Langer SZ, Enero MA. The potentiation of responses to adrenergic nerve stimulation in the presence of cocaine: Its relationship to metabolic fate of released norepinephrine. *J. Pharmacol. Exp. Ther.* 1974; **191**: 431–443.

25 Billman GE, Hoskins RS. Time series analysis of heart rate variability during submaximal exercise: Evidence for reduced cardiac vagal tone in animals susceptible to ventricular fibrillation. *Circulation* 1989; **80**: 146–157.

26 Corr PB, Yamada KA, Witkowski RX. Mechanisms controlling cardiac autonomic function and their relationships to arrhythmogenesis: In: Fozzard HA, Haber E, Jennings RB *et al.* (Eds.). *The Heart and Cardiovascular System.* Raven Press, New York 1986; p. 1597.

27 Garfinkel A, Raltz SL, Harper RM. Heart rate dynamics after acute cocaine administration. *J. Cardiovasc. Pharmacol.* 1992; **19**: 453–459.

28 Stambler BS, Morgan JP, Mietus J *et al.* Cocaine alters heart rate dynamics in conscious ferrets. *Yale J. Biol. Med.* 1991; **64**: 143–153.

29 Billman GE, Lappi MD. The effects of cocaine on cardiac vagal tone before and during coronary artery occlusion: Cocaine exacerbates the autonomic response to myocardial ischemia. *J.Cardiovasc. Pharmacol.* 1993; **22**: 869–876.

30 Gay GR. Clinical management of acute and chronic cocaine poisoning. *Ann. Emerg. Med.* 1982; **11**: 562–572.

31 Pollan S, Tadjziechy M. Esmolol in the management of epinephrine and cocaine-induced cardiovascular toxicity. *Anesth. Analg.* 1989; **69**: 663–664.

32 Rappolt RT, Gay GR, Inaba DS. Propranolol: A specific antagonist of cocaine. *Clin. Toxicol.* 1977; **10**: 265–271.

33 Tella SR, Korupolu GR, Schindler CW *et al.* Pathophysiological and pharmacological mechanisms of acute cocaine toxicity in conscious rats. *J. Pharmacol. Exp. Ther.* 1992; **262**: 936–946.

34 Branch CA, Kneupfer MM. Adrenergic mechanisms underlying cardiac and vascular responses to cocaine in conscious rats. *J. Pharmacol. Exp. Ther.* 1992; **263**: 742–751.

35 Schindler CW, Tella SR, Goldberg SR. Adrenoreceptor mechanisms in the cardiovascular effects of cocaine in conscious squirrel monkeys. *Life Sci.* 1992; **51**: 653–660.

36 Stambler BS, Komamura K, Shara T *et al.* Acute intravenous cocaine causes transient depression followed by enhanced left ventricular function in conscious dogs. *Circulation* 1993; **87**: 1687–1697.

37 Gantenberg NS, Hageman GR. Cocaine enhanced arrhythmogenesis: Neural and non-neural mechanisms. *Can. J. Physiol. Pharmacol.* 1992; **70**: 240–246.

38 Catravas JD, Waters IW. Acute cocaine intoxication in the conscious dog: Studies on the mechanism of lethality. *J. Pharmacol. Exp. Ther.* 1981; **217**: 350–356.

39 Guinn MM, Bedford JA, Wilson MC. Antagonism of intravenous cocaine lethality in non-human primates. *Clin. Toxicol.* 1980; **16**: 499–508.

40 Terzic A, Puceat M, Vassort G *et al.* Cardiac β-1 adrenoreceptors: An overview. *Pharmacol. Rev.* 1993; **45**: 147–175.

41 Kurtz T, Yamada KA, Da Torre SD *et al.* Alpha-adrenergic systems and arrhythmias in ischemic heart disease. *Eur. Heart. J.* 1991; **12**(Suppl. F): 88.

42 Billman GE. The effect of adrenergic antagonists on cocaine-induced ventricular fibrillation: Alpha-adrenergic, but not β-adrenergic antagonists prevent malignant arrhythmias independent of heart rate. *J. Pharmacol. Exp. Ther.* 1994; **269**: 409–416.

43 Billman GE. The intracellular chelator, BAPTA-AM, prevents cocaine-induced ventricular fibrillation. *Am. J. Physiol.* 1993b; **265**(Heart Circ. Physiol. 34): H1529–H1535.

44 Robin ED, Wong RJ, Ptashne KA. Increased lung water after massive cocaine overdose in mice and improved survival related to Beta-adrenergic blockade. *Ann. Intern. Med.* 1989; **110**: 202–207.

45 Billman GE. Cellular mechanisms for ventricular fibrillation. *NIPS* 1992; **7**: 254.

46 Evans DB. Modulation of cAMP: Mechanism for positive inotropic action. *J. Cardiovasc. Pharmacol.* 1986; **8**(Suppl. 9): S22–S29.

47 Berridge MJ. Inositol triphosphate and diacylglycerol: Two interacting second messengers. *Annu. Rev. Biochem.* 1987; **56**: 159–193.

48 Del Balzo U, Rosen MR, Malfatto G *et al.* Specific β-1 adrenergic receptor subtypes modulate catecholamine-induced increases and decreases in ventricular automaticity. *Circ. Res.* 1990; **67**: 1535–1551.

49 Billingham ME. Direct and indirect morphological markers of cocaine toxicity in the human heart. *NIDA Res. Mongr.* 1991; **108**: 202–219.

50 Levy MN. Role of calcium in arrhythmogenesis. *Circulation* 1989; **80**(Suppl. IV): IV30–IV31.

51 Perreault CL, Hague NL, Ransil B *et al.* The effects of cocaine on intracellular Ca^{2+} handling and myofilament Ca^{2+} responsiveness of ferret ventricular myocardium. *Br. J. Pharmacol.* 1990; **101**: 679–685.

52 Tomita F, Bassett AL, Myerburg RJ *et al.* Effects of cocaine on sarcoplasmic reticulum in skinned rat heart muscle. *Am. J. Physiol.* 1993; **264**: H845–H850.

53 Kimura S, Bassett AL, Xi H *et al.* Early afterdepolarizations and triggered activity induced by cocaine: A possible mechanism of cocaine arrhythmogenesis. *Circulation* 1992; **85**: 2227–2235.

54 Tazelaar HD, Karch SB, Stephens BG *et al.* Cocaine and the heart. *Human Pathol.* 1987; **18**: 195–199.

55 Billman GE. Effect of calcium channel antagonists on cocaine-induced malignant arrhythmias: Protection against ventricular fibrillation. *J. Pharmacol. Exp. Ther.* 1993; **266**: 407–416.

56 Weidmann S. Effect of calcium ions and local anaesthetics on electrical properties of Purkinje fibers. *J. Physiol. (Lond.)* 1955; **129**: 568–582.

57 Grossie J. Ca-dependent action of cocaine on K current in freshly dissociated dorsal root ganglia from rats. *Am. J. Physiol.* 1993; **265**: C674–C679.

58 Kabas JS, Blanchard SM, Matsuyama Y *et al.* Cocaine-mediated impairment of cardiac conduction in the dog: A potential mechanism for sudden death after cocaine. *J. Pharmacol. Exp.Ther.* 1990; **252**: 185–191.

59 Schwartz AB, Janzen D, Jones RT *et al.* Electrocardiographic and hemodynamic effects of intravenous cocaine in awake and anesthetized dogs. *J. Electrocardiol.* 1989; **22**: 159–166.

60 Temesy-Armos PN, Fraker TD Jr., Brewster PS *et al.* The effects of cocaine on cardiac electrophysiology in conscious, unsedated dogs. *J. Cardiovasc. Pharmacol.* 1991; **19**: 883–891.

61 Watt TB, Pruitt RD. Cocaine-induced incomplete bundle branch block in dogs. *Circ. Res.* 1964; **15**: 234–239.

62 Pryzwara DA, Dambach GE. Direct actions of cocaine on cardiac cellular electric activity. *Circ. Res.* 1989; **65**: 185–192.

63 Janse MJ, Wit AS. Electrophysiological mechanisms of ventricular arrhythmia resulting from myocardial ischemia and infarction. *Physiol. Rev.* 1989; **69**: 1049–1169.

64 Kasten GW. Amide local anesthetic alterations of effective refractory period temporal dispersion: Relationship to ventricular arrhythmias. *Anesthesiology* 1986; **65**: 61–66.

65 Hale SL, Alker KJ, Rezkalla S *et al*. Adverse effects of cocaine in cardiovascular dynamics, myocardial blood flow, and coronary artery diameter in an experimental model. *Am. Heart J.* 1989; **118**: 927–933.

66 Fraker TD, Temesy-Armos PN, Brewster PS *et al*. Mechanism of cocaine-induced myocardial depression in dogs. *Circulation* 1990; **81**: 1012–1016.

67 Hale SL, Alker KJ, Rezkalla SH *et al*. Nifedipine protects the heart from the acute deleterious effects of cocaine if administered before but not after cocaine. *Circulation* 1991; **83**: 1437–1443.

68 Egashira K, Pipers FS, Morgan JP. Effects of cocaine on epicardial coronary artery reactivity in miniature swine after endothelial injury and high cholesterol feeding: *In vitro* and *in vivo* analysis. *J. Clin. Invest.* 1991; **88**: 1307–1314.

69 Egashira K, Morgan KG, Morgan JP. Effects of cocaine on excitation-contraction coupling of aortic smooth muscle from the ferret. *J. Clin. Invest.* 1991; **87**: 1322–1328.

70 Kalsner S. Cocaine sensitization of coronary artery contraction: Mechanism of drug-induced spasm. *J. Pharmacol. Exp. Ther.* 1993; **264**: 1132–1140.

71 Mueller PJ, Kneupfer MM. Coronary vascular effects of cocaine in rats. *J. Pharmacol. Exp. Ther.* 1994; **268**: 97–103.

72 Shannon RP, Stambler BS, Komamura K *et al*. Cholinergic modulation of the coronary vasoconstriction induced by cocaine in conscious dogs. *Circulation* 1993; **87**: 939–949.

73 Vargas R, Gillis RA, Ramwell PW. Propranolol promotes cocaine-induced spasm of porcine coronary artery. *J. Pharmacol. Exp. Ther.* 1991; **257**: 644–646.

74 Hayes SN, Moyer TP, Morley D *et al*. Intravenous cocaine causes epicardial coronary vasoconstriction in the intact dog. *Am. Heart J.* 1991; **121**: 1639–1648.

75 Moliterno DJ, Willard JE, Hillis LD *et al*. Coronary-artery vasoconstriction induced by cocaine, cigarette smoking, or both. *New Engl. J. Med.* 1994; p. 454–459.

76 Pirwitz MJ, Willard JE, Hillis LD *et al*. Influence of cocaine, ethanol, or their combination on epicardial coronary arterial dimensions in humans. *Arch. Intern. Med.* 1995; **155**: 1186–1191.

Chapter 21

Alcohol and reflex regulation of the cardiovascular system

Abdel A. Abdel-Rahman

INTRODUCTION

There is considerable epidemiological evidence that suggests a positive relationship between ethanol consumption and arterial blood pressure [1–5]. However, the mechanism by which ethanol elevates blood pressure is not known. We have performed a number of studies to test the hypothesis that ethanol-associated hypertension may be a consequence of ethanol-evoked attenuation of baroreflex activity. Our earlier findings in animals [6–8] were the first to describe the effect of ethanol on the baroreflex mediated bradycardic response. An earlier clinical study showed that moderate amounts of ethanol enhanced the reflex tachycardic response triggered by the Valsalva maneuver and body tilt [9]. This effect of ethanol was observed in the absence of any change in blood pressure and in spite of an increased basal heart rate [9]. In this chapter, we will discuss the acute and chronic effects of ethanol on baroreflex activity in normotensive humans and rats. Furthermore, based on our data and reported findings, we will identify the major neuroanatomical targets for ethanol action on baroreflexes and discuss a pivotal role for ethanol-evoked inhibition of glutamatergic neurotransmission in its depressant action on baroreflexes.

The baroreceptor heart rate response, which has been used in experimental and clinical studies [7,10–16] has provided definitive evidence that this reflex response is attenuated in the hypertensive state [15,16]. More importantly, this attenuation precedes and may contribute to the development of some forms of hypertension including ethanol-induced hypertension [7,8,17–19]. Assessment of the baroreceptor heart rate response can be made either by the ramp or by the steady state method [14]. As discussed below, most of the reported findings on the effect of ethanol on baroreflexes were based on the ramp method.

THE ACUTE EFFECT OF ETHANOL ON BAROREFLEX ACTIVITY

Moderate amounts (0.1–1 g/kg) of ethanol administered to anesthetized [6,20–23] or conscious [24–26] rats caused little if any change in baseline blood pressure. However, the associated heart rate response depended on the route of administration and varied from no change, following i.v. administration, to dose-related increases, following oral or i.p. administration [7,20,22,27]. It is imperative to note that the effects of ethanol on baroreflex sensitivity were investigated in the absence of significant changes in baseline blood pressure, which rules out a potential confounding factor for data interpretation. The first finding that demonstrated a dose-related inhibition in baroreflex sensitivity was obtained in anesthetized rats [22]. Subsequent studies replicated this finding in conscious rats [26,28,29] and, therefore, ruled out the possibility that an additive or synergistic interaction between ethanol and the anesthetic contributed to the observed attenuation of baroreflex activity. Nonetheless, it seems that an interaction between ethanol and the anesthetic agent affected the responsiveness of vascular α_1-adrenergic receptor. In anesthetized rats, ethanol caused a significant rightward shift in the dose–pressor response curve constructed with phenylephrine, which suggested that ethanol exhibits alpha-receptor blocking activity [23]. Notably, this effect of ethanol was absent in conscious rats [22,26] and in normotensive humans [27], which supports the notion that anesthesia alters the effects of ethanol on vascular reactivity.

IS THE RAT AN APPROPRIATE MODEL FOR STUDIES ON ETHANOL ACTIONS ON BAROREFLEXES?

It is important to highlight the clinical relevance of our findings, which pertained to ethanol-evoked attenuation of the baroreflex sensitivity. Therefore, we investigated the effects of moderate amounts (0.5, 1 and 1.5 g/kg) of ethanol on baseline blood pressure and heart rate as well as on the baroreflex-mediated bradycardia in young human volunteers [27]. While none of the doses of ethanol significantly affected baseline blood pressure, a dose-related increase in heart rate was evident [27]. These findings are compatible with reported observations [9,31]. The findings demonstrated, for the first time, that ethanol caused a dose-related attenuation of the baroreflex-mediated bradycardia when the ramp (bolus) method was used [27]. On the other hand, when the steady-state (infusion) method was used, the baroreflex sensitivity (slope of the relationship between evoked increases in blood pressure and heart rate responses) was not influenced by ethanol [27]. Nonetheless, it was noted that the baroreflex curve generated after ethanol was shifted to the right, which suggested resetting of baroreceptors by ethanol [27]. Interestingly, the magnitude of resetting, expressed as a shift in MAP_{50}, was related to blood ethanol concentration [27]. Together these findings suggest the following. First, the effect of ethanol on baroreflex sensitivity depends on the method of measurement of the reflex response. Since, the baroreflex-evoked heart rate response observed following abrupt increases in blood pressure (the ramp method) reflects the vagal contribution more than does the steady state method [11,14], the findings suggest that ethanol attenuates the cardiac vagal component [27]. The findings of more recent studies, which employed power spectral analysis, [31–35] support this conclusion. Second, the similarity between the findings in humans and earlier findings in rats support the appropriateness of the rat as a model for mechanistic studies on the effects of ethanol on baroreceptor function.

SELECTIVE INTERACTION BETWEEN ETHANOL AND AORTIC BARORECEPTORS

In this series of experiments, we addressed the question whether ethanol-evoked attenuation of the baroreflex bradycardic response is dependent on either or both sets of the baroreceptor afferents. In the first study, bilateral transection of the aortic nerves in the cervical region,

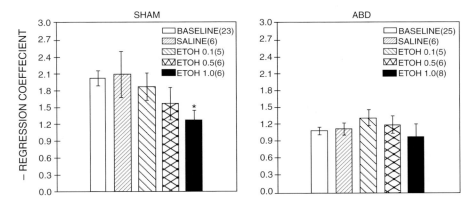

Figure 21.1 Bar graphs showing that ethanol (0.1, 0.5 and 1.0 g/kg) produces graded decreases in regression coefficient (baroreflex slopes; beats/min/mmHg) in SO, but not in aortic barodenervated (ABD) rats. Values are expressed as mean ± S.E.M.; *$p < 0.05$ compared to base-line value. Number of rats in each group is shown in parentheses; with permission [28].

or sham operation, was conducted under methohexital anesthesia. Post-operative care was performed as described in accordance with the institutional guidelines [28]. Following a 2–3 day recovery, the baroreflex sensitivity was significantly attenuated in aortic denervated as compared with sham operated rats [28]. As in our previous studies [21,22], ethanol caused a dose-related attenuation of the baroreflex-mediated bradycardia in sham operated rats (Figure 21.1) [28]. However, such an effect of ethanol was absent in aortic barodenervated rats (Figure 21.1). These findings suggest that ethanol selectively acts on the aortic baro-reflex arc to depress the baroreflex-mediated bradycardia in intact rats [28]. It was important to consider the possibility that consequent changes in body functions caused by aortic

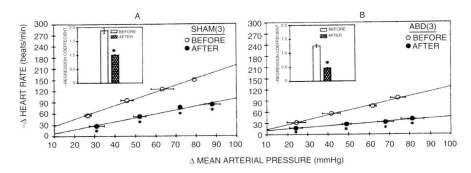

Figure 21.2 Baroreflex curves relating decreases in HR to PE-induced elevations in BP obtained in conscious freely moving ABD or SO rats before and after i.v. administration of an anesthetizing dose of pentobarbital (30 mg/kg). In either group, pentobarbital produced a downward shift in the curve as evident by a reduction in the regression coefficient (baroreflex slope; inset). Values are expressed as mean ± S.E.M.; *$p < 0.05$ compared to prepentobarbital values (ANOVA). Number of rats in each group is shown in parentheses; with permission [28].

barodenervation may have contributed to the lack of ethanol action on baroreflexes in this animal model. An expected effect of aortic barodenervation is the increase in blood pressure, which we observed while the rats were under anesthesia and for the following 24 hrs after recovery [28]. If it persisted, a higher blood pressure in aortic barodenervated rats may have confounded the data interpretation. However, by 48–72 hrs after barodenervation, the time at which the effect of ethanol was investigated, blood pressure had subsided to control levels [28].

Another possibility that needed to be considered was the significantly lower baseline baroreflex sensitivity in aortic barodenervated rats, which persisted even after blood pressure subsided to control levels [28]. The depressant effect of ethanol on baroreflex sensitivity may be obscured by the lower baseline BRS value, which may not be lowered any more by any intervention. To address this issue, an anesthetizing dose of pentobarbital was administered to aortic barodenervated and control rats. As shown in Figure 21.2, pentobarbital depressed the baroreflex sensitivity to a similar degree in both preparations [28]. These results ruled out the low baroreflex sensitivity, in aortic barodenervated rats, as a cause for the absence of ethanol action. Therefore, the results of this investigation, in conscious rats, suggest a major role for the aortic baroreceptors in the ethanol-evoked attenuation of baroreflex sensitivity [28].

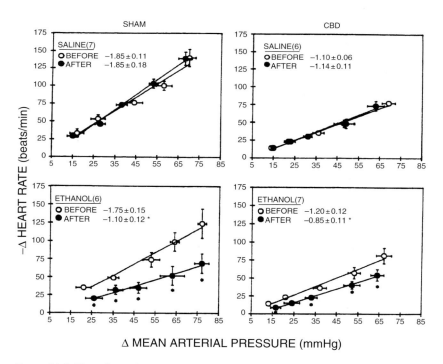

Figure 21.3 The effect of ethanol (1 g/kg) on baroreflex curves relating changes in HR to rises in BP evoked by PE in conscious unrestrained CBD and SO rats. Note that ethanol, but not saline, causes a significant (*$p < 0.05$, ANOVA) downward shift in the baroreflex curves in both groups of rats as compared to pre-ethanol values. Values shown are the regression coefficients of baroreflex curves in beats per minute per millimeter of mercury; the number of rats in each group is shown in parentheses; with permission [29].

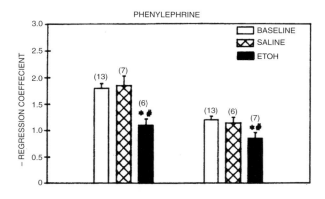

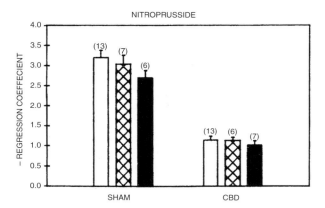

Figure 21.4 Bar graphs showing the capacity of ethanol (1 g/kg) to produce a significant reduction in the regression coefficient (baroreflex slopes; beats/min/mmHg) of PE-baroreflex curves. Values are expressed as mean ± S.E.M.; # and *$p < 0.05$ compared to base-line and after-saline values, respectively. CBD, carotid barodenervation. The number of rats in each group is shown in parentheses; with permission [29].

Direct evidence was sought to further support the pivotal role of the aortic baroafferents in ethanol-evoked attenuation of baroreflex mediated bradycardia. In this study, the rats were subjected to carotid barodenervation and the aortic nerves were left intact [29]. Similar pressor and tachycardic responses to those observed following aortic barodenervation were obtained during the first 24 hr [28,29]. These hemodynamic responses subsided to control levels by 2–3 days after carotid barodenervation but the baroreflex sensitivity remained significantly attenuated [29]. In effect, the latter was similar in magnitude to the level obtained in aortic barodenervated rats [28,29]. In support of the hypothesis, ethanol attenuated the baroreflex sensitivity in carotid barodenervated rats in spite of the low basal value (Figures 21.3, 21.4) [29]. Taken together, these findings provide evidence that implicates the aortic baroreceptors and their projections in the depressant action of ethanol of baroreceptor-mediated bradycardia [28,29].

NEUROANATOMICAL TARGETS FOR ETHANOL ACTION ON BAROREFLEXES

We have previously shown that systemically administered ethanol attenuated the brady-cardic and depressor responses to stimulation of the aortic nerve in sinaortic denervated rats [36]. These findings provided indirect evidence of a possible ethanol-evoked impairment of the central pathways that mediate the baroreceptor reflex control of heart rate. In a subsequent study, we examined the effects of microinjection of ethanol in some CNS sites that are possibly involved in the baroreceptor reflex arc [20]. Since our previous findings also showed that systemic ethanol administration augmented preganglionic sympathetic discharge [21], we expanded our study to include the effects of centrally administered ethanol on the baroreceptor reflex control of heart rate and sympathetic efferent discharge [20]. In this latter study, we identified the potential sites within the CNS at which ethanol may influence cardiovascular variables controlled by baroreceptor reflexes [20]. We initially chose the nucleus tractus solitarius (NTS) because we have already shown that systemic ethanol administration attenuated baroreceptor reflex activity and because the NTS is the first relay station in the baroreceptor reflex arc. The amounts of ethanol microinjected were based on calculations of the amount of ethanol expected to reach this area after systemic injection of 0.33, 0.66, and 1 g/kg ethanol, which were administered systemically in our previous studies [22,23,28]. Further, we microinjected ethanol into the anterior and posterior hypothalamus and the rostral ventrolateral medulla (RVLM) to determine if the effects of ethanol were specific to one or more of these areas [20].

Microinjection of either artificial CSF or ethanol into the NTS, DMV, posterior hypothalamus, or RVLM did not cause any change in baseline MAP or heart rate [20]. The only change was a 30% and 40% increase in sympathetic efferent discharge that occurred at 12 and 20 minutes, respectively, after microinjection of ethanol into the RVLM [20]. Further, a 15 mmHg increase in MAP associated with a corresponding increase in sympathetic efferent discharge when ethanol was microinjected into the anterior hypothalamus [20]. This effect of ethanol was related to the distance from the bregma where ethanol was injected [20]. Microinjection of 5.5, 11, or 16 μg ethanol into the NTS produced a dose-related attenuation of the baroreceptor heart rate response but had no effect on the reflex response of the sympathetic efferent discharge to baroreceptor activation [20]. Thus, for a comparable rise in MAP evoked by phenylephrine, the reflex decrease in heart rate was significantly smaller after ethanol [20]. Microinjection of artificial CSF into the NTS had no effect on the reflex responses of heart rate and sympathetic efferent discharge [20] eliminating the possibility that the changes observed were volume related. To eliminate the possibility that the observed changes were due to leakage of ethanol from the NTS or DMV, 16 μg ethanol was microinjected 0.5 mm lateral to the NTS/DMV complex. Ethanol microinjection outside of the NTS had no effect on the baroreceptor reflex variables [20].

Routine histological verification of the site of injection showed that the DMV was stained by the dye microinjected into the NTS [20]. Because of the close proximity of the NTS to the DMV and because the DMV contributes to the control of central vagal tone, we decided to investigate the effect of low doses (6.4 μg) of ethanol in the DMV. This dose produced a greater inhibition of the baroreceptor heart rate response than did the dose of 16 μg in the NTS [20]. This effect was solely due to ethanol since an equivalent volume of artificial CSF had no effect on the baroreceptor reflex control of heart rate. Ethanol microinjected into the DMV had no effect on the baroreceptor reflex control of sympathetic efferent discharge similar to the results obtained when ethanol was administered into the NTS [20]. Similar findings were obtained when ethanol (6.4 µg) was microinjected into the RVLM. However, the inhibition of baroreceptor reflex-mediated bradycardia was much less than that obtained after microinjection of the same amount into the DMV (90% vs. 62%, respectively). Finally, microinjection of 16 µg ethanol into the anterior or the posterior hypothalamus had no effect on baroreceptor reflex control of heart rate or sympathetic efferent discharge [20].

Ethanol microinjected into the RVLM also attenuated the baroreceptor heart rate response but did not affect baroreceptor reflex control of sympathetic efferent discharge. These data suggest the involvement of the RVLM in the baroreceptor reflex-mediated bradycardia observed after systemic administration of ethanol [20,26,28,29]. Injection of ethanol into the anterior and posterior hypothalamus had no effect on baroreceptor reflex-mediated bradycardia. However, ethanol injection into the anterior, but not the posterior hypothalamus, was associated with a modest but significant increase in baseline MAP, which was associated with an excitatory effect on sympathetic efferent discharge [20]. These data highlight the anterior hypothalamus as the possible site of action of enhanced sympathetic efferent activity observed after systemic ethanol administration [36]. This finding is consistent with a pressor effect of ethanol of central origin [20]. It is interesting that the effect of ethanol on baroreceptor reflex-mediated bradycardia was specific to the medullary areas (NTS, DMV, and the RVLM). However, since the baroreceptor reflex control of sympathetic efferent discharge was not altered by ethanol [20], the data suggest that the baroreceptor reflex-mediated bradycardia did not involve significant changes in the sympathetic component of the reflex. Therefore, this effect of ethanol is mediated at the NTS, the DMV, or the RVLM, or on interneurons that connect the areas and seems to involve the efferent vagal component.

The selective action of ethanol on baroreceptor reflex control of heart rate deserves a comment. First, leakage of ethanol to the DMV and nucleus ambiguous, which control central vagal tone, may explain the effect of ethanol on heart rate responses. However, the finding that ethanol increased sympathetic efferent discharge after its administration into the anterior hypothalamus indicates its ability to interact with central sympathetic structures as well. Second, it is possible that ethanol attenuates the baroreceptor reflex control of sympathetic activity in some sympathetic nerves and not in others [20]. Other investigators have shown that the baroreceptor reflex control of splanchnic nerve activity was preserved while that of renal nerve activity was impaired under the same conditions [37,38]. Third, the selective effect of ethanol may suggest that potentially different physiological processes be involved in the baroreceptor reflex control of heart rate and sympathetic efferent discharge. These processes include transmitters or cotransmitters (e.g., glutamate and norepinephrine), different receptors or subreceptor mechanisms, or a combination of both. Finally, the results rule out the possibility that ethanol-evoked nonspecific cell damage contributed to the observed effect. However, our data could not determine whether ethanol acted on the cell bodies or the fibers of passage. The excitatory amino acid, L-glutamate, has been shown to have a selective effect on cell bodies and not fibers of passage. Since an ethanol effect was observed in those areas in which the excitatory amino acid L-glutamate produced the expected cardiovascular responses, we believe that the effect of ethanol is on cell bodies in the areas studied [20,30].

ETHANOL INTERACTION WITH MEDULLARY L-GLUTAMATE NEUROTRANSMISSION

The following experiments addressed two questions that pertained to the hypothesis that ethanol impairs BRS by blockade of EAA receptors in the lower brainstem. First, does systemic administration of ethanol concomitantly attenuate the BRS and the hemodynamic responses elicited by L-glutamate microinjected into the brainstem nuclei? Second, does ethanol-evoked attenuation of BRS involve an interaction with the NMDA receptor in the NTS? Evidence suggests selectivity of ethanol toward NMDA receptors [39,40]. Therefore, in this study we examined the effects of systemic and intra-NTS ethanol administration on NMDA and non-NMDA mediated hemodynamic responses and on BRS in anesthetized Sprague-Dawley rats [30].

The base-line MAP and HR for all ethanol- and vehicle-treated groups were similar [30]. The site of microinjection within the NTS was chemically identified at the beginning of each experiment by microinjection of a test dose of L-glutamate (2 nmol). Depressor responses of 20 to 40 mmHg were obtained when the micropipette was placed in the caudal or intermediate regions of the NTS, which was confirmed by post-mortem histological verification [30]. The hemodynamic responses evoked by ethanol varied and depended on the dose used and the route of administration. Systemic ethanol (0.1 g/kg) had no influence on MAP but slightly increased the HR [30]. A higher dose, (1 g/kg) of ethanol, modestly increased MAP and decreased HR [30]. Intra-NTS ethanol (10 μg) had no effect on MAP

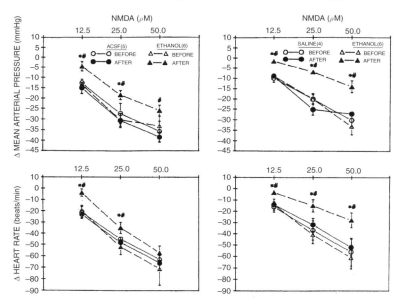

Figure 21.5 Effect of ethanol on depressor and bradycardic responses elicited by unilateral microinjection of graded doses of NMDA into the NTS of urethane-anesthetized rats. Ethanol was administered either into the NTS (10 μg, left panels) or systematically (1 g/kg, right panels). The values are expressed as the mean ± S.E.M. *and# p< 0.05 (ANOVA) compared with corresponding pre-ethanol and after-vehicle (ACSF or saline) values, respectively. The number of rats in each group is shown in parentheses; with permission [30].

or HR [20,30]. The blood ethanol concentration measured 10 min after i.v. administration of 0.1 and 1.0 g/kg of ethanol was 14.7 ± 2.8 and 174.2 ± 16.8 mg/dl, respectively [30].

We tested the hypothesis that ethanol attenuates the BRS by selective blockade of the NMDA receptor in the NTS. Our studies, therefore, sought evidence to determine whether doses of ethanol that attenuate BRS also selectively attenuate the hemodynamic responses elicited by NMDA microinjected into the NTS. Reported studies have implicated the EAA receptors in the NTS in BRS modulation [41–43]. The doses of ethanol used for systemic and intra-NTS administration have attenuated BRS in reported studies [28,29,44]. The results of this study showed that systemic administration of ethanol depressed the BRS and attenuated the hemodynamic responses elicited by NMDA (Figure 21.5) and non-NMDA agonists but the effect was more evident on NMDA-mediated responses [30]. Three findings established a link between ethanol-evoked attenuation of BRS and its selective blockade of NMDA receptors in the NTS. First, intra-NTS ethanol attenuated BRS and the hemodynamic responses elicited by NMDA but not non-NMDA (kainic acid or AMPA) agonists (Figures 21.6, 21.7). Second, intra-NTS microinjection of the selective NMDA antagonist, AP-5, elicited similar effects to those evoked by ethanol on BRS and the hemodynamic responses evoked by NMDA [30]. Third, a small dose of ethanol (0.1 g/kg i.v.) that had no effect on BRS did not influence the hemodynamic responses elicited by NMDA [30]. The depressant effect of systemically administered ethanol on BRS was associated with an attenuation of the depressor and bradycardic responses elicited by microinjection of NMDA and non-NMDA agonists into the NTS. These findings implicate the EAA receptors in the NTS in the depressant effect of ethanol on BRS [30]. However, because ethanol was administered systemically, it was not possible to determine whether the ethanol-evoked attenuation of BRS and the hemodynamic responses to EAA were linked and involved local glutamatergic pathways in the NTS. The possibility had to be considered that the actions of ethanol on other brain areas [45] might have contributed to these effects. The finding that intra-NTS ethanol caused a significant attenuation of the BRS (Figure 21.7) suggests that the NTS is involved, at least partly, in this action of ethanol [30]. Furthermore, the concomitant reductions by intra-NTS ethanol of the BRS and the NMDA but not on non-NMDA mediated responses (Figures 21.6, 21.7) implicated the NMDA receptor in the depressant effect of ethanol on BRS [30]. This notion was supported by the observation that the selective blockade of NMDA receptor by intra-NTS AP-5 attenuated BRS and the hemodynamic responses elicited by NMDA but not L-glutamate [30]. It is important to note that the enhancement of GABA receptor-mediated responses in the NTS is also involved in the depressant effect of ethanol the BRS [44]. It is possible that ethanol induced inhibition of BRS involves an interaction between glutamatergic and GABAergic pathways. Consistent with this view is the finding that ethanol-mediated attenuation of BRS was associated with opposite changes in GABA (enhancement) and L-glutamate (attenuation)-mediated neuronal responses in the rostral ventrolateral medulla [45]. Nevertheless, the nature of such an interaction remains to be elucidated.

ETHANOL INTERACTION WITH THE NMDA AND VASOPRESSIN RECEPTORS IN CONSCIOUS RATS

Reported studies including our own that dealt with the identification of the neuroanatomical sites of ethanol action on baroreflexes and the role of the NMDA receptor in this action of

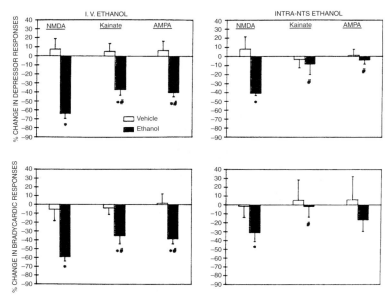

Figure 21.6 Bar graphs showing the depressant effects of ethanol (i.v., 1 g/kg; intra-NTS, 10 µg) or respective vehicle (saline, i.v.; ACSF, intra-NTS) treatment on hemodynamic responses elicited by NMDA (25 pmol) and non-NMDA (kainate, 3 pmol and AMPA, 1 pmol (expressed as the percent reduction in these responses compared with pre-treatment responses. The values are the means ± S.E.M. * and # $p < 0.05$ (ANOVA) compared with corresponding vehicle and NMDA (after ethanol) values, respectively; with permission [30].

ethanol were undertaken in anesthetized rats [20,30,44–46]. Because anesthesia alters glutamatergic neurotransmission and attenuates baroreflexes [28,47], it was imperative to rule out the possibility that the interpretation of our previous findings [20,30] was not confounded by the presence of anesthesia. Two studies were performed to address this issue. We investigated the effects of ethanol microinjection into the rostral ventrolateral medulla (RVLM) on the glutamatergic modulation of baroreflexes in conscious rats [24]. An important finding of our studies was the clear cause-and-effect relationship between the level of the glutamatergic neurotransmission in the RVLM and baroreflex sensitivity [24,48]. We demonstrated that intra-RVLM microinjection of the selective NMDA antagonist AP-5 produces significant reductions of the hemodynamic responses elicited by NMDA microinjection into the same site and the baroreflex sensitivity [24]. Furthermore, simultaneous enhancements of glutamatergic neurotransmission and baroreflex activity were caused by the inhibition of L-glutamate uptake with p-chloromercuriphenylsulphonic acid (PCMS) [24,48]. Therefore, this model system allowed us to investigate the effects of ethanol on the glutamatergic (NMDA) neurotransmission and baroreflex sensitivity at the basal as well as the stimulated conditions. The finding that intra-RVLM ethanol attenuated the baroreflex sensitivity and the NMDA-evoked hemodynamic responses [24] confirms and extends our previous findings on similar effects in the NTS of anesthetized rats [30]. Equally important, we demonstrated, for the first time, that intra-RVLM ethanol counteracted the enhancements of the glutamatergic neurotransmission in the RVLM and the baroreflex

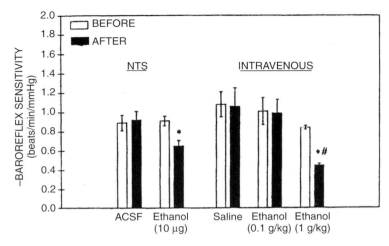

Figure 21.7 Bar graphs showing the depressant effect of ethanol on BRS (Δ/HR/ΔMAP) tested by i.v. PE (16 μg/kg) in urethane-anesthetized rats. Ethanol was administered either unilaterally into the NTS (10 μg) or systemically (0.1 or 1.0 g/kg). The values are expressed as the mean ± S.E.M. * and # $p < 0.05$ (ANOVA) compared with corresponding pre-ethanol and after intra-NTS ethanol values, respectively; with permission [30].

sensitivity caused by the L-glutamate uptake blocker PCMS [24]. Together, these findings provide direct evidence that implicates the NMDA receptor in the RVLM in ethanol-evoked attenuation of the baroreflex sensitivity [24]. This evidence was obtained, for the first time, in conscious unrestrained rats in the absence of the confounding effects of anesthesia [45,46].

Our earlier studies focused on the role of the brainstem EAA receptors in the depressant action of ethanol on baroreflex sensitivity. Notably, ethanol gains access to all brain areas and may interact with different neuronal signaling pathways. Therefore, we sought evidence to support the hypothesis that ethanol-vasopressin (AVP) interaction in the area postrema (AP) may contribute to the ethanol-evoked attenuation of the baroreflex sensitivity [25]. The following findings provided the basis for this hypothesis: (i) Vasopressin, even when administered systemically, activates neurons in the AP and causes enhancement of baroreflexes [49,50]; (ii) Ethanol inhibits AVP release [51,52] and some of its neurobiological actions [53]. Therefore, the following experiments were undertaken in conscious unrestrained rats to determine if ethanol microinjection into the AP will selectively inhibits the baroreflex sensitivity measured by AVP [25]. Appropriate control groups were included to support the selectivity of ethanol-AVP interaction and to rule out the possibility that ethanol diffusion to the anatomically close NTS contributed to ethanol action. The data showed that intra-AP ethanol (10 μg) attenuated the baroreflex sensitivity measured by AVP but not by phenylephrine [25]. Further, the effect of ethanol on AP neurons was replicated by a selective AVP antagonist and histological and functional evidence limited the action of ethanol on AVP neurons to the AP [25]. These results highlight a new neurobiological action of ethanol that may contribute to its deleterious effects on central structures that control blood pressure and cardiovascular reflexes [25].

DEPENDENCE OF ETHANOL-EVOKED ATTENUATION OF BAROREFLEX SENSITIVITY ON THE OVARIAN HORMONES

Very few studies dealt with the acute effects of ethanol on cardiovascular reflexes in the female population. Even when female subjects were included [27], the small sample size did not permit conclusions of whether the action of ethanol on baroreflexes is sexually dimorphic. Our recent studies have demonstrated that ethanol causes a dose-related attenuation of baroreflex-mediated bradycardia in female rats [54], even though the baseline baroreflex sensitivity was significantly lower in female rats compared with age-matched male rats [55]. These findings suggest that ethanol-evoked attenuation of the baroreflex-mediated bradycardia is independent of gender [54]. Interestingly, ethanol-evoked attenuation of the baroreflex sensitivity was abolished in ovariectomized rats [54]. These latter findings suggest the dependence of ethanol action on the ovarian hormones [54]. Whether ethanol interacts with estrogen or progesterone to attenuate the baroreflex sensitivity in female rats remains to be investigated.

CONCLUSIONS

Ethanol causes a dose-dependent attenuation of baroreflex sensitivity in both genders. The findings in rats are consistent with clinical findings, which makes the rat an appropriate model for studies intended to delineate the mechanisms that underlie the depressant action of ethanol on baroreflexes. Our results provided evidence that suggests that ethanol interaction with the aortic baroreceptors or their central projections contributes to its depressant action on baroreflexes. We have identified the neuroanatomical targets for ethanol action on baroreflexes to be mainly located in the brainstem. In addition, we have established a causal role for the disruption of the glutamatergic (NMDA) neurotransmission in the nucleus tractus solitarius and the rostral ventrolateral medulla in the depressant action of ethanol on baroreflexes. Another potential central site is the area postrema in which ethanol selectively counteracts the facilitatory action of vasopressin on baroreflex sensitivity. Finally, ethanol-evoked attenuation of the baroreflex-mediated bradycardia in female rats involves its interaction with the ovarian hormones or their receptors. The findings reported in this chapter have clinical significance because our earlier studies have suggested that the attenuation of baroreflex activity seems to be a predisposing factor in ethanol-evoked hypertension.

ACKNOWLEDGEMENT

Supplemented by NIH grants AA07839 and AA10257. The author thanks Ms. Barbara Davis and Ms. Rani Vadlamudi for their excellent technical assistance.

ABBREVIATIONS

MAP   mean arterial pressure
HR   heart rate

BRS   baroreflex sensitivity
AP   area postrema
NTS   nucleus tractus solitarius
RVLM   rostral ventrolateral medulla
CSF   cerebrospinal fluid
DMV   dorsal motor nucleus of the vagus
EAA   excitatory amino acid

REFERENCES

1 Puddey IB, Beilin LJ, Vandongen R, Rouse IL, Rogers P. Evidence for a direct effect of alcohol on blood pressure in normotensive men: a randomized controlled trial. *Hyperten.* 1985; **7**: 707–713.

2 Arkwright PD, Beilin LJ, Rouse IL, Armstrong BK, Vandongen R. Effects of alcohol use and other aspects of lifestyle on blood pressure levels and prevalence of hypertension in working populations. *Circ.* 1982; **66**: 60–66.

3 Klatsky AL, Friedman GD, Siegelaub AB, Gerald MJ. Alcohol consumption and blood pressure: Kaiser-Permanente multiphasic health examination data. *New Engl. J. Med.* 1977; **296**: 1194–1200.

4 Friedman GD, Klatsky AL, Siegelaub AB. Alcohol, tobacco and hypertension. *Hypertens.* 1982; **4** (Suppl. 3): 143–150.

5 Potter JF, Beevers DG. Pressor effect of alcohol in hypertension. *Lancet*, **i**, 1984; 119–122.

6 Zhang X, Abdel-Rahman A-RA, Wooles WR. A differential action for ethanol on baroreceptor reflex control of heart rate and sympathetic efferent discharge in rats. *Proc. Soc. Biol. Med.* 1988; **187**: 14–21.

7 Abdel-Rahman A-RA, Dar MS, Wooles WR. Effect of chronic ethanol administration on arterial baroreceptor function and pressor and depressor responsiveness in rats. *J. Pharmacol. Exptl. Ther.* 1985; **232**: 194–201.

8 Abdel-Rahman A-RA. Differential effects of ethanol on baroreceptor heart rate responses of conscious spontaneously hypertensive and normotensive rats. *Alcohol. Clin. Exp. Res.* 1994: **18**(6): 1515–1522.

9 Zsoter TT, Sellers EM. Effect of alcohol on cardiovascular reflexes. *J. Studies on Alcohol* 1977; **38**: 1–10.

10 Coleman TG. Arterial baroreflex control of heart rate in the conscious rat. *Amer. J. Physiol.* 1980; **238**: H515–H520.

11 Korner PJ, Shaw J, West MJ, Oliver JR. Central nervous system control of baroreceptor reflexes in the rabbit. *Circ. Res.* 1972; **31**: 639–652.

12 Guo GB, Abboud FM. Angiotensin II attenuates baroreflex control of heart rate and sympathetic activity. *Amer. J. Physiol.* 1984; **246**: H80–H89.

13 Smyth HS, Sleight P, Pickering GW. Reflex regulation of arterial pressure during sleep in man: a quantitative method for assessing baroreflex sensitivity. *Circ. Res.* 1969; **24**: 109–121.

14 Korner PI, West MJ, Shaw J, Uther JB. 'Steady-state' properties of the baroreceptor-heart rate reflex in essential hypertension in man. *Clin. Exptl. Pharmacol. Physiol.* 1974; **1**: 65–76.

15 Goldstein DS. Arterial baroreflex sensitivity, plasma catecholamines, and pressor responsiveness in essential hypertension. *Circ.* 1983; **68**: 234–240.

16 Bristow SD, Honour AS, Pickering GW, Sleight P, Smyth HS. Diminished baroreflex sensitivity in high blood pressure. *Circ.* 1969; **38**: 48–54.

17 Gordon FJ, Matsuguchi H, Mark AL. Abnormal baroreflex control of heart rate in prehypertensive and hypertensive Dahl genetically salt-sensitive rats. *Hypertens.* 1981; **3**: 1135–1141.

18 Gordon FJ, Mark AL. Impaired baroreflex control of vascular resistance in prehypertensive Dahl S rats. *Amer. J. Physiol.* 1983; **245**: H210–H217.

19 Gordon FJ, Mark AL. Mechanism of impaired baroreflex control in prehypertensive Dahl salt-sensitive rats. *Circ. Res.* 1984; **54**: 378–387.

20 Zhang X, Abdel-Rahman AA, Wooles WR. Impairment of baroreceptor reflex control of heart rate but not sympathetic efferent discharge by central neuroadministration of ethanol. *Hypertens.* 1989; **14**: 282–292.

21 Russ R, Abdel-Rahman A-RA, Wooles WR. Role of the sympathetic nervous system in ethanol-induced hypertension in rats. *Alcohol* 1991; **8**(4): 301–307.

22 Abdel-Rahman A-RA, Russ R, Strickland JA, Wooles WR. Acute effects of ethanol on barore-ceptor reflex control of heart rate and on pressor and depressor responsiveness in rats. *Can. J. Physiol. Pharmacol.* 1986; **65**: 834–841.

23 Russ R, Abdel-Rahman A-RA, Wooles WR. Ethanol exhibits α-receptor blocking-like properties in anesthetized rats (42821). *Soc. Exptl. Biol. Med.* 1989; **190**: 1–6.

24 Mao L, Abdel-Rahman AA. Blockade of L-glutamate receptors in the rostral ventrolateral medulla contributes to ethanol-evoked impairment of baroreflexes in conscious rats. *Brain Res. Bull.* 1995; **37**(5): 513–521.

25 Mao L, Abdel-Rahman AA. Ethanol microinjection into the area postrema selectively attenuates baroreflex sensitivity measured by vasopressin in conscious rats. *Neurosci. Lett.* 1996; **220**: 13–16.

26 Abdel-Rahman AA. Differential effects of ethanol on baroreceptor heart rate responses of conscious spontaneously hypertensive and normotensive rats. *Alcoholism: Clin. Exptl. Res.* 1994; **18**(6): 1515–1522.

27 Abdel-Rahman A-RA, Merrill RH, Wooles WR. Effect of acute ethanol administration on the baroreceptor reflex control of heart rate in normotensive human volunteers. *Clin. Sci.* 1987; **72**: 113–122.

28 El-Mas MM, Abdel-Rahman AA. Role of aortic baroreceptors in ethanol-induced impairment of baroreflex control of heart rate in conscious rats. *J. Pharmacol. Exptl. Ther.* 1992; **262**(1): 157–165.

29 El-Mas MM, Abdel-Rahman AA. Direct evidence for selective involvement of aortic baroreceptors in ethanol-induced impairment of baroreflex control of heart rate. *J. Pharmacol. Exptl. Ther.* 1992; **264**(3): 1198–1205.

30 El-Mas MM, Abdel-Rahman AA. Role of NMDA and non-NMDA receptors in the nucleus tractus solitarius in the depressant effect of ethanol on baroreflexes. *J. Pharmacol. Exptl. Ther.* 1993; **266**(2): 602–610.

31 Koskinen P, Virolainen J, Kupari M. Acute alcohol intake decreases short-term heart rate variability in healthy subjects. *Clin. Sci.* 1994; **87**(2): 225–230.

32 Gonzalez GJ, Mendez LA, Mendez NA, Cordero VJJ. Effect of acute alcohol ingestion on short-term heart rate fluctuations. *J. Stud. Alcohol* 1992; **53**(1): 86–90.

33 Weise F, Kressl D, Brinkhoff N. Acute alcohol ingestion reduces heart rate variability. *Drug. Alcohol Depend.* 1986; **17**(1): 89–91.

34 Murata K, Araki S, Yokoyama K, Sata F, Yamashita K, Ono Y. Autonomic neurotoxicity of alcohol assessed by heart rate variability. *J. Auton. Nerv. Syst.* 1994; **48**(2): 105–111.

35 Maki T, Toivonen L, Koskinen P, Naveri H, Harkonen M, Leinonen H. Effect of ethanol drinking, hangover, and exercise on adrenergic activity and heart rate variability in patients with a history of alcohol-induced atrial fibrillation. *Am. J. Cardiol.* 1998; **82**(3): 317–322.

36 Zhang X, Abdel-Rahman A-RA, Wooles WR. Impairment of central mediation of the arterial baroreflex by acute ethanol administration. *Alcohol* 1988; **5**: 221–228.

37 Richsten SE, Thoren PN. Reflex inhibition of sympathetic nerve activity during volume load in awake normotensive and spontaneously hypertensive rats. *Acta Physiol. Scand.* 1980; **110**: 77–82.

38 Judy WV, Farrell SK. Arterial baroreceptor reflex control of sympathetic nerve activity in spontan-eously hypertensive rat. *Hypertension* 1979; **1**: 605–614.

39 Lovinger DM, White G, Weight FF. Ethanol inhibits NMDA-activated ion current on hippocampal neurons. *Science* 1989; **243**: 1721–1724.

40 Hoffman PL, Rabe CS, Moses F, Tabakoff B. N-methyl-D-aspartate receptors and ethanol: inhibition of calcium flux and cyclic GMP production. *J. Neurochem.* 1989; **52**: 1937–1940.

41 Talman WT, Perrone MH, Scher P, Kwo S, Reis DJ. Antagonism of baroreceptor reflex by glutamate diethyl ester, an antagonist to L-glutamate. *Brain Res.* 1981; **217**: 186–191.

42 Galloudec EL, Merahi N, Laguzzi R. Cardiovascular changes induced by local application of glutamate-related drugs in the rats nucleus tractus solitarii. *Brain Res.* 1989; **503**: 322–325.

43 Talman WT. Kynurenic acid microinjected into the nucleus tractus solitarius of rat blocks the arterial baroreflex but not responses to glutamate. *Neurosci. Lett.* 1989; **102**: 247–252.

44 Varga K, Kunos G. Inhibition of baroreflex bradycardia by ethanol involves both $GABA_A$ and $GABA_B$ receptors in the brainstem of the rats. *Eur. J. Phamacol.* 1992; **214**: 223–232.

45 Sun MK, Reis DJ. Effects of systemic ethanol on medullary vasomotor neurons and baroreflexes. *Neurosci. Lett.* 1992; **137**: 232–236.

46 Sun M-K, Reis DJ. Ethanol inhibits chemoreflex excitation of reticulospinal vasomotor neurons. *Brain Res.* 1996; **730**: 182–192.

47 Colombari E, Menani JV, Talman WT. Commissural NTS contributes to pressor responses to glutamate injected into the medial NTS of awake rats. *Am. J. Physiol.* 1996; **270** (6 Pt 2): R1220–R1225.

48 Mao L, Abdel-Rahman A-RA. Inhibition of glutamate uptake in the rostral ventrolateral medulla enhances baroreflex-mediated bradycardia in conscious rats. *Brain Res.* 1994; **654**: 343–348.

49 Cox BF, Hay M, Bishop VS. Neurons in area postrema mediate vasopressin-induced enhancement of the baroreflex. *Am. J. Physiol.* 1990; **258**: H1943–H1946.

50 Hasser EM, Bishop VS. Reflex effect of vasopressin after blockade of V1 receptors in the area postrema. *Circ. Res.* 1990; **67**: 265–271.

51 Eisenhower G, Johnson RH. Effect of ethanol ingestion on plasma vasopressin and water balance in humans. *Am. J. Physiol.* 1982; **242**: R522–R527.

52 Wang XM, Dayanithi G, Lemos JR, Nordmann JJ, Treistman SN. Calcium currents and peptide release from neurohypophysial terminals are inhibited by ethanol. *J. Pharmacol. Exp. Ther.* 1991; **259**: 705–711.

53 Bottoms GD, Fessler JF, Jognson M, Coatney RW, Voorhees W. Effects of acute alcohol intake on tolerance to hypotension. *Alcohol Clin. Exp. Res.* 1990; **14**: 776–780.

54 El-Mas MM, Abdel-Rahman A-RA. Ovariectomy abolishes ethanol-induced impairment of baroreflex control of heart rate in conscious rats. *Eur. J. Pharmacol.* 1998; **349**: 253–261.

55 Abdel-Rahman A-RA. Gender differences in baroreflex-mediated bradycardia in young rats: Role of the sympathetic and parasympathetic components. *Can. J. Physiol. Pharmacol.* 1999; **77**: 1–9.

Chapter 22

Alcohol's accentuation of AIDS' nutritional and immune damage, a cofactor in heart disease

R. Tomas Sepulveda and Ronald R. Watson

INTRODUCTION

Infection with Human Immunodeficiency Virus (HIV) results, in the vast majority of cases, in the development of the Acquired Immune Deficiency Syndrome (AIDS). A great number of papers have been published that analyze the affect of alcohol consumption on numerous aspects of HIV infection. Some of the questions examined have been: alcohol use and the likelihood of sexual practices with high risk behavior for HIV infection; alcohol consumption and susceptibility to HIV infection; and alcohol consumption and disease progression in HIV infected persons [1]. Also, the effect that micronutrient deficiency has on immune system development and viral disease progression is well known. In this chapter, we will examine a different question: are the influences of ethanol and micronutrients on HIV infection merely defined and distinct or do they interact together to produce additive and/or synergistic effects on the immune system? Early studies *in vitro* have shown that addition of alcohol to lymphocyte cell cultures corresponding to intoxication levels *in vivo* significantly suppress the proliferation of HIV recombinant antigens [2]. Interestingly enough, the study also indicates that while high levels of ethanol will suppress proliferation of lymphocytes in healthy individuals, it does not have the same effect in lymphocytes from AIDS patients. Lower levels of ethanol (EtOH) will suppress proliferation of lymphocytes from AIDS patients [2]. Studies have shown that micronutrient deficiencies are common during HIV infection. Insufficient dietary intake, malabsorption, diarrhea, excessive urinary secretion, impaired storage and altered metabolism of micronutrients can contribute to the development of these deficiencies. Low plasma or serum levels of vitamins A, E, B6, B12 and C, carotenoids, Se, and Zn are common in many HIV-infected populations. The effect of micronutrient deficiencies is clearly seen in the increase in oxidative stress and this in turn may contribute to the pathogenesis of HIV infection. Low levels or intakes of micronutrients such as vitamins A, E, B6 and B12, Zn and Se have been associated with a poor prognosis in the symptomology and progression of HIV infection, and new studies are emerging which suggest that micronutrient supplementation may help reduce the morbidity and mortality of patients suffering from this disease.

ALCOHOL AND THE IMMUNE SYSTEM

NK cells are important because they play a role in natural immunity against tumor and infected cells. In fact, advanced aging is associated with functional impairment of NK cells and increased susceptibility to nutritional deficiencies. Studies from human and experimental animals have proven that EtOH acts as a co-carcinogen, and suppression of the immune system has been considered as one mechanism by which EtOH could increase the incidence or progression of cancers [3], like Kaposi's sarcoma. A recent report regarding HIV-related cancers compared cancer incidences in Zimbabwe, Africa between 1990–1992 to those in 1993–1995. It showed an increase in the incidence of Kaposi's sarcoma with a doubling of the rates in both men and women. A significant increase in the incidence of squamous cell tumours, as well as non-Hodgkin's lymphoma in women was also observed [4]. Research shows a relationship between increased ethanol levels and a decrease in natural killer cells. Decreased natural killer (NK) activity is observed in cancer patients with EtOH consumption [5]. Animal models clearly support an important role for NK cells in preventing the growth and metastasis of several types of cancers [6,7]. Substances like epinephrine and norepinephrine, which are markedly increased in acute EtOH exposure, have also been associated with suppression of NK-cell activity [8–10]. Collectively, these observations suggest that NK cells may play an important role in resistance to EtOH-related cancers in humans.

Micronutrients affect the function of NK cells as well. NK cell cytotoxicity is diminished in vitamin E and ubiquinone-10 deficiencies. Also, low plasma levels of selenium and zinc have been associated with total percentages of NK cells [49].

Alterations of the immune system due to alcohol consumption have been a focus of multiple studies that have revealed impaired delayed-type hypersensitivity responses and ameliorated host defense against infections. Acute alcohol use has been associated with increased susceptibility to infections, posttrauma immunosuppression, and a decrease in antigen-specific T-cell proliferation response [13,16]. Malnutrition and cirrhosis are two of the conditions that develop with chronic ethanol consumption that affect the efficiency of the immune system to combat infections [11,12]. Ethanol influences the function of lymphocytes, monocytes and polymorphonuclear cells [13–15].

Lipid emulsions provided parentally have been associated with mononuclear phagocytic system functional changes. Supplementation with fish oil increases macrophage numbers as well as phagocytosis [17].

Glutamine-enriched diets influence the production of TNF-α, IL-1, and IL-6. Studies in mice have concluded that glutamine enriched diets enhance the ability of macrophages to respond to cytokine stimulation, produced via the autocrine system [18].

MICRONUTRIENTS AND AIDS

There is abundant evidence that micronutrient deficiencies can deeply affect immunity; micronutrient deficiencies are widely seen in HIV, even in asymptomatic patients. Direct relationships have been found between deficiencies of specific nutrients, such as vitamins A and B12, and a decline in CD4 counts [22–24]. Deficiencies in vitamin A influence vertical transmission of HIV [26–29] and may affect progression to AIDS (vitamin A, B12, zinc). Correction of deficiencies has been shown to affect symptoms and disease manifestation (AIDS dementia complex and B12; diarrhea, weight loss, and zinc), and certain micronutrients have demonstrated a direct anti-viral effect *in vitro* (vitamin E and zinc). Some studies suggest that micronutrient deficiencies probably have few direct effects on the functioning of immune cells. The main effect appears to be a reduction in cell mass that may indirectly affect immune cell function [42]. Although the results published appear contradictory, some of these inconsistencies may be accounted for by the fact that the disease itself may lower concentrations of micronutrients in plasma that may be misinterpreted as deficiency due to intake. However, low plasma vitamin A concentrations appear to affect immune responsiveness and has degenerative effects on membrane integrity and mucosal immunity. Zinc may have similar effects on gut integrity. Low concentrations of other nutrients such as ascorbate and iron can affect cellular immune effector functions involving cytokines and nitric oxide [48]. Low plasma ascorbate increases the removal of iron from plasma. These low iron concentrations appear to increase the *cytotoxicity* of macrophages [42].

VITAMIN A

Individuals with HIV and patients with AIDS present a variety of pathologic alterations that influence their nutritional status during various stages of the disease. Some studies have revealed a greater level of malnutrition and an elevated excretion of vitamin A in the urine of AIDS patients. Secretion of vitamin A in urine has been associated with infection, fever, and acute diarrhea. Therefore, the monitoring of nutritional status, especially in relation to vitamin A is recommended for patients with HIV and AIDS. Studies show that around 10–40% of HIV-positive women will give birth to children who are also infected. However, the risk factors for transmission from mother to child are not well understood and the effects of maternal nutritional status on fetal transmission are unknown. Vitamin A is an essential micronutrient for normal immune function. Vitamin A deficiency is common among HIV-infected pregnant women and is associated with higher mother-to-child transmission of HIV-1 and increased infant mortality. The biological mechanisms by which vitamin A deficiency could influence mother-to-child transmission of HIV-1 include impairment of immune responses in both mother and infant (specifically the CD4 T cell count), abnormal placental and vaginal pathology, and increased HIV viral burden in breastmilk and blood. Some clinical trials have demonstrated that daily micronutrient supplementation, including vitamin A, should be considered during pregnancy to reduce mother-to-child transmission of HIV-1 [30]. Severe vitamin A deficiency (<20 micrograms/Dl) has been associated with a 20-fold increased risk of having HIV-1 DNA in breast milk among women with <400 CD4 cells/mm^3 [28]. Women with CD4 cell depletion, especially those with vitamin A deficiency, may be at increased risk of transmitting HIV-1 to their infants through breast milk.

The relationship between ethanol and vitamin A has been clear for quite some time now. In adults, ethanol ingestion appears to alter vitamin A metabolism and tissue distribution [31]. Associations have also been made between fetal alcohol syndrome and malformations induced by toxicity and deficiency of vitamin A [32].

One explanation for this may be the role alcohol plays in altering retinoic acid levels. Studies show that retinoic acid appears to curb the adverse effects of alcohol [31]. Ethanol has been found to inhibit alcohol dehydrogenase, an enzyme that normally converts retinal to retinoic acid. The resulting decrease in retinoic acid may negatively alter the development and maturation of the immune system. The associations between retinoic acid and alcohol are further strengthened by other studies. Retinoic acid and ethanol reverse or block each others effects in studies on isolated neuroblastoma cells [33], and ethanol treatment has been found to promote deficits in vitamin A. Although these studies clarify the effects of ethanol on vitamin A levels, further studies are needed to determine how these factors contribute to immune system damage and an increased likelihood of mother to child transmission of HIV-1.

VITAMIN E

Excessive alcohol consumption is a major health problem in the United States. Prolonged consumption of alcohol results in alterations of immune responses, ultimately manifested by increasing susceptibility to infectious agents. Vitamin E supplementation has been associated with enhancement of immune response and improvement of host defense, and may provide a useful therapeutic approach for treatment of alcoholics to improve host defense [34–38].

Much literature has addressed the close relationship between cellular immunity and vitamins. In the case of water-soluble vitamins it is well known that a deficiency induces a marked decrease in cellular immunity, although supplementation of these vitamins has little effect. In contrast, lipid-soluble vitamins such as vitamin A and E markedly affect cellular immunity in both deficient and excess state. Vitamin A supplementation induces the enhancement of cellular immunity such as phagocytic and tumoricidal activities in human monocytes and mouse peritoneal macrophages. In the elderly, a high intake of vitamin E is able to improve decreased cellular immunity, which appears to be associated with production of prostaglandin E2. In summary, since vitamins are important to maintain and promote cellular immunity, the beneficial use of vitamins to enhance the health of humans should be seriously considered [40].

Vitamin E supplementation has also been shown to improve some aspects of immune function in aged animals and human subjects. The protective effect of vitamin E against viral or bacterial infections in experimentally challenged young animals has been reported [41]. In a study with young and old animals supplemented with vitamin E after injection with influenza, vitamin E young mice showed only a modest reduction in lung viral titer, while supplemented old mice exhibited a high significant reduction in the viral titer [41].

Ethanol feeding markedly decreases both alpha- and gamma-tocopherol in the livers of normal and vitamin E-deficient rats, but only decreases plasma levels of tocopherols in normal rats. High serum levels of the enzyme transaminase in vitamin E-deficient animals suggest that enhanced lipid peroxidation is associated with greater severity of liver injury induced by ethanol in vitamin E-deficient rats [39]. Evidence is accumulating that intermediates of oxygen reduction may in fact be associated with the development of alcoholic liver disease. In a study with rats fed a diet deficient or supplemented with vitamin E and treated with ethanol, chronic ethanol feeding enhanced hepatic consumption of vitamin E in both groups. Also, both EtOH-fed groups exhibited increased manganese superoxide dismutase gene expression, although the enzyme activity was enhanced only in the vitamin E-deprived group of EtOH-treated animals [50]. It seems that superoxide dismutase is produced to counteract the effects of oxidative stress induced by ethanol. Therefore, vitamin E supplementation may reduce the hepatotoxic effects of ethanol. Previous studies have reported a reduction in plasma vitamin E levels in patients is associated with a higher production of free radicals [19,20].

It has been reported that urinary excretion may play a significant role in the reduction of plasma vitamin E levels. A group of 16 patients with AIDS were measured by chromatography for their urinary and plasma vitamin E levels. Patients with AIDS presented reduced plasma vitamin E levels as compared with HIV and controls, which correlated with a higher urinary excretion in the AIDS group. Supplementation of this micronutrient will be essential to avoid vitamin E deficiency in AIDS patients [21,51].

SELENIUM

Selenium (Se) is required for the activity of the enzyme glutathione peroxidase, and selenium deficiency may be associated with myopathy, cardiomyopathy and immune dysfunction including oral candidiasis, impaired phagocytic function and decreased CD4 T-cell counts. When a host is malnourished, the immune system is compromised and there is an increased susceptibility to viral infections. Research published points about the importance of host nutrition during a viral disease, not only from the perspective of the host, but from the perspective of the viral pathogen as well. When a benign strain of coxsackievirus B3 is injected into Selenium (Se)-deficient or vitamin E-deficient mice, it evolves to become virulent. Studies have shown that in addition to immunosuppression due to micronutrient deficiency, the virus itself becomes altered [43]. Beck *et al.* have shown in a mouse model of coxsackievirus-induced myocarditis, that host deficiency in either selenium or vitamin E leads to a change in viral phenotype such that an avirulent strain of the virus becomes virulent and a virulent strain becomes more virulent. The change in phenotype was shown to be due to point mutations in the viral genome. Once the mutations occur, the phenotype change is stable and can now be expressed even in well nourished mice. These results suggest that nutrition can affect not only the host, but the pathogen as well, and show a new model of relating host nutritional effects to viral pathogenesis [44].

In a study done with AIDS patients, plasma and red blood cell levels of Se were found to be less than half of those in healthy individuals [45]. A correlation between Se and glutathione perioxidase and the total lymphocyte count was also established. This occurred in both homosexuals and drug users with AIDS and was irrespective of the presence or absence of diarrhea or GI malabsorption. Interestingly, cardiac tissue Se levels in AIDS patients was also found to be low [45].

One reason for the decreased selenium levels in HIV infected patients may have to do with the virus itself. The virus uses selenoproteins to regulate its replication, which deplete the Se levels of the host. Supplementation trials with individual antioxidants have shown improvement in immunological parameters and decreased evidence of lipid peroxidation when selenium is added [46]. Recent investigations indicate that supplementation with Se may help to increase the enzymatic defense systems in HIV-infected patients [47,48]. These studies help support the assertion that increased Se levels help to decrease morbidity and prolong survival in HIV infected hosts.

Micronutrient deficiency is common in HIV positive patients as documented by low plasma and red blood cell levels of Se, diminished activity of glutathione peroxidase, and low cardiac Se levels in AIDS infected hearts. This worsens with time since AIDS patients tend to have more severe vitamin deficits than those with earlier stages of HIV infection. The Se deficit in blood correlates with serum albumin levels and total lymphocyte counts, which in turn accetuates the conditions to predispose the AIDS patients to secondary infections.

MURINE AIDS (MAIDS) AND MICRONUTRIENT DEFICIENCY

LP-BM5 Murine leukemia virus (MuLV) infection of C57BL/6 mice causes a disease that has many features in common with human AIDS, in particular abnormal lympho-proliferation and severe immunodeficiency. Thus, this murine AIDS (MAIDS) model is useful for evaluation of antiviral agents as well as deficiency in antioxidant micronutri-ents such as selenium (Se), vitamin A, vitamin E, zinc (Zn), cooper (Cu), and glu-tathione. In one study using MAIDS, the effect of Se as sodium selenite was used to evaluate immunological and oxidative effects. The results indicated that Se treatment inhibited splenomegaly, which is characteristic of chronic murine AIDS. In addition to detecting abnormal immune function, oxidative imbalance possibly existed in the MAIDS model, as lipid peroxide increased significantly in the spleen and whole blood glutathione peroxidase (GSH-Px) activity decreased markedly. Se supplementation had a good protective effect [54]. In another study using MuLV, ethanol administration sig-nificantly increased Fe concentration in the liver, yet significantly decreased the con-centration of Cu in the heart. MuLV alone, which had not proceeded to murine AIDS, resulted in a significant increase in heart Cu and Zn concentration as compared with uninfected mice. Retrovirus infection in C57BL/6 mice significantly increased Iron (Fe) and Zn levels/g of muscle. Early retrovirus infection alters tissue micronutrient levels, and may thus contribute to immunological changes [55].

CONCLUSIONS

Infection by HIV is one of the most aggressive pandemics of our time, with high econom-ical, social, and health care costs. In the last few years the development of new, highly effective therapies has made it possible to change the prognosis, the quality of life, and the survival of many patients. However, nutrition has long been known to affect the ability of the host to respond to infectious disease. Widespread famines are often accompanied by increased morbidity and mortality due to infectious diseases. The currently accepted view of the relationship between nutrition of the host and its susceptibility to infectious disease is one of a direct relationship with host immune status. That is, if the host has nutrient deficiencies, then the functioning of the host immune system is compromised. This impairment of the immune response will lead to an increased susceptibility to infectious disease. Clearly, the immune response has been shown to be weakened by inadequate nutrition in many model systems and in human studies. In sub-Saharan Africa, studies have shown that 25% of children with malnutrition have HIV infection. Vitamin A, E, and B12 deficiency accelerated the development of AIDS with low T cells, whereas their normalization retarded the development of immune dysfunction. Decreased cellular immunity with aging or during the development of AIDS is markedly improved by the intake of micronutrients like vitamins E, A, and C, and minerals like Se and Zn. Also, vitamin supplementation induces higher rates of differentiation of immature T cells in the thymus which results in the improvement of cellular immunity in the aged, and the early recovery of thymic atrophy following X-ray irradiation. Taken together, micronutrients are an important factor maintaining the immune system, especially in the aged and those suffering from HIV infection.

ACKNOWLEDGEMENTS

Supported by NIH grant, HL63667.

REFERENCES

1 Laso FJ, Iglesias-Osma C, Ciudad J, Lopez A, Pastor I, Orfao A. Chronic Alcoholism is associated with an imbalanced production of Th-1/Th2 cytokines by peripheral blood T cells. *Alcohol. Clin. Exp. Res.* 1999; **23**: 1306–1311.

2 Balla AK, Lischner HW, Pomerantz RJ, Bagasra O. Human Studies on Alcohol and Susceptibility to HIV Infection. *Alcohol* 1994; **11**: 99–103.

3 Garro AJ, Espina N, Lieber CS. Ethanol and cancer. *Alcohol Hlth. Res. Wld.* 1992; **16**: 81–86.

4 Chokunoga E, Levy LM, Bassett MT, Borok MZ, Mauchaza BG, Chirenje MZ, Parkin DM. Aids and cancer in Africa: the evolving epidemic in Zimbabwe. *AIDS* 1999; **13**: 2583–2588.

5 Gonzalez FM, Vargas JA, Lacoma F, Gea-Banacloche JC, Vergara J, Fernandez-Corugedo A, Durantez A. Natural killer cell activity in laryngeal carcinoma. *Arch. Otolaryngol.* 1993; **119**: 69–72.

6 Mather GG, Talcott PA, Exon JH. Characterization of a chemically induced tumor model and the effects of natural killer cell depletion by antiasialo GM-1. *Immunobiology* 1994; **190**: 333–345.

7 Seaman WE, Sleisenger M, Eriksson E, Koo GC. Depletion of natural killer cells by monoclonal antibody to NK-1.1: reduction in host defense against malignancy without loss of cellular or humoral immunity. *J. Immunol.* 1987; **138**: 4539–4544.

8 Pruett SB, Collier SD, Wu W-J. Ethanol-induced activation of the hypothalamic-pituitary-adrenal axis in a mouse model for binge drinking: role of Ro15-4513-sensitive gamma aminobutyric acid receptors, tolerance, and relevance to humans. *Life Sci.* 1998; **63**: 1137–1146.

9 Wu W-J, Pruett SB. Involvement of catecholamines and glucocorticoids in ethanol-induced suppression of splenic natural killer cell activity in a mouse model for binge drinking. *Alcohol. Clin. Exp. Res.* 1997; **21**: 1030–1036.

10 Wu W-J, Pruett SB. Ethanol decreases host resistance to pulmonary metastases in a mouse model:role of natural killer cells and the ethanol-induced stress response. *Int. J. Cancer* 1999; **82**: 866–892.

11 Hirsch S, de la Maza MP, Gattas V, Barrera G, Petermann M, Gotteland M, Munoz C, Lopez M, Bunout D. Nutritional support in alcoholic cirrhotic patients improves host defenses. *J. Am. Coll. Nut.* 1999; **18**(5): 434–441.

12 Sopena B, Fernandez-Rodriguez CM, Martinez Vazquez C, Mendez MX, de la Fuente J, Freire M, Arnillas E, Outon A. Serum levels of soluble interleukin-2 receptor in alcoholic patients. *Anal. Med. Int.* 1998; **15**: 189–193.

13 Padgett EL, Sibley DA, Jerrells TR. Effect of adrenalectomy on ethanol-associated changes in lymphocyte cell numbers and subpopulations in thymus, spleen, and gut-associated lymphoid tissues. *Int. J. Immunopharmacol.* 2000; **22**: 285–298.

14 Szabo G. Monocytes, Alcohol use, and altered immunity. *Alcohol Clin. Exp. Res.* 1998; **22**: 216S–219S.

15 Greenberg SS, Zhao X, Hua L, Wang JF, Nelson S, Ouyang J. Ethanol inhibits lung clearance of Pseudomonas aeruginosa by a neutrophil and nitric oxide-dependent mechanism, *in vivo. Alcohol Clin. Exp. Res.* 1999; **23**: 735–744.

16 Hunt JD, Robert EG, Zieske AW, Bautista AP, Bukara M, Lei D, Shellito JE, Nelson S, Kolls JK, Skrepnik N. Orthotopic human lung carcinoma xenografts in BALB/c mice immunosuppressed with anti-CD4 monoclonal antibodies and chronic alcohol consumption. *Cancer* 2000 **88**: 468–479.

17 Cukier C, Waitzber DL, Logullo AF, Bacchi CE, Trayassos VH, Torrinhas RS, Soares SR, Saldiva PH, Oliveira TS, Heymsfield S. Lipid and lipid-free total parenteral nutrition: differential effects on macrophage phagocytosis in rats. *Nutrition* 1999; **15**: 885–889.

18 Wells SM, Kew S, Yaqoob P, Wallace FA, Calder PC. Dietary glutamine enhances cytokine production by murine macrophages. *Nutrition* 1999; **15**: 881–884.

19 Jordao Junior AA, Silveira S, Figueiredo JF, Vannucchi H. Urinary excretion and plasma vitamin E levels in patients with AIDS. *Nutrition* 1998; **14**: 423–426.

20 Liang B, Chung S, Araghinikam M, Watson R. Vitamins and Immunomodultation in AIDS. *Nutrition* 1996; **12**: 1–7.

21 Wang Y, Watson RR. Potential therapeutics of vitamin E (tocopherol) in AIDS and HIV. *Drugs* 1994; **48**: 327–338.

22 Dawson HD, Ross AC. Chronic marginal vitamin A status affects the distribution and function of T cells and natural T cells in aging Lewis rats. *J. Nutr.* 1999; **129**: 1782–1790.

23 Erf GF, Bottje WG, Bersi TK. Effects of dietary vitamin E on the immune system in broilers: altered proportions of CD4 T cells in the thymus and spleen. *Poult. Sci.* 1998; **77**: 529–537.

24 Fawzi WW, Msamanga GI, Spiegelman D. Randomised trial of effects of vitamin supplements on pregnancy outcomes and T cell counts in HIV-1-infected women in Tanzania. *Lancet* 1998; **351**: 1477–1482.

25 Pike J, Chandra RK. Effect of vitamin and trace element supplementation on immune indices in healthy elderly. *Int. J. Vitam. Nutr. Res.* 1995; **65**: 117–121.

26 Semba RD. Overview of the potential role of vitamin A in mother-to-child transmission of HIV-1. *Acta. Paediatr. Suppl.* 1997; **421**: 107–112.

27 Greenberg BL, Semba RD, Vink PE. Vitamin A deficiency and maternal-infant transmissions of HIV in two metropolitan areas in the United States. *AIDS* 1997; **11**: 325–332.

28 Nduati RW, John GC, Richardson BA. Human immunodeficiency virus type 1-infected cells in breast milk: association with immunosuppression and vitamin A deficiency. *J. Infect. Dis.* 1995; **172**: 1461–1468.

29 Semba RD, Miotti PG, Chiphangwi JD. Maternal vitamin A deficiency and mother-to-child transmission of HIV-1. *Lancet* 1994; **343**: 1593–1597.

30 Wiratchai A, Phuapradit W, Sunthornkachit R. Maternal and umbilical cord serum vitamin A, E levels and mother-to-child transmission in the non-supplemented vitamin A, E HIV-1 infected parturients with short-course zidovudine therapy. *J. Med. Assoc. Thai.* 1999; **82**: 885–890.

31 Duester G. Alcohol dehydrogenase as a critical mediator of retinoic acid synthesis from vitamin A in the mouse embryo. *J. Nutr.* 1998; **128**: 459S–462S.

32 De Jonge MH, Zachman RD. The effect of maternal ethanol ingestion on fetal rat heart vitamin A: a model for fetal alcohol syndrome. *Pediatr. Res.* 1995; **37**: 418–423.

33 Haidar NE, Andriamampandry C, Carrara M. The conversion of ethanolamine and of its metabolites to choline in human neuroblastoma clones: effect of differentiation induced by retinoic acid. *Neurochem. Res.* 1994; **19**: 457–462.

34 Wang Y, Watson RR. Ethanol, immune responses, and murine AIDS: the role of vitamin E as an immunostimulant and antioxidant. *Alcohol* 1994; **11**: 75–84.

35 Wang Y, Liang B, Watson RR. The effect of alcohol consumption on nutritional status during murine AIDS. *Alcohol* 1994; **11**: 273–278.

36 Wang Y, Watson RR. Potential therapeutics of vitamin E (tocopherol) in AIDS and HIV. *Drugs* 1994; **48**: 327–338.

37 Wang JY, Liang B, Watson RR. Alcohol consumption alters cytokine release during murine AIDS. *Alcohol* 1997; **14**: 155–159.

38 Lee J, Sepulveda RT, Jiang S, Watson RR. Immune dysfunction during alcohol consumption and murine AIDS: the protective role of dehydroepiandrosterone sulfate. *Alcohol Clin. Exp. Res.* 1999; **23**: 856–862.

39 Sadrzadeh SM, Nanji AA, Meydani M. Effect of chronic ethanol feeding on plasma and liver alpha- and gamma-tocopherol levels in normal and vitamin E-deficient rats. Relationship to lipid peroxidation. *Biochem. Pharmacol.* 1994; **47**: 2005–2010.

40 Meydani SN, Beharka AA. Recent developments in vitamin E and immune response. *Nutr. Rev.* 1998; **56**: S49–S58.

41 Han SN, Meydani SN. Vitamin E and infectious diseases in the aged. *Proc. Nutr. Soc.* 1999; **58**: 697–705.

42 Thurnham DI. Micronutrients and immune function: some recent developments. *J. Clin. Pathol.* 1997; **50**: 887–891.

43 Beck MA. Selenium and host defence towards viruses. *Proc. Nutr. Soc.* 1999; **58**: 707–711.

44 Beck MA. Increased virulence of coxsackievirus B3 in mice due to vitamin E or selenium deficiency. *J. Nutr.* 1997; **127**: 966S–970S.

45 Dworkin BM. Selenium deficiency in HIV infection and the acquired immunodeficiency syndrome (AIDS). *Chem. Biol. Interact.* 1994; **91**: 181–186.

46 Patrick L. Nutrients and HIV: part one – beta carotene and selenium. *Altern. Med. Rev.* 1999; **4**: 403–413.

47 Delmas-Beauvieux MC, Peuchant E, Couchouron A. The enzymatic antioxidant system in blood and glutathione status in human immunodeficiency virus (HIV)-infected patients: effects of supplementation with selenium or beta-carotene. Published erratum appears in *Am. J. Clin. Nutr.* 1996; **64**: 971.

48 Constans J, Delmas-Beauvieux MC, Sergeant C. One-year antioxidant supplementation with beta-carotene or selenium for patients infected with human immunodeficiency virus: a pilot study. *Clin. Infect. Dis.* 1996; **23**: 654–656.

49 Baum MK, Shor-Posner G. Micronutrient status in relationship to mortality in HIV-1 disease. *Nutr. Rev.* 1998; **56**: S135–S139.

50 Weiss G, Wachter H, Fuchs D. Linkage of cell-mediated immunity to iron metabolism. *Immunol. Today* 1995; **16**: 495–500.

51 Ravaglia G, Forti P, Maioli F. Effect of micronutrient status on natural killer cell immune function in healthy free-living subjects aged ≥90 y. *Am. J. Clin. Nutr.* 2000; **71**: 590–598.

52 Koch O, Farre S, De Leo ME. Regulation of manganese superoxide dismutase (MnSOD) in chronic experimental alcoholism: effects of vitamin E-supplemented and -deficient diets. *Alcohol Alcohol.* 2000; **35**: 159–163.

53 Jordao Junior AA, Figueiredo JF, Silveira S. Urinary excretion of vitamin A and thiobarbituric acid reactive substances in AIDS patients. *Rev. Hosp. Clin. Fac. Med. Sao Paulo* 1998; **53**: 11–15.

54 Chen C, Zhou J, Xu H, Jiang Y, Zhu G. Effect of selenium supplementation on mice infected with LP-BM5 MuLV, a murine AIDS model. *Biol. Trace Elem. Res.* 1997; **59**: 187–193.

55 Shahbazian LM, Wood S, Watson RR. Ethanol consumption and early murine retrovirus infection influence liver, heart, and muscle levels of iron, zinc, and copper in C57BL/6 mice. *Alcohol Clin. Exp. Res.* 1994; **18**: 964–968.

Index